Protocols in
Pediatric
Nephrology

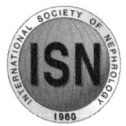

Supported by the International Society of Nephrology
Sister Renal Center Program

Protocols in
Pediatric
Nephrology

Arvind Bagga MD, FIAP, FAMS
Professor of Pediatrics
All India Institute of Medical Sciences, New Delhi

Aditi Sinha MD, DNB, MNAMS
Senior Research Associate, Department of Pediatrics
All India Institute of Medical Sciences, New Delhi

Ashima Gulati MD, MNAMS
Senior Research Associate, Department of Pediatrics
All India Institute of Medical Sciences, New Delhi

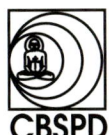

CBSPD

CBS Publishers & Distributors Pvt Ltd

New Delhi • Bengaluru • Chennai • Kochi • Kolkata • Lucknow • Mumbai
Hyderabad • Jharkhand • Nagpur • Patna • Pune • Uttarakhand

Protocols in
Pediatric Nephrology

ISBN: 978-81-239-2059-7 (Hardcover)
ISBN: 978-81-239-2058-0 (Softcover)

Copyright © Authors and Publishers

First Edition 2012
Reprint 2013, 2015, 2017, 2019, 2023, **2025**

Published by Satish Kumar Jain and produced by Varun Jain for

CBS Publishers & Distributors Pvt Ltd
4819/XI Prahlad Street, 24 Ansari Road, Daryaganj, New Delhi 110 002, India.
Ph: 011-23289259, 23266838   Website: www.cbspd.com
                                    e-mail: delhi@cbspd.com

Corporate Office: 204 FIE, Industrial Area, Patparganj, Delhi 110 092
Ph: 011-4934 4934   Fax: 011-4934 4935   e-mail: publishing@cbspd.com;
                                               publicity@cbspd.com

Branches

• **Bengaluru:** Seema House 2975, 17th Cross, KR Road, Banasankari 2nd Stage, Bengaluru 560 070, Karnataka, India
  Ph: +91-80-26771678/79   Fax: +91-80-26771680   e-mail: bangalore@cbspd.com
• **Chennai:** 7, Subbaraya Street, Shenoy Nagar, Chennai 600 030, Tamil Nadu, India
  Ph: +91-44-26680620, 26681266   Fax: +91-44-42032115   e-mail: chennai@cbspd.com
• **Kochi:** 42/1325, 1326, Power House Road, Opp KSEB, Power House, Ernakulum Kochi 682 018, Kerala, India
  Ph: +91-484-4059061-65,67   Fax: +91-484-4059065   e-mail: kochi@cbspd.com
• **Kolkata:** 147, Hind Ceramics Compound, 1st Floor, Nilgunj Road, Belghoria, Kolkata-700056, West Bengal, India
  Ph: +033-25633055, 033-25633056   e-mail: kolkata@cbspd.com
• **Lucknow:** Basement, Khushnuma Complex, 7 Meerabai Marg (Behind Jawahar Bhawan), Lucknow-226001, UP, India
  Ph: +0522-4000032   e-mail: tiwari.lucknow@cbspd.com
• **Mumbai:** PWD Shed, Gala no 25/26, Ramchandra Bhatt Marg, Next to JJ Hospital Gate no. 2, Opp. Union Bank of India,
  Noorbaug, Mumbai-400009, Maharashtra, India
  Ph: 022-66661880/89   e-mail: mumbai@cbspd.com

Representatives

• Hyderabad   0-9885175004   • Jharkhand   0-9811541605   • Nagpur   0-8692091830
• Patna   0-9334159340   • Pune   0-9664372571   • Uttarakhand   0-9716462459

Printed at HT Media Ltd., Greater Noida, UP, India

Foreword

I am very happy to write about the book *Protocols in Pediatric Nephrology.* This important text is a welcome addition to the available literature on renal diseases in children. Major advances have taken place in the understanding, evaluation and treatment of a variety of disorders of kidney and urinary tract. Across specialties, management protocols are shown to improve patient outcomes and are being used increasingly. In a large country like India the necessary expertise is often not widely available and clear diagnostic and management guidelines serve a very useful purpose.

The authors of the present book have presented standardized approaches to management of common acute and chronic renal diseases utilizing an easily understandable format. The text is richly illustrated and includes several informative flow diagrams and tables which add to the clarity of diagnostic investigations. The management of complex disorders is presented using a practical approach that synthesizes contemporary recommendations from across the world, thus conforming to global practices. Using a syndrome-based approach, the authors discuss the evaluation and management of all common presentations.

With increasing recognition of acute and chronic renal conditions in children, I have no doubt this book will satisfy a huge and growing need. *Protocols in Pediatric Nephrology* should be extremely helpful to practicing pediatricians and trainees. I strongly recommend this book to all health care personnel involved in taking care of children with renal diseases.

Dr RN Srivastava
Senior Consultant Pediatric Nephrologist
Apollo Indraprastha Hospitals
New Delhi

Foreword

It is my honor and great pleasure to present *Protocols in Pediatric Nephrology* which has been written and edited by Dr Arvind Bagga of the All India Institute of Medical Sciences.

The last few decades have seen rapid progress in the field of pediatric nephrology, with advances in understanding of pathophysiology translating into an improved management of childhood renal diseases. Across the world, the number of healthcare professionals involved in the multidisciplinary care for children with kidney diseases continues to grow. Since trained personnel in pediatric nephrology are scarce, particularly in settings of limited resources, pediatricians in training and practice require a practical resource that summarizes approaches to diagnosis and management of common renal diseases.

Thus *Protocols in Pediatric Nephrology* successfully fulfills the above requirement. While a number of excellent textbooks are available that provide detailed information on the various topics in the field, the current tract is a clinically oriented text. It provides the reader with a concise and up-to-date overview of the evaluation and therapy of specific childhood kidney diseases. The simple language and an extensive use of clinical algorithms, tables and illustrations focuses the content and allows for greater assimilation of the information provided. The addition of a CD complements this book by allowing in-depth understanding of the practical nuances of common procedures and presentation of algorithms, graphs, histological photomicrographs and X-rays.

Through our long-standing commitment to the Sister Renal Center Program of the International Society of Nephrology, I have closely observed the growth in Pediatric Nephrology in India. Enhancement of educational activities has been a major aim of our partnership with the Division of Pediatric Nephrology at AIIMS, and the *Protocols in Pediatric Nephrology* has been a mandate of this relationship. It is expected that this compilation of clinical practices shall be useful to pediatricians, pediatric nephrologists and pediatric urologists across the country, thus enabling improved care of children with renal diseases. We are very proud of our relationship with AIIMS and the advancements it has help engender. We look forward to many more years of productive interactions.

Stanley C Jordan MD
Professor of Pediatrics and Medicine
David Geffen School of Medicine at UCLA
Director, Nephrology and Transplant Immunology
Cedars-Sinai Medical Center, Los Angeles, CA

Preface

Rapid advances have taken place in the diagnosis and management of renal disorders in children. The availability of biochemical, serological and radiological investigations have improved our understanding of various disorders and contributed to ascertainment of diagnosis. The genetic basis of many inherited tubular and glomerular disorders has been elucidated, allowing accurate diagnoses. Recent decades have also seen advances in therapeutics, with availability of focused immunosuppressive agents for management of patients with glomerulonephritis, nephrotic syndrome and following transplantation. Expertise in application of chronic hemodialysis and peritoneal dialysis, and the use of erythropoietin, growth hormone, vitamin D analogs and nutritional supplements have considerably improved the prognosis and quality of life for children with progressive kidney failure.

This concise text aims to provide practical guidelines on evaluation and therapy for children with acute and chronic disorders of the kidney and urinary tract. We have consciously avoided a review of the pathophysiologic basis of diseases or details of strength of evidence favoring specific therapies. The focus, instead, is on syndrome-based approaches to evaluation and management, based on current evidence and practice. However, brevity has not been at the expense of continuous text, which is easier to assimilate than a telegraphic format usual with lecture or bedside notes.

The book has eleven sections that detail major renal disorders encountered in practice. Each section has between 2–8 chapters that include definitions, tools for evaluation, diagnosis and monitoring, and therapeutic strategies. The contents of each chapter are enhanced through liberal use of illustrations, algorithms and tables. Where necessary, concepts of pathophysiology have been discussed using line diagrams. Each chapter includes resources for Support Reading that shall be a valuable supplement which readers can refer to for detailed understanding. An exhaustive list of appendices offers a handy reference for bedside patient management. An accompanying DVD demonstrates common procedures, including kidney biopsy and insertion of catheters for peritoneal dialysis. It also includes a ready pictorial resource of histological slides, radiographs, line diagrams and algorithms used in the text.

The preparation of this text was supported in substantial measure through interactions with Cedars Sinai Medical Center, under the aegis of the Sister Renal Center Program (SRC) of the International Society of

Nephrology. Augmentation of educational activities is an important aim of this partnership, and the *Protocols in Pediatric Nephrology* is an outcome of this affiliation. The support of the ISN through its Sister Renal Center program is thankfully acknowledged. It is our hope that the book reflects the commitment of the SRC program towards building partnerships across regions to promote sharing of scientific advances that enable provision of high quality care for kidney diseases.

We are grateful to our colleague Dr Pankaj Hari for constant guidance, cooperation and unstinted support in enabling completion of this project. We thank Prof Amit Dinda and Dr Geetika Singh for providing the histological pictures, and Prof Arun Gupta and Prof CS Bal for illustrations on imaging. The help of Mr Yogesh Kumar, Center for Medical Education and Technology, AIIMS in preparation of video films on dialysis and kidney biopsy is acknowledged. The completion of this book would not have been possible without the support and sagacious advice of Mr YN Arjuna, CBS Publishers.

This book is expected to be a useful practical resource for inpatient and outpatient management, and serve the needs for pediatric residents, fellows and advanced trainees in nephrology, urology and critical care medicine in India and the region. We trust that the readers shall find this inaugural edition of *Protocols in Pediatric Nephrology* useful in improving the care for children with kidney disease.

Arvind Bagga
Aditi Sinha
Ashima Gulati

Contents

RENAL REPLACEMENT THERAPY

SPECIFIC THERAPY

APPENDICES

Protocols in
Pediatric
Nephrology

Diagnostic Evaluation

1 Evaluation of Kidney Function

URINALYSIS

Urine examination is an important step in the diagnosis of renal disease. The urine specimen should be fresh and relatively concentrated. Microscopic examination of uncentrifuged as well as a centrifuged specimen should be done. The presence of red cells and their morphologic characteristics, white cells, cellular and hyaline casts and various types of crystals should be noted.

Sample Collection

The first morning specimen is preferred as it is the most concentrated. It can be collected in a sterile container by one of the following methods:

Midstream urine: A clean-catch midstream specimen can be collected after proper local cleaning to minimize contamination by peri-urethral and prepucial organisms. The initial part of urine, which may be contaminated, is discarded.

Bag collection: In neonates and infants, urine can be collected in sterile bags applied after cleaning of skin, and removed immediately once the baby has voided. While a negative culture often helps to exclude urinary tract infection, a positive bag specimen should be confirmed by testing a specimen obtained by bladder aspiration.

Suprapubic bladder aspiration: The most reliable way to obtain a urine specimen in neonates and young infants is by suprapubic aspiration. This is unlikely to be contaminated and is therefore most suitable for a definitive diagnosis of infection. A 5 to 10 mL syringe with a thin needle is vertically inserted 1 to 2 cm above the pubic symphysis to a depth of 2 to 3 cm. A full bladder should be confirmed by percussion or ultrasonography before the procedure.

Bladder catheterization: A urine specimen can also be obtained by bladder catheterization under strict aseptic precautions.

Specific Gravity

The specific gravity should be measured with a refractometer. The early morning urine specific gravity should exceed 1015.

pH

Urine is collected in a capped syringe and pH measured promptly. It is not necessary to collect the urine under paraffin. Fasting, early

Diagnostic Evaluation

I

morning urine pH is low (below 5.5) and increases following meals.

Protein

Proteinuria is an important marker of glomerular or tubular pathology. The detection of 3–4+ albuminuria suggests the presence of glomerular disease. Low molecular weight proteinuria, including lysozyme, beta-2 microglobulin, neutrophil gelatinase associated lipocalin (NGAL) and retinol binding protein, suggest the presence of tubular injury. The evaluation of proteinuria is detailed in Chapter 2.

Glucose

The dipstick test produces a graded color change and is specific for glucose. It has replaced older methods (e.g. Benedict test) that detect the presence of reducing substances.

Microscopic Examination

A fresh urine sample (10 mL) is centrifuged in a test tube at 1500 rpm for 10 minutes; the urine is decanted and the cell pellet resuspended in 0.3–0.5 mL of urine. The urine is examined for presence of formed elements (red and white cells), and for casts and crystals. Examination for red cell morphology and for red cell casts is useful in determining the cause of hematuria (Chapter 3). The presence of leukocyturia does not always indicate urinary tract infection as it might also be seen in interstitial nephritis, stones and high fever . Examination of crystals might be helpful in determining the etiology of urinary tract stones, e.g. presence of hexagonal crystals of cystine help in the diagnosis of cystinuria.

EVALUATION OF GLOMERULAR FUNCTION

Urea, Creatinine

Blood urea is not a reliable marker of kidney function. It might be raised in patients with volume depletion, high protein intake and excessive protein catabolism, trauma and corticosteroid therapy. Creatinine is chiefly excreted by glomerular filtration and a small amount is also secreted by the tubules. Despite limitations of fallaciously low serum creatinine values in undernourished children, laboratory measurement of creatinine provides a satisfactory and practical estimate of glomerular filtration rate (GFR).

Glomerular Filtration Rate

Radionuclide techniques for measuring GFR are accurate, though determination of the precise values of GFR is not necessary in clinical practice. For practical purposes, plasma creatinine and endogenous creatinine clearance are commonly used as more convenient though less accurate methods for GFR assessment. Normal age-related values of serum creatinine and GFR are given in the Appendix 8. The GFR may be directly estimated using the following equations:

1. Modified Schwartz formula

$$GFR = \frac{k \times \text{height (cm)}}{\text{serum creatinine (mg/dL)}}$$

where, predicted GFR (mL/min/1.73 m^2) is the product of height (cm) and a constant, k (empirically derived constant relating height to muscle mass), divided by the serum creatinine.

The value of k varies from 0.33 in preterm and 0.45 in term infants, to 0.55 for children and adolescent girls and 0.70 for adolescent boys. With more accurate estimation of creatinine (through modified Jaffe reaction, ELISA and HPLC techniques), reports suggest that the value of the constant (k) should be derived locally. In most recent reports the value of k ranges between 0.41 and 0.43.

2. Cockcroft Gault equation, which is used to estimate GFR in adults, may be used in children over 12 years of age.

$$GFR = \frac{(140 - \text{age}) \times \text{body weight (kg)}}{72 \times \text{serum creatinine (mg/dL)}}$$

For females, a correction factor of 0.85 is applied.

3. Chronic Kidney Disease in Children (CKiD) formula

   Estimated GFR= 39.1 $[Ht/SCr]^{0.516}[1.8/CysC]^{0.294}[30/BUN]^{0.169}[1.099]^{male}[Ht/1.4]^{0.188}$

   Ht height (in m); SCr serum creatinine; Cysc eystatia C; BUN blood urea nitrogen.

Cystatin C

Cystatin C is a low molecular weight non-glycosylated protein produced at a constant rate by all nucleated cells in the body, freely filtered by the glomeruli, not secreted but totally reabsorbed and catabolized by the renal tubules. Serum levels of this product are proposed as a marker of GFR. It has been suggested that serum cystatin C has an advantage over creatinine with a better correlation with measured GFR as it is independent of age, gender, body composition and muscle mass. Cystatin C can be estimated in blood by kit-based enzyme immunoassays or by immunoturbidometry.

EVALUATION OF TUBULAR FUNCTION

A renal tubular disorder should be suspected in children presenting with symptoms listed in (Table 1.1). The diagnosis of a primary tubular disorder implies that there is no significant impairment of glomerular filtration or tubulointerstitial inflammation. Thus,

Table 1.1: Presenting features in tubular disorders

Growth retardation, failure to thrive
Delayed gross motor milestones
Polyuria, excessive thirst
Recurrent episodes of dehydration, vomiting, fever
Rickets, bone pains
Episodic weakness
Constipation
Craving for salt and savory foods

Table 1.2: Investigations for evaluation of suspected tubular diseases

Substrate	Test
Phosphate	Tubular reabsorption of phosphate
	Tubular maximum for reabsorption/GFR
	Blood parathormone
Glucose	Renal threshold and tubular maximum for glucose reabsorption
Amino acids	Clearance of amino acid; in relation to GFR
Bicarbonate	Blood anion gap
	Fractional excretion of bicarbonate
H^+	Minimum urinary pH
	Urine anion gap; urine osmolal gap
	U-B CO_2 gradient
Water	Maximum urine osmolality
	Water deprivation test
	Plasma ADH
Sodium	Urinary sodium excretion
	Plasma renin, aldosterone

ADH antidiuretic hormone; GFR glomerular filtration rate

tubular dysfunction observed in various glomerular diseases (e.g. in some patients with focal segmental glomerulosclerosis, cystic diseases of the kidney) is regarded as secondary. A tubular disorder may be congenital or acquired. It may involve a single function of the tubule (e.g. renal glucosuria, nephrogenic diabetes insipidus) or multiple functions (e.g. Fanconi syndrome).

A primary tubulopathy is usually congenital and hereditary and often involves a single tubular function. Secondary derangement of tubular function is usually acquired, being due to endogenous or exogenous toxic substances, and involves multiple functions. A list of laboratory investigations used for diagnosis of common tubular disorders is shown in Table 1.2 and detailed in Section III.

SUPPORT READING

Schwartz GJ, Munoz A, Schneider MF, *et al.* New equations to estimate GFR in children with CKD. J Am Soc Nephrol 2009; 20: 629–37

Bagga A, Bajpai A, Menon S. Approach to renal tubular disorders. Indian J Pediatr 2005; 72: 771–76

2 Approach to Proteinuria

Proteinuria is usually associated with progressive renal disease, but may sometimes be a transient finding occurring during stress, including exercise, fever and dehydration. Excess urinary protein loss can result from (i) increased permeability of the glomeruli to the passage of serum proteins (glomerular proteinuria); (ii) decreased reabsorption of proteins by the renal tubules (tubular proteinuria); (iii) increased secretion of tissue protein into the urine (secretory proteinuria).

Detection of Proteinuria

Normal protein excretion in urine is less than $4 \, mg/m^2$ per hour or less than $150 \, mg/1.73 \, m^2$ per day. Abnormal proteinuria is defined as protein excretion of $>4 \, mg/m^2$ per hr. Proteinuria $>40 \, mg/m^2$ per hr is considered *nephrotic range*.

Urine Dipstick

The urine dipstick (impregnated with tetrabromophenol blue) is a screening test for the presence of proteinuria. Based on the intensity of the color change (proportionate to the amount of protein present), the dipstick can be read as negative or trace; 1+ (30 mg/dL protein), 2+ (100 mg/dL), 3+ (300 mg/dL) and 4+ (2 g/dL).

False positive tests can occur if the dipstick is kept in the urine too long and the buffer leaches out. It may also occur in the presence of hematuria, pyuria and bacteriuria, if the urine is contaminated with antiseptics such as chlorhexidine and also after administration of radiographic contrast, penicillin or cephalosporins. Highly concentrated urine (specific gravity >1025) and very alkaline urine (pH >8.0) can also show false positive results.

False negative tests may be seen if the urine is very dilute (specific gravity less than 1002) or very acidic (pH less than 4.5). This may also occur in non-albumin proteinuria because albumin binds better to the dye than do other proteins.

Sulfosalicylic Acid Test

An alternative method for measuring urine protein is the sulfosalicylic acid precipitation of protein in urine. This technique estimates all the proteins present, including albumin and low molecular weight proteins. The test is performed by mixing one part urine supernatant with three parts 3% sulfosalicylic acid. The resultant turbidity is graded as: no turbidity [0]; slight turbidity [0.01–0.1 g/L]; turbidity through which print can be read [0.15–0.3 g/L]; white cloud without precipitate through which heavy black lines on a white background are seen [0.4–1 g/L]; white cloud with precipitate through which heavy black lines cannot be seen [1–3 g/L]; flocculent precipitate [>5 g/L].

Quantitation of Proteinuria

Quantitative methods detect all proteins including low molecular weight proteins. A

24-hr urine collection is cumbersome in children because of difficulties of collection and the need to correct the protein excretion rate for body surface area. Urine dipstick testing correlates with 24-hr urinary protein estimation.

Another method is to measure the concentration of protein and creatinine in *single voided sample* and express as a ratio (Up/Uc). The first morning sample is the most suitable as it eliminates any effect of posture (orthostatic proteinuria).

Etiology

When proteinuria is detected, it is important to determine whether it is intermittent or persistent. Isolated proteinuria is benign in the majority and can be transient and postural. Table 2.1 lists important conditions presenting with proteinuria.

Intermittent Proteinuria

In intermittent proteinuria, protein is detected in only some urine samples. Intermittent proteinuria can also occur after exercise or in association with stress, dehydration, or fever.

Orthostatic (postural) proteinuria is defined as an elevated protein excretion when the child is upright but normal protein excretion during recumbency. It is related to alterations in renal or glomerular hemodynamics and is benign. No treatment is required for children with orthostatic proteinuria.

Persistent Proteinuria

Persistent proteinuria is defined as proteinuria of ≥1+, on multiple occasions over 4 weeks or more. The presence of persistent proteinuria requires evaluation. It is important to exclude acute nephritic or nephrotic syndrome as these are distinct clinical entities which require specific management.

EVALUATION

A step-by-step approach is recommended to evaluate isolated proteinuria in an asymptomatic child. However, if the child has signs and symptoms that suggest renal disease,

---

Table 2.1: Conditions presenting with proteinuria

Glomerular proteinuria
Nephrotic syndrome: minimal change disease, focal segmental glomerulosclerosis, congenital nephrotic syndrome, membranous nephropathy
Hepatitis B and C nephropathy, HIV nephropathy
Reflux nephropathy
Amyloidosis
Associated hematuria: Membranoproliferative glomerulonephritis, postinfectious glomerulonephritis, IgA nephropathy, Henoch Schonlein nephritis, lupus nephritis, Alport syndrome

Tubular proteinuria
Drugs (analgesics) induced nephropathy
Heavy metal nephropathy (e.g. gold, lead, cadmium)
Renal tubular acidosis
Interstitial nephritis, pyelonephritis

Intermittent or transient proteinuria
Postural (orthostatic)
Fever
Exercise

detailed investigation should be initiated. An approach to evaluation is detailed below.

History

History is taken for clues that suggest an underlying etiology.

1. Edema, hematuria, polyuria or nocturia; symptoms of glomerulonephritis or renal failure
2. Rashes and joint pain; history of connective tissue disorders
3. History of recurrent urinary tract infections
4. Family history of polycystic kidney disease, renal failure or deafness

Physical Examination

Important signs include:

1. Evidence of renal failure, such as growth failure, anemia, hypertension and bone disease
2. Signs of acute nephritic or nephrotic syndrome
3. Signs of systemic illnesses: palpable purpuric rash, arthritis
4. Palpable flank masses: hydronephrosis or polycystic kidneys

Investigations

In an asymptomatic child, the first step is to determine whether the proteinuria is persistent. Patients with persistent proteinuria ($\geq$1+ on multiple occasions over 4 weeks or more) need further investigations. If proteinuria is absent on subsequent testing, the initial proteinuria may be *transient* and related to fever or severe exercise, and no further investigations required. The patient should be reassured and a urine dipstick test for protein repeated at 3 to 6 months.

For orthostatic proteinuria, the urine is examined two times a day for 1 week, with the first sample voided in the morning as soon as the child wakes up and the last voided in mid-afternoon or evening. No further investi-

gations are required, and the urine should be rechecked for proteinuria in 1 year.

If proteinuria on dipstick *recurs* or is *persistent*, the next step is to quantify the amount of proteinuria. This may be done either as spot urine protein to creatinine ratio or a 24-hr protein excretion. A spot urine protein to creatinine ratio that exceeds 0.2 mg/mg or 24-hour urinary total protein greater than 150 mg/1.73 m^2 confirms the presence of significant proteinuria, which requires evaluation for the presence of kidney disease.

Urinalysis

Patients with the combination of hematuria with proteinuria require evaluation for an underlying glomerular disorder. Microscopic examination of a fresh specimen is necessary. Urine culture is done in patients with suspected urinary tract infection. Measurement of excretion of low-molecular proteins such as β_2-microglobulin and retinol-binding protein indicate tubular proteinuria.

Blood Examination

These include, wherever necessary, one or more of the following investigations: *(i)* renal function tests, electrolytes, total protein and albumin, lipid profile; *(ii)* serum complement C3 and C4; *(iii)* antistreptolysin O, anti DNAse B titers; *(iv)* serology for hepatitis B, hepatitis C and HIV; and *(v)* antinuclear antibodies (ANA); anti-double stranded DNA antibodies; antineutrophil cytoplasmic antibodies (ANCA).

Renal Imaging

Ultrasonography is useful in identifying congenital or acquired anatomic abnormalities of the kidneys or urinary tract. A dimercaptosuccinic acid (DMSA) scan is a sensitive test for detecting reflux nephropathy that might be due to an underlying vesicoureteric reflux. Doppler sonography may be useful for detecting the nutcracker syndrome, a rare cause of proteinuria in children.

Confirmation may require magnetic resonance venography.

Audiometry and Eye Examination

Audiometry is recommended in patients with family history of nephritis, renal failure or sensorineural deafness. Eye examination may show lenticonus, keratoconus and macular degeneration in patients with Alport syndrome.

Indications for Renal Biopsy

A kidney biopsy is required in patients with:

1. Persistent significant proteinuria >1 g/ 1.73 m² per day, except in patient with steroid sensitive nephrotic syndrome
2. Persistent proteinuria associated with urinary sediment abnormalities (microscopic hematuria)
3. Elevated serum creatinine; decreased glomerular filtration rate except in patients with resolving glomerulonephritis

4. Persistent low C3 levels for more than 3 months
5. Clinical or serological evidence of collagen vascular disease or vasculitis (systemic lupus, Henoch-Schönlein purpura or ANCA-associated vasculitis)

SUPPORT READING

Rademacher ER, Sinaiko AR. Albuminuria in children. Curr Opin Nephrol Hypertens 2009; 18: 246–51

Quigley R. Evaluation of hematuria and proteinuria: how should a pediatrician proceed? Curr Opin Pediatr 2008; 20: 140–44

Hogg RJ. Adolescents with proteinuria and/or the nephrotic syndrome. Adolesc Med Clin 2005; 16: 163–72

Caring for Australians with Renal Impairment (CARI). The CARI guidelines. Urine protein as diagnostic test: evaluation of proteinuria in children. Nephrology (Carlton) 2004; 9 Suppl 3: S15–19

3 Evaluation of Hematuria

Hematuria is defined as a urine microscopy showing red blood cells (RBC) more than 10/µL in a fresh uncentrifuged midstream urine specimen, or more than 5 RBC/high power field in the centrifuged sediment from 10 ml of freshly voided midstream urine.

False positive results (an absence of red blood cells in the urine with a positive dipstick reaction) can occur in the following conditions: *(i)* hemoglobinuria following intravascular hemolysis; *(ii)* myoglobinuria after rhabdomyolysis; and *(iii)* presence of oxidizing agents in the urine, such as microbial peroxidases associated with urinary tract infection. Table 3.1 lists conditions causing discoloration of urine. *False negative results* can be due to the presence of large amounts of reducing agents such as ascorbic acid or urine with high specific gravity, in which case the dipstick test is less sensitive.

Etiology

Hematuria may originate from the glomeruli, renal tubules and interstitium, or the urinary tract (including collecting systems, ureters, bladder, and urethra). In children, the source of bleeding is more often the glomeruli than from the urinary tract. The causes of hematuria in children are listed in Table 3.2.

Table 3.1: Causes of discoloration of urine

Dark yellow, orange urine
    Normal concentrated urine
    Drugs such as rifampicin

Dark brown, black urine
    Bile pigments
    Methemoglobinemia
    Alanine, cascara, resorcinol
    Alkaptonuria, melanin, thymol, tyrosinosis

Red, pink urine
    Red blood cells
    Free hemoglobin
    Myoglobin
    Porphyrins
    Urates in high concentration
    Foods: beetroot, blackberries, red dyes
    Drugs: benzene, chloroquine, desferoxamine, phenazopyridine, phenolphthalein

Table 3.2: Causes of hematuria

Glomerular	Nonglomerular
Postinfectious glomerulonephritis (GN)	Hypercalciuria
IgA nephropathy, Henoch-Schönlein nephritis	Renal calculi
Membranoproliferative GN	Urinary tract infection
Rapidly progressive GN	Hemorrhagic cystitis
Familial benign hematuria	Trauma, exercise
(thin basement membrane disease)	Cystic renal disease
Uncommon	*Uncommon*
Lupus nephritis	Vascular malformations
Other vasculitides, e.g. microscopic polyangiitis	Coagulation disorder, thrombocytopenia
Membranous nephropathy	Nutcracker syndrome
Alport syndrome	Malignancy (renal or bladder)

EVALUATION

The first step is to confirm the presence of hematuria by urine microscopy. It is important to determine if the hematuria is of glomerular or non-glomerular origin (Table 3.3). A careful history and physical examination, followed by urinalysis is crucial. Fig. 3.1 provides an approach to evaluation of hematuria.

History

History is taken for (*i*) duration and timing of hematuria; (*ii*) recent trauma, exercise, or passage of stones; (*iii*) recent respiratory or skin infections; intake of medications or herbal compounds; (*iv*) fever, dysuria, urinary frequency and urgency, back pain, skin rashes, joint symptoms, and face and leg swelling; and (*v*) family history of hematuria,

Table 3.3: Features that distinguish glomerular from non-glomerular hematuria

Features	Glomerular causes	Non-glomerular causes
Dysuria	–	Suggests urethritis or cystitis
Systemic complaints	Edema, pharyngitis, rash, arthralgia (postinfectious glomerulonephritis, lupus, Henoch-Schönlein purpura)	Fever (UTI), loin pain (calculi)
Family history	Deafness, renal failure (Alport syndrome)	Calculi (hypercalciuria)
Hypertension, edema	Common	Rare
Abdominal mass	Absent	Wilms tumor, obstructive uropathy
Urine color	Brown, tea, cola	Bright red, clots
Proteinuria	2+ or more	Trace, 1+
Dysmorphic RBCs	>20%	<15%
RBC casts	Common	Absent
Crystals	Absent	May suggest calculi

UTI urinary tract infection; RBC red blood cells

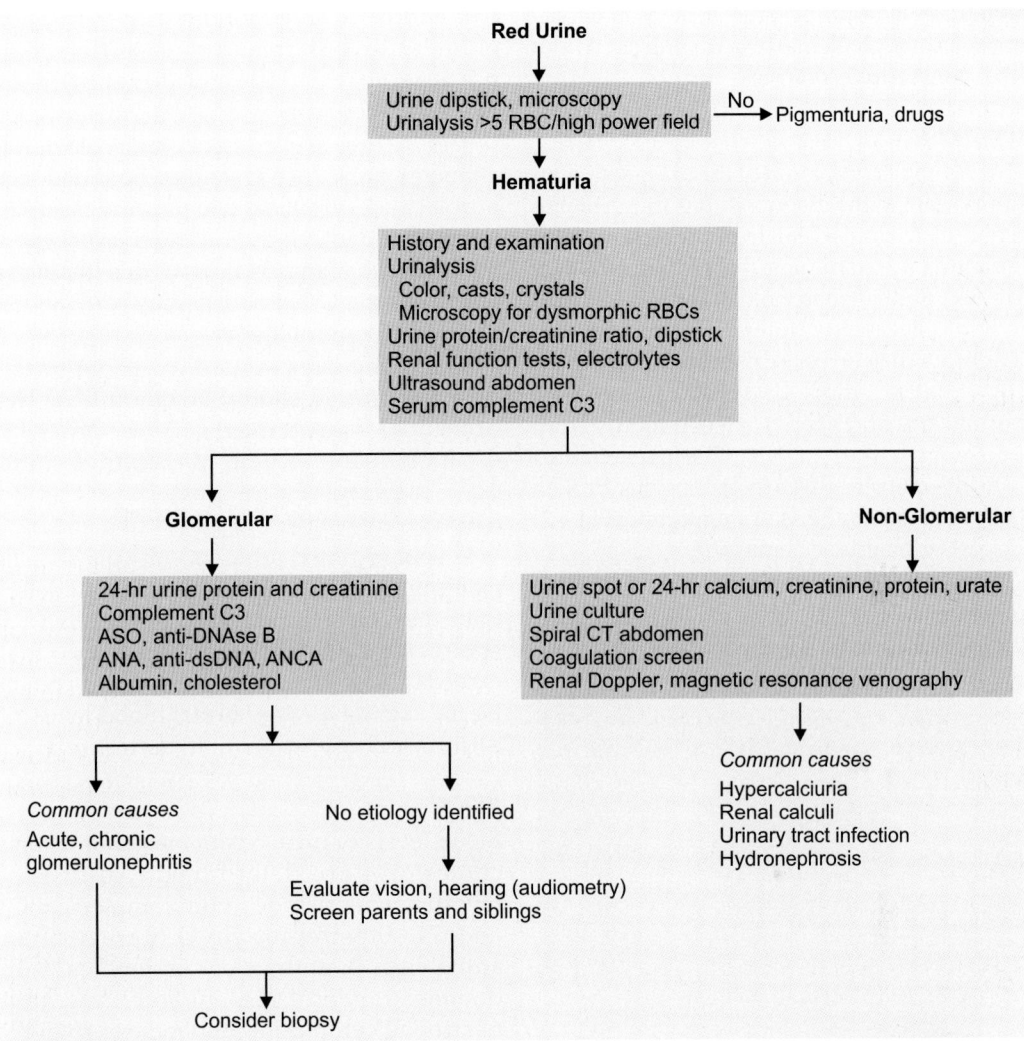

Red Urine

↓

Urine dipstick, microscopy
Urinalysis >5 RBC/high power field → **No** → Pigmenturia, drugs

↓

Hematuria

↓

History and examination
Urinalysis
  Color, casts, crystals
  Microscopy for dysmorphic RBCs
Urine protein/creatinine ratio, dipstick
Renal function tests, electrolytes
Ultrasound abdomen
Serum complement C3

Glomerular   **Non-Glomerular**

24-hr urine protein and creatinine
Complement C3
ASO, anti-DNAse B
ANA, anti-dsDNA, ANCA
Albumin, cholesterol

Urine spot or 24-hr calcium, creatinine, protein, urate
Urine culture
Spiral CT abdomen
Coagulation screen
Renal Doppler, magnetic resonance venography

Common causes
Hypercalciuria
Renal calculi
Urinary tract infection
Hydronephrosis

Common causes
Acute, chronic
glomerulonephritis

No etiology identified

↓

Evaluate vision, hearing (audiometry)
Screen parents and siblings

Consider biopsy

Fig. 3.1: Approach to evaluation of a patient with hematuria. The initial evaluation attempts to distinguish glomerular from non-glomerular causes of hematuria. Estimation of C3 is an important screening test for postinfectious glomerulonephritis. Patients with persistent glomerular hematuria might require kidney biopsy and/or screening for familial causes. ASO antistreptolysin O, ANA antinuclear antibody, anti dsDNA anti-double stranded DNA antibody, ANCA antineutrophil cytoplasmic antibody

hypertension, renal stones, renal failure, deafness and coagulopathy.

Physical Examination

The presence of hypertension and edema suggests acute nephritic syndrome. Patients with systemic lupus erythematosus or Henoch-Schönlein purpura show rash or arthritis. The abdomen should be examined for renal masses.

Investigations

Microscopic hematuria may incidentally occur during illness or after exertion. Further evaluation is required only if there is persistent microscopic hematuria on at least two of three consecutive samples.

Urinalysis

Microscopic examination of the urine sediment is important in the diagnosis. It is important to distinguish glomerular from nonglomerular hematuria by examining red cell morphology (Fig. 3.2). Red cell morphology can be identified on light microscopy (following staining with Wright stain) or on phase contrast microscopy. RBCs that are more than 80% isomorphic (normal size and shape) are commonly from the lower urinary tract. The presence of >20% dysmorphic RBCs (acanthocytes, broken RBCs or segmental loss of membrane; Fig 3.2) suggests glomerular hematuria.

The detection of *red cell casts* (Fig. 3.2) in fresh urine is always pathological and suggests glomerulonephritis. Co-existence of *white blood cells* indicates infection and interstitial or glomerular inflammatory disorders, e.g. poststreptococcal glomerulonephritis or interstitial nephritis.

Hyaline casts signify associated proteinuria, although a few such casts may be found in a normal concentrated early morning sample. While abundant *calcium oxalate crystals* suggest the presence of hypercalciuria, this finding is not diagnostic. Other crystals may be identified in cases of nephrolithiasis.

The urine is examined for proteinuria, which if present should be quantified. The presence of proteinuria (2+ or more by dipstick; urine protein to creatinine ratio >0.2 mg/mg; 24-hr protein excretion >100 mg/m^2) suggests a glomerular etiology.

A spot or timed urine specimen is done to determine urine calcium excretion and determine the ratio of urine calcium to creatinine. A spot urine calcium to creatinine ratio that exceeds 0.2 mg/mg or urine calcium excretion >4 mg/kg/day, with normal blood levels of calcium is characteristic of hypercalciuria.

Blood

Blood levels of urea, creatinine, albumin and cholesterol are determined. Additional investigations include serum complement C3 and C4, antistreptolysin O titer (ASO) or antiDNAse B, antinuclear antibodies, anti-double-stranded DNA antibody, and anti-neutrophil cytoplasmic antibodies (ANCA).

Imaging

Renal ultrasound and abdominal X-ray are indicated if urinary tract calculi are suspected. Renal ultrasound is useful in determining the size of the kidneys, and diagnosing polycystic kidneys and tumors.

Cystoscopy

Cystoscopy should be done when preliminary investigations fail to find a cause and when a bladder or urethral pathology is suspected because of accompanying voiding symptoms.

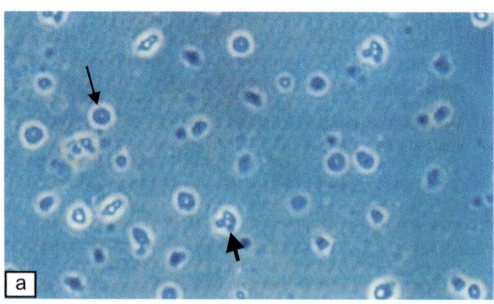

a

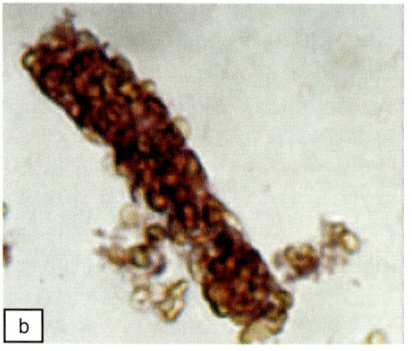

b

Fig. 3.2: (a) Phase contrast microscopy showing dysmorphic red cells (arrowhead). Normal red cells are also seen (arrow). (b) Light microscopy showing red cell cast

Initial hematuria suggests a urethral origin, whereas terminal hematuria is indicative of a bladder cause. Vascular malformations in the bladder or a bladder mass can be detected by cystoscopy.

Family Screening

Family members should be screened for microscopic hematuria in patients with benign familial hematuria and suspected Alport syndrome.

Audiometry

This is useful in detecting high frequency sensorineural hearing deficit, as in Alport syndrome.

Renal Biopsy

A renal biopsy should be considered in patients with persistent microscopic hematuria and:

1. Nephrotic range proteinuria persisting beyond >2 weeks
2. Persistent (>12 weeks) low serum complement C3
3. Azotemia lasting beyond 7–10 days
4. Suspected systemic disorder, e.g. systemic lupus erythematosus, Henoch-Schönlein purpura, and ANCA-associated vasculitis
5. Family history suggestive of Alport syndrome, chronic kidney disease
6. Recurrent gross hematuria of unknown etiology
7. Microscopic hematuria of unknown etiology persisting beyond 2 years

Renal histology should be examined by light microscopy and immunofluorescence. Electron microscopy is required for the diagnosis of Alport syndrome (Fig. 3.3), thin basement membrane disease and membranoproliferative glomerulonephritis.

SUPPORT READING

Higashihara E, Nishiyama T, Horie S, et al; Working Group for the Creation of Hematuria Guidelines.

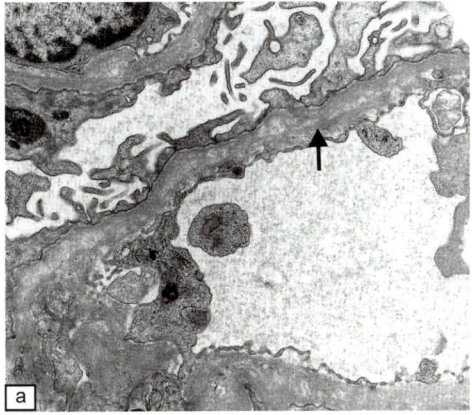
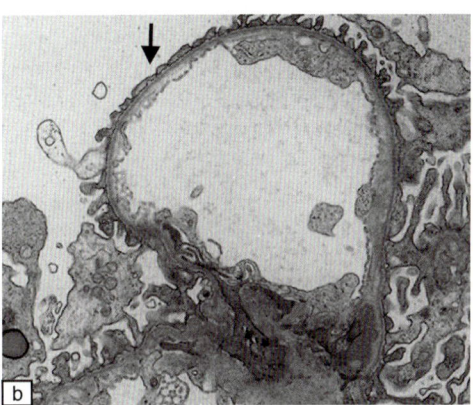

Fig. 3.3: Electron microscopy showing (a) thickening of the glomerular basement membrane with splitting and fragmentation (arrow) of the lamina densa characteristic of Alport syndrome; and (b) diffuse thinning of the basement membrane with focal fusion of foot processes (arrow) characteristic of thin basement membrane disease

Hematuria: definition and screening test methods. Int J Urol. 2008; 15: 281–84

Quigley R. Evaluation of hematuria and proteinuria: how should a pediatrician proceed? Curr Opin Pediatr 2008; 20: 140–44

Phadke KD, Vijayakumar M, Sharma J, Iyengar A; Indian Pediatric Nephrology Group. Consensus statement on evaluation of hematuria. Indian Pediatr 2006; 43: 965–73

Pan CG. Evaluation of gross hematuria. Pediatr Clin North Am 2006; 53: 401–12

Meyers KE. Evaluation of hematuria in children. Urol Clin North Am 2004; 31: 559–73

4 Renal Biopsy

Examination of the renal histology is an important investigation, particularly in a proportion of patients with renal diseases. A final histological diagnosis is based on synthesis of information on light, immuno-fluorescence and electron microscopy.

Indications

Identification of the underlying etiology has implications for understanding the course of the illness and guiding its management. The indications for renal biopsy are listed in Table 4.1. A kidney biopsy is useful in ascertaining the underlying diagnosis in patients with unexplained chronic kidney disease, since this may have implications in management and counseling regarding transplantation.

Contraindications

While there are no absolute contraindications to performing a renal biopsy, caution should be exercised in presence of the following:

1. Uncontrolled high blood pressure: increases risk of bleeding
2. Bleeding disorders: hemophilia, thrombocytopenia; or recent use of medications that increase the risk of bleeding
3. Solitary kidney: Transplant kidneys are often biopsied, but the biopsy procedure is safe since the kidney is closer to the surface
4. Active kidney infection

Pre-Biopsy Work up

Before biopsy, the medical history, examination and investigations are reviewed.

History

Cardiac or respiratory illness; bleeding tendencies; allergy to povidone or iodine, ketamine, midazolam and lidocaine

Examination

Blood pressure; anatomic abnormalities of the spine, chest or abdomen; subcutaneous infection over biopsy site; ascites

Laboratory evaluation

The level of hemoglobin should be more than 8 g/dL and platelet count more than $75,000/mm^3$. Blood levels of urea and creatinine are estimated. Studies are performed to measure the prothrombin time (PT), bleeding time and clotting time. PT should be normal (international normalized ratio, INR <1.5) at least 24-hr prior, particularly if the patient has been receiving treatment with oral anticoagulants.

Radiology

Ultrasonography is done to examine the anatomy, position and size of both kidneys.

Precautions

1. Treatment with aspirin, non-steroidal anti-inflammatory drugs, or warfarin

Table 4.1: Indications for renal biopsy

Acute glomerulonephritis (Chapter 20)
Systemic features: fever, rash, joint pain
Lack of serologic evidence of streptococcal infection; normal C3
Rapidly progressive GN
Delayed resolution
 (i) Oliguria, hypertension and/or azotemia persisting past 7 days
 (ii) Gross hematuria persisting past 3–4 weeks
 (iii) Nephrotic range proteinuria beyond 2 weeks or persistent proteinuria beyond 6 months
 (iv) Low C3 levels beyond 12 weeks
 (v) Persistent microscopic hematuria beyond 12–18 months

Nephrotic syndrome (Section IV)
Onset below 1-yr; late adolescence
Associated persistent hematuria, stage II hypertension, elevated blood creatinine; low C3
Steroid resistance
Suspected systemic disorder
Screen for calcineurin inhibitor nephrotoxicity

Hematuria (Chapter 3)
Persistent glomerular hematuria (2+ or more proteinuria, red cell casts, dysmorphic red cells; or
   azotemia)
Microscopic hematuria of unknown etiology persisting beyond 2 years

Asymptomatic proteinuria (Chapter 2)
Nephrotic range proteinuria (>1000 mg/m^2 per day, except in patients with steroid sensitive nephrotic
   syndrome
Persistent non-nephrotic range proteinuria (100–1000 mg/m^2 per day) with hematuria

Acute renal failure (Chapter 31)
Unremitting ARF lasting longer than 2 to 3 weeks
Suspected drug-induced renal failure; acute interstitial nephritis
Etiology of renal failure not identified

Following renal transplantation (Chapter 43)
Protocol biopsies
Distinguish rejection, acute tubular necrosis, drug toxicity

Systemic diseases (Section V)
Henoch-Schönlein syndrome; systemic lupus erythematosus; microscopic polyarteritis
Monitor course; assess histological activity

should be discontinued 5–7 days before the biopsy
2. Ketamine should be avoided in patients with respiratory tract infections or in young infants (<3-month-old).

3. In patients on hemodialysis who require a renal biopsy, the procedure should be performed at least 6-hr after the hemodialysis. The use of anticoagulants should be avoided for the next 24-hr.

4. In patients with azotemia or prolonged bleeding time (>8–10 minutes), the risk of post-biopsy bleeding is reduced by the administration of IV desmopressin (DDAVP 0.3 μg/kg) 30 minutes prior, or nasal DDAVP (2–4 μg/kg) 2 hr before the procedure.

PROCEDURE

Percutaneous renal biopsies are usually outpatient procedures, except in infants, children with solitary kidney and those with chronic kidney disease. The renal biopsy may be performed under imaging (ultrasound or CT) guidance or as a blind procedure, with conscious sedation.

A video showing the procedure of renal biopsy is enclosed.

The patient should be fasting 4–6 hours prior; clear liquids are allowed until 2 hr before the biopsy. *A written consent is taken from either of the parents or the legal guardian.*

Biopsy Needles

A semi-automatic kidney biopsy needle (e.g. Bard Biopsy gun) is used (Fig. 4.1). Alternatively, a Trucut biopsy needle is used. Either 16 or 18 gauge needle or gun may be used. The internal diameter of the 18 gauge needle (300–400 μm) is only barely larger than the adult glomeruli (200–250 μm). Hence, pathology departments prefer larger cores, such as those provided by the 16 gauge needle (700–800 μm diameters). The 18 gauge needles are preferred for biopsies in

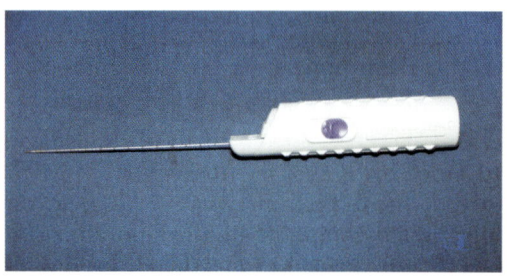

Fig. 4.1: Semi-automatic guns used for kidney biopsy

newborns and infants, and from the allograft kidney.

Positioning

Native kidneys are most easily biopsied with the patient lying in a prone position, with support under the lower chest and epigastrium. Alternatively, the patient may be positioned ipsilateral side down to splint the normal motion of the kidney due to respiration. Typically, a transplanted kidney is positioned in the right or left lower pelvis and the most direct access is via an anterior approach.

Sedation and Anesthesia

The choice between conscious sedation versus local anesthetic alone depends on institutional policies. Most children would require conscious sedation with monitoring of vital signs as described below. However, transplant biopsies in older cooperative children may be performed under ultrasound guidance using only local lidocaine.

An IV access with wide bore cannula should be established. The patient's heart rate, saturation and blood pressure are closely monitored during sedation and the procedure. Medications administered for purpose of sedation are listed in Table 4.2.

Midazolam 0.05–0.1 mg/kg IV (maximum 2 mg) is given until speech slurs or eyes become "glassy" to a total dose of 0.2 mg/kg (maximum 5 mg). For cooperative patients >8 years old, midazolam with local anesthesia may be sufficient (conscious sedation). The dose of midazolam should not be repeated within 1 hour.

Atropine (0.01 mg/kg IV) is administered 1–2 minutes prior to midazolam to reduce excessive secretions (due to ketamine).

Ketamine (0.5 mg/kg) is given 3–5 minutes after midazolam, just before the biopsy. The dose may be repeated at 3 minute intervals, until there is a reduced response to verbal or painful stimuli, or to a maximum dose of 4 mg/kg. Repeat doses of ketamine may be

Table 4.2: Medications for deep sedation; administered intravenously (IV)

Agent	Dose, mg/kg	Maximum dose	Onset, minutes	Duration of action, minutes
Midazolam	0.05 – 0.1	0.2 mg/kg; 5 mg total	2–3	30–60
Ketamine	0.5	2 mg/kg	1–2	10–30
Atropine	0.01	0.5 mg total		
Flumazenil	0.02 q 60 sec	1 mg/dose		

required every 10–20 minutes if patient becomes responsive. Ketamine is contra-indicated in children with poorly controlled hypertension and raised intraocular pressure. Doses above 2 mg/kg may cause apnea.

Surface Preparation

Betadine and spirit (70% alcohol) are used in successive order to clean the site and adjoining area centrifugally. Drapes are applied. Lidocaine is injected locally (IV preparation, 1%) (maximum 0.5 mL/kg).

Ultrasonic Localization

The lower pole of the kidney is located at the midaxillary line. The probe is then moved to the back, determining the depth and marking a 2 mm wheal at the proposed site of insertion. Then the probe is repositioned at the midaxillary line. If real time guidance is desired, the probe can be kept at the site when procedure is performed.

The needle is inserted from a posterior approach in a trajectory that avoids the lungs, adjacent organs, and central renal collecting system. A trajectory that passes vertically down to the lower pole cortex, avoiding the central echogenic hilum, is chosen (Fig. 4. 2a). Alternatively a trajectory that allows one to enter the cortex with the needle lying flat on the surface, such that the hilum is not entered, may be used (Fig. 4. 2b). A route directed towards the central hilum is associated with risk of vascular injury and should be avoided (Fig. 4. 2c).

If USG localization not available

A probing needle (1½ inch, 23 guage; or 9 cm 20 guage spinal needle) is used to locate the renal capsule at lower pole (below 12th rib, lateral to the sacrospinalis muscle). While withdrawing the needle, the tract should be anaesthesized.

A stab incision is given at the proposed site with a 11 gauge surgical blade. The needle biopsy is passed to the required depth, and cores are taken.

Specimen Collection

With either method of biopsy, two or three cores are taken for processing for light microscopy, immunofluorescence and electron microscopy. Preferably, a pathologist should be present throughout the procedure to confirm the adequacy of samples.

Post Biopsy Monitoring

The heart and respiratory rate and blood pressure are monitored every 15 minutes for one hr, then every 30 minutes for the next 2-hr and then every hr for 4–6 hr. Each urine specimen is inspected for presence of hematuria. The patient is kept supine and oral fluids are allowed once conscious.

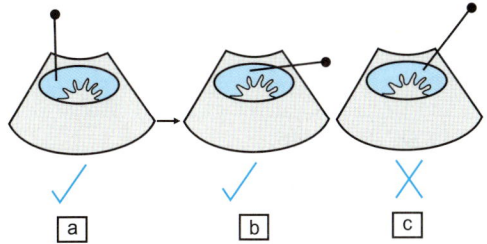

Fig. 4.2: Panels a and b indicate suitable trajectory, while panel c indicates a path that carries a high risk of vascular injury

Discharge

Patients should stay in the hospital for 8–24 hr after the procedure. Bed rest is advised for 24 hr. Contact sports, cycling or lifting of heavy objects should be avoided for 1 week. Oral paracetamol is given for pain relief. Treatment with aspirin and warfarin can be restarted after 48–72 hr if the procedure was uncomplicated.

At discharge the vital signs should be normal and there should be no gross hematuria. Patients should not be discharged early until resolution of sedation related complications, circulatory compromise and gross hematuria.

Complications

Renal biopsy is a safe procedure. The most common complication is hemorrhage, which may be perinephric or into the collecting system. Rare complications include infection and formation of arteriovenous fistula.

Gross Hematuria

Microscopic or gross hematuria may be noted in one-third patients. However, blood loss is usually insignificant and less than 1% of patients require blood transfusion; renal loss is rare (<0.1%). Large perinephric hematomas particularly those extending into the pelvis, require close monitoring for hemodynamic instability.

In presence of gross hematuria, an ultrasound is done to examine for bleeds, clots or for perinephric hematoma. Packed cells should be arranged and transfused if the hemoglobin declines by 10–15% from the baseline. An adequate intake of fluids is ensured; either orally or parenterally. If coagulation is deranged, fresh frozen plasma (FFP), cryoprecipitate or DDAVP should be administered. If hematuria persists, an AV fistula should be suspected. Such patients require radiographic transcatheter embolization or surgical intervention.

Sedation Related Complications

Administration of sedation may occasionally result in brief hypoxia, transient airway complications, vomiting, minor aspiration or laryngospasm. Management includes repositioning, suction and oxygen administration.

Antidote for midazolam: Flumazenil (500 µg/5 mL) 5–10 µg/kg/dose every 60 sec (to a maximum of 40 µg/kg) with monitoring for further 2-hr. Since flumazenil is short-acting and respiratory depression may recur.

Processing Biopsy Specimens

Two cores of tissue are obtained; one core each is processed for light microscopy (LM) and immunofluorescence (IF) examination respectively. Tissue for electron microscopy (EM) may be obtained either with a third core or by incising off 2 mm tissue at each end of the two cores. The tissue for LM is transported either in 10% formalin or paraformaldehyde, for IF in special media (e.g. Michel) and snap frozen in the laboratory, and for EM in glutaraldehyde.

An adequate biopsy should contain representative portions of the cortex and medulla to enable comment on the morphology of glomeruli, tubules, interstitium and blood vessels. A focal and segmental lesion may be missed in a biopsy containing fewer than 8–10 glomeruli.

Appropriate stains are required for proper interpretation of histological findings. Hematoxylin and eosin are useful for general evaluation, and cellular characterization; periodic Schiff for staining glomerular basement membranes and the mesangium; silver methenamine for details of basement membranes; Masson Trichrome and Sirus red for fibrosis; and Congo red for amyloid.

SUPPORT READING

Uppot RN, Harisinghani MG, Gervais DA. Imaging-guided percutaneous renal biopsy: rationale and approach. Am J Roent 2010; 194: 1443–49

Walker PD. The renal biopsy. Arch Pathol Lab Med 2009; 133: 181–88

Structural Diseases

5 Antenatal Hydronephrosis

Hydronephrosis is commonly diagnosed on antenatal ultrasonography, with an incidence of 1–5% among all pregnancies. Antenatally detected dilatation, which persists after birth is labeled as *neonatal hydronephrosis*. Evaluation aims to identify fetuses that require prompt perinatal evaluation and management. In addition, it allows us to distinguish them from those with benign dilatation of the urinary tract, where undue parental anxiety may be avoided.

Etiology and Differential Diagnosis

Important conditions associated with antenatal hydronephrosis (ANH) are listed in Table 5.1. Physiological narrowing of the pelviureteric junction (PUJ) and natural kinks account for a large proportion of cases. Of all hydronephrosis identified prenatally, 50% cases are transient, resolving before birth. Pelviureteric junction (PUJ) obstruction accounts for 15–25% cases of persistent unilateral ANH without ureteral dilatation. No specific anomaly is detected in 15% cases.

Bilateral ANH is more severe than unilateral disease. The combination of bilateral ANH with a dilated, thick-walled bladder that fails to empty, dilated posterior urethra and decreased amniotic fluid suggest lower urinary tract obstruction. The most common cause of hydroureteronephrosis with a normal bladder is vesicoureteric reflux (VUR). Upper

Table 5.1: Causes of antenatal hydronephrosis

Pelviureteric junction (PUJ) anomalies	*Vesicourethral anomalies*
Transient dysfunction of the PUJ	Posterior urethral valves
PUJ obstruction	Urethral atresia
Ureteral and vesicoureteric junction (VUJ) anomalies	Urogenital sinus and cloacal anomalies
Vesicoureteral reflux	*Miscellaneous disorders*
Megaureter	Prune belly syndrome
Ureterocele	Tumors
Ectopic ureter	Neurogenic bladder

pole hydroureteronephrosis and duplex draining system suggests the presence of ureterocele or ectopic ureter. The ultrasound finding of a thin walled cystic structure at the base of the bladder suggests ureterocele.

ANTENATAL MANAGEMENT

Evaluation of Severity

The anteroposterior diameter of renal pelvis is used to assess the severity of ANH. The diameter varies by gestation, hydration, and degree of bladder distension (Table 5.2). About 50–85% of ANH is classified as mild, 10–30% as moderate and 2–15% as severe. The risk of postnatal pathology is estimated at 5–12% for mild, 45% for moderate and 88–90% for severe ANH. Measurements in the third trimester have the highest predictive value. Most fetuses with anteroposterior diameter below 6 mm during the second trimester, or less than 8 mm during the third trimester have transient hydronephrosis. Those with pelvic

Table 5.2: Severity of antenatal hydronephrosis based on anteroposterior pelvic diameter in second and third trimester

Degree	Second trimester	Third trimester
Mild	4 to 6 mm	7 to 9 mm
Moderate	7 to 9 mm	10 to 14 mm
Severe	≥10 mm	≥15 mm

diameter <10 mm usually do not require surgery later.

Other features on ultrasonography: Antenatal ultrasonography provides additional information that is useful in understanding the etiology and severity of antenatal hydronephrosis (Table 5.3).

Ultrasound is an unsatisfactory screening investigation for vesicoureteric reflux. The incidence and severity of reflux does not correlate with the severity of antenatal hydronephrosis.

Management

Serial ultrasound evaluations are required to monitor the change in severity of ANH, and to screen for oligohydramnios and other abnormalities. The frequency of evaluation is 2–4 weekly, depending on the severity of hydronephrosis (Fig. 5.1). Additionally, at least one level II-III ultrasound should be performed to screen for other systemic abnormalities.

1. *Unilateral hydronephrosis* does not require fetal intervention, regardless of its severity. Patients with isolated, unilateral hydronephrosis are carefully followed and delivered at term. Their postnatal evaluation is given below.

2. *Mild to moderate bilateral hydronephrosis* is similarly followed with sequential ultra-

Table 5.3: Features on antenatal ultrasound suggesting an organic cause

Oligohydramnios*
Multiple systemic malformations
Dilated bladder
Ureteral and/or calyceal dilation
Duplex kidney
Loss of renal parenchyma, cortical thinning
Poor corticomedullary differentiation, non-visualized renal pyramids
Increased renal echogenicity
Renal cysts (suggest renal dysplasia)

*Early onset of oligohydramnios (<20-wk gestation) is likely to be associated with pulmonary hypoplasia

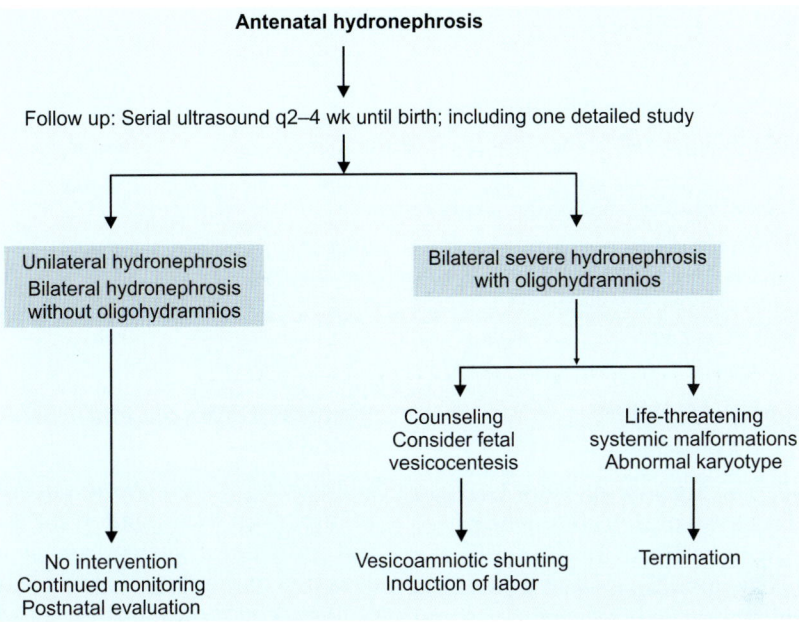

Antenatal hydronephrosis

Follow up: Serial ultrasound q2–4 wk until birth; including one detailed study

| Unilateral hydronephrosis Bilateral hydronephrosis without oligohydramnios | Bilateral severe hydronephrosis with oligohydramnios |

Counseling Consider fetal vesicocentesis

Life-threatening systemic malformations Abnormal karyotype

No intervention Continued monitoring Postnatal evaluation

Vesicoamniotic shunting Induction of labor

Termination

Fig. 5.1: Antenatal management of hydronephrosis. No fetal intervention is required for patients with unilateral hydronephrosis and the majority of those with bilateral hydronephrosis. These patients are evaluated postnatally. Patients with severe bilateral hydronephrosis and oligohydramnios are at considerable risk for adverse outcomes. Parents are counseled about the options of fetal intervention *versus* induction of early labor and postnatal intervention. Termination of pregnancy may be indicated in patients with associated congenital abnormalities, as detected by level II/III ultrasound or abnormal karyotype

sound evaluations till term. Monitoring for worsening of hydronephrosis and amniotic fluid volume is essential since these may indicate presence of lower urinary tract obstruction.

3. *Bilateral (or solitary kidney with) severe ANH with or without oligohydramnios* requires careful follow up. Patients with normal amniotic fluid volume should be followed to term, and evaluated postnataly for vesicoureteric reflux or obstruction. Patients with progressive oligohydramnios may require early termination of pregnancy beyond 32 weeks gestation or vesicoamniotic shunting. The decision to intervene should be a counseled one, weighing the risks of intervention (prematurity, fetal loss) against possible benefits. Before intervention, extrarenal abnormalities are excluded by a level II-III ultrasound and karyotyping. An estimate of fetal renal function may be made by examining electrolytes in urine obtained by serial percutaneous bladder puncture. However, the utility of these measurements is unclear.

Vesicoamniotic shunting is useful in correcting oligohydramnios, which might prevent pulmonary hypoplasia and delay need for induction of labor. However, the procedure is also associated with a high risk of fetal loss due to risks of infection and preterm labor, and the results of long-term outcome are not encouraging. Early delivery at a centre with pediatric surgery expertise is preferred, since it allows immediate postnatal intervention (catheterization and surgery).

Structural Diseases

II

Table 5.4: Society for Fetal Urology (SFU) Hydronephrosis Grading System

Grade	Renal sinus status	Cortical thickness
0	No splitting of renal sinus (intact sinus)	Normal
1	Urine in pelvis barely splits sinus (mild splitting)	Normal
2	Urine fills intrarenal pelvis ± major calyces dilated (moderate splitting, confined to renal border)	Normal
3	Urine fills extrarenal pelvis; minor calyces uniformly dilated (marked splitting, extending beyond renal border and with calyceal involvement)	Normal
4	Same as SFU grade 3	Thin

POSTNATAL MANAGEMENT

Modalities for Assessment

Ultrasound: The Society for Fetal Urology (SFU) grading system is recommended for reporting the severity of hydronephrosis (Table 5.4). This grading system guides the management, helps predict the outcome and allows comparisons between consecutive evaluations. Additional features to be noted on ultrasound include renal length, anteroposterior diameter of the renal pelvis, renal parenchymal thickness, ureteral dilatation and presence of renal or bladder cyst.

Nuclear scintigraphy: Nuclear scintigraphy assesses total and differential function and is a useful test to identify an obstructed urinary tract. It is performed at 6 weeks after birth to allow for renal maturation. Technetium labeled *mercaptotriacetylglycine* (MAG3), an agent principally excreted by tubular secretion, defines the parenchyma and collecting system while providing functional assessment. *Tc-diethylene triamine penta-acetic acid* (DTPA) is cleared by glomerular filtration, providing excellent visualization of the pelvicalyceal system, but delineates parenchymal abnormalities poorly. By binding to renal tubular cells, *Tc-dimercaptosuccinic acid* (DMSA) provides excellent visualization of the parenchymal structure, but provides inferior functional assessment. Where available, Tc-MAG3 is preferred over Tc-DTPA for the assessment of differential renal function, particularly in infants. Tc-DMSA is useful in the evaluation of cortical scars.

Micturating cystourethrogram (MCU): This is an important investigation for the diagnosis and grading of vesicoureteric reflux, and detection of the abnormalities of bladder and urethra. The indications for an MCU are: *(i)* significant bilateral hydronephrosis; *(ii)* suspected infravesical obstruction; *(iii)* suspected vesicoureteric reflux; *(iv)* dilated ureter (s); and *(v)* duplex kidney.

Children undergoing MCU are at risk of urinary tract infection following catheterization. It is necessary that the procedure be performed under aseptic precautions. The risk of UTI may be reduced by administration of oral amoxicillin (50 mg/kg within 1-hr prior to the procedure, and 25 mg/kg 6-hr later) or a single intramuscular or intravenous injection of gentamicin (1.5 mg/kg) 30 minutes prior to MCU.

Magnetic resonance urography: MRU provides satisfactory functional assessment as well as superior imaging details without the risk of radiation injury. Utilization of this technique is currently low because of non-availability at most centers, cost, need for anesthesia and limited data on efficacy in infants.

Management

Figure 5.2 provides a scheme for postnatal evaluation of antenatal hydronephrosis. All newborns with ANH should undergo an

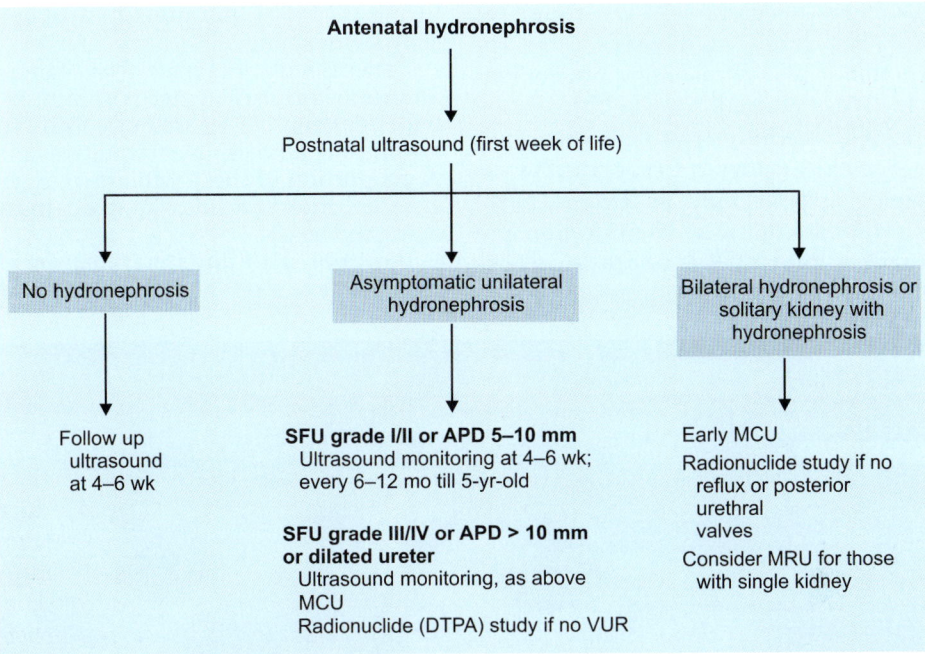

Fig. 5.2: Postnatal evaluation of antenatally detected hydronephrosis. The majority of mild unilateral hydronephrosis is benign but requires follow up to rule out progression. Newborns with unilateral hydronephrosis are evaluated for obstruction at pelviureteric or vesicoureteric junction by post diuretic radionuclide scan. In patients with bilateral hydronephrosis or in those with solitary kidney, micturating cystourethrography (MCU) is a useful test to rule out or confirm lower urinary tract obstruction or significant vesicoureteric reflux (VUR). Where available, magnetic resonance urography (MRU) is the modality of choice for assessment of differential function

ultrasound evaluation, including fetuses with mild ANH, and those in whom pelvic dilation had resolved on later antenatal ultrasounds.

Timing of ultrasound: In most cases the ultrasound is performed at 48–72 hours. An earlier ultrasound within 24–48 hours of life is necessary in newborns with bilateral hydronephrosis, hydronephrosis in solitary kidney, oligohydramnios, or those with suspected obstructive uropathy (bladder wall thickening, dilated posterior urethra). In neonates with unilateral hydronephrosis and a normal contralateral kidney, a delayed ultrasound at day 3–7 of life may be more sensitive for detection of abnormalities.

Follow up ultrasound: A single postnatal ultrasound is insensitive for detecting all

anomalies. Late worsening and recurrent hydronephrosis are seen in 1–5% cases. Hence, a second evaluation should be done in all newborns with ANH at 4–6 weeks to ensure that patients with significant VUR or worsening hydronephrosis are not missed. *Patients with two normal ultrasounds (within the first week, at 4–6 weeks) do not require further evaluation.* Patients with persistent hydronephrosis (SFU 1–4) on postnatal ultrasound require follow up examinations every 6–12 months till 5-yr of age.

Further Evaluation

The majority of hydronephrosis of *SFU grade 1 and 2* (approximate anteroposterior diameter <10 mm) resolves by 18 months of age. Patients with minimal unilateral dilation on postnatal ultrasonography (APD <10 mm) are unlikely to have significant VUR or obstruction if two ultrasonographic exams after birth are normal. *Such patients do not require MCU or scintigraphy.* This is because there is no clear evidence to support the use of imaging to detect mild VUR alone, particularly since the utility of identification and treatment of mild VUR is unproven. These patients are followed with ultrasound moni-

toring till 5-yr-old, unless hydronephrosis shows worsening.

Patients with *SFU grades 3 and 4* or a pelvic anteroposterior diameter >10 mm or those with dilated ureter(s) are more likely to have significant pathology that requires evaluation. A proportion of these patients may require surgical intervention. Their evaluation is discussed below.

Patients with *unilateral hydronephrosis* require nuclear scintigraphy at 6–8 weeks to

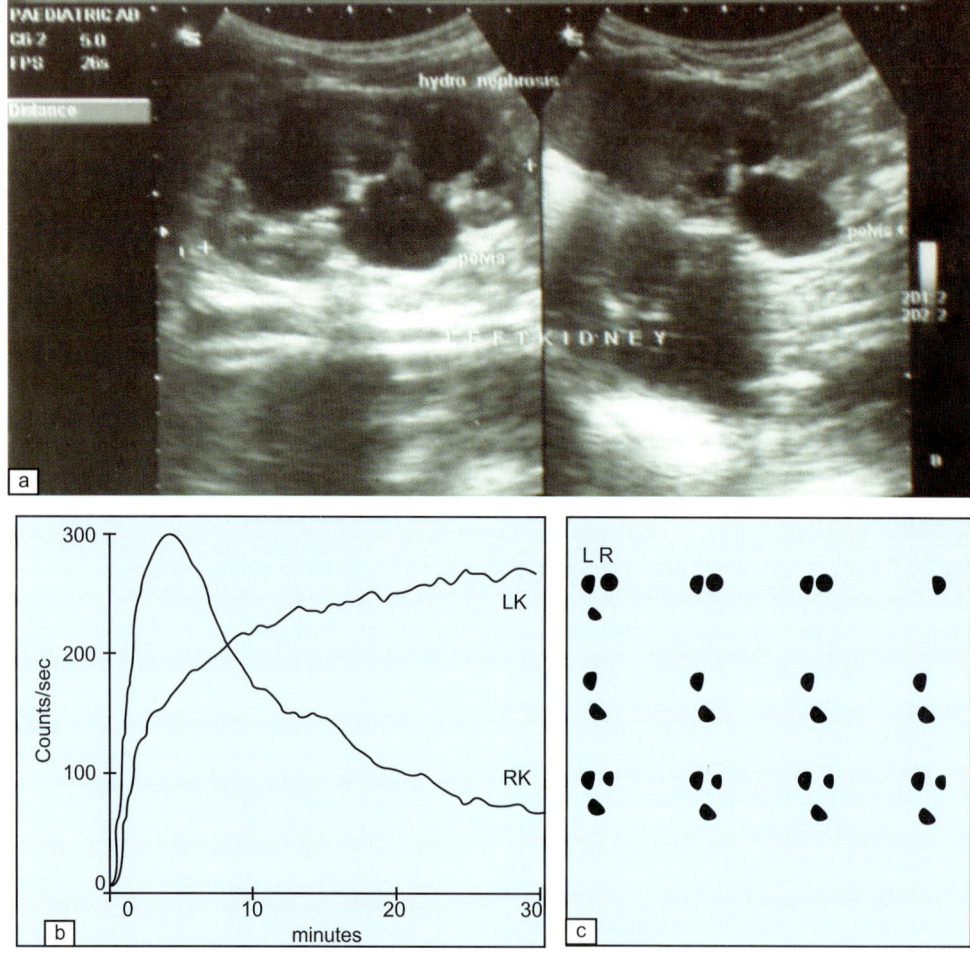

Fig. 5.3: Pelviureteric junction obstruction. (a) Postnatal ultrasonography suggests unilateral hydronephrosis of the left kidney; the other kidney was normal. (b) Renal dynamic scan at 6 weeks shows that the excretion of the tracer on the left side is sluggish and unchanged with administration of diuretic, suggesting an obstructive pattern of excretion. (c) Scan images showing pooling of tracer in the left kidney, most marked in the lower panels

rule out obstruction. Scintigraphic demons-tration of differential renal function of <40% indicates significant pelviureteric junction (PUJ) obstruction and the need for pyeloplasty (Fig. 5.3). Normally, the time required for clearance of 50% of the accumulated radio-nuclide (t½) is less than 10 minutes. Evidence of impaired drainage (t½ >20 min) is another indication for pyeloplasty. Repeat scinti-graphy is required at 4–6 months to evaluate the success or failure of conservative or surgical management. A decline in split renal function by >10% or a fall to <40% requires consideration for surgery.

In patients with unilateral hydronephrosis, an MCU is performed to evaluate for vesicou-reteric reflux if: *(i)* obstruction has been ruled out by nuclear scintigraphy at 6–8 weeks; *(ii)* hydronephrosis is associated with a dilated ureter.

Patients with *significant bilateral hydro-nephrosis* (or *single kidney with significant hydronephrosis*) require an early MCU to evaluate for vesicoureteric reflux or lower

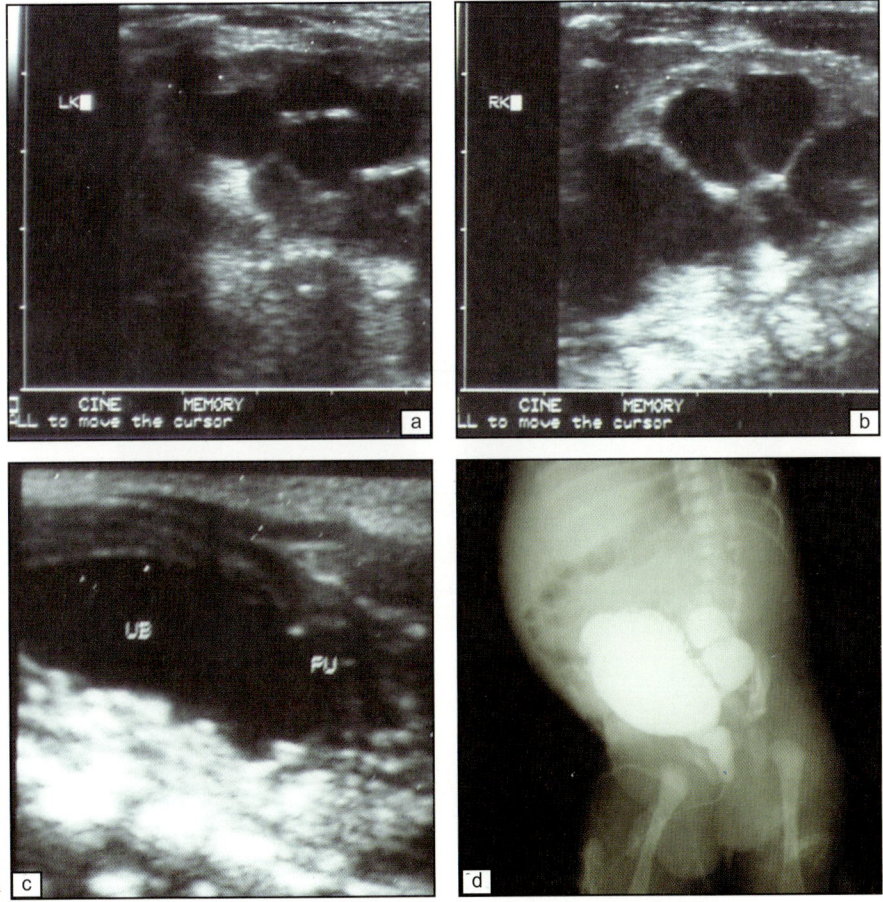

Fig. 5.4: Evaluation in a male newborn with antenatally detected bilateral hydronephrosis and oligohydramnios, delivered at 36 weeks gestation by induction of labour. Day 1 ultrasound shows severe hydronephrosis of the (a) left and (b) right kidneys, along with (c) dilatation of the posterior urethra. Panel (d) shows micturating cysturethrography performed at 48 hours of life. A diagnosis of posterior urethral valves was made

Structural Diseases

II

urinary tract obstruction. Patients with vesicou-reteric reflux require a DMSA scan to rule our reflux associated scarring. Patients showing bilateral hydroureteronephrosis with oligohy-dramnios, large thick-walled bladder, bladder diverticuli or dilated posterior urethra are likely to have lower urinary tract obstruction (Fig. 5.4). These patients are catheterized at birth and an MCU is performed at 24–72 hours. Patients showing posterior urethral valves require early surgical intervention.

Patients with bilateral hydronephrosis (or single kidney with hydronephrosis) with a normal MCU should undergo nuclear scinti-graphy at 6–8 weeks to estimate total GFR and differential renal function, and to rule eva-luate for obstruction. Split renal function may be inaccurate because of over-representation of the renal function in the large hydro-nephrotic kidney. If required, the kidney which shows the least function should un-dergo repair first.

Antibiotic Prophylaxis

The presence of vesicoureteric reflux places an infant at an increased risk of urinary tract infections. Prophyaxis is administered to infants with (i) moderate to severe antenatal hydronephrosis (APD >10 mm) while awai-ting results of MCU, and (ii) grade III-V reflux on MCU. Agents used include amoxicillin (5–8 mg/kg/day) or a first-generation cepha-losporin (cefadroxil 5 mg/kg/day).

Surgical Intervention

Almost half the cases of antenatal hydro-nephrosis resolve spontaneously without complications. Most infants require only observation and periodic monitoring. Surgical intervention is indicated for: (i) posterior urethral valve; (ii) ureterocoele (Fig. 5.5); (iii) ectopic ureter with significant reflux or obstruction; (iv) PUJ obstruction: unilateral obstructed hydronephrosis with either diffe-rential renal function <40%, or a follow up study

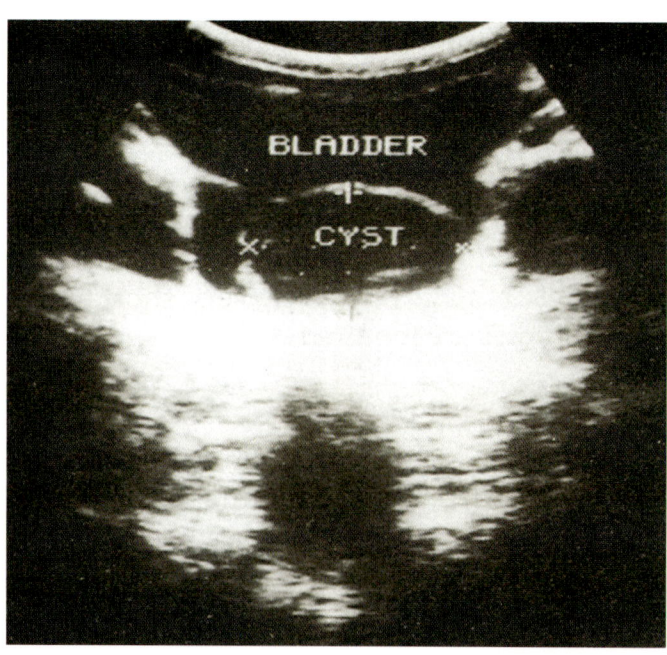

Fig. 5.5: Postnatal ultrasound showing ureterocele as a cystic thin walled structure at the base of the urinary bladder

showing increasing renal pelvic dilatation or >10% decline in differential renal function; *(v)* solitary kidney with obstructive hydronephrosis; *(vi)* bilateral obstructive hydronephrosis (the kidney with the lower GFR undergoes repair first); and *(vii)* grade III-V vesicoureteric reflux with breakthrough febrile urinary infections or the appearance of new scars despite antibiotic prophylaxis (*see* Chapter 28).

Monitoring of Renal Dysfunction

All newborns with neonatal hydronephrosis should undergo assessment of renal function (blood urea, creatinine) and urinalysis by the end of the first week of life. Oscillometric blood pressure should be recorded. Patients with hydronephrosis are followed with ultrasound evaluations every 6–12 months till at least 5-yr-old. Monitoring also includes physical examination for anthropometry and blood pressure at every visit, and annual urinalysis and estimation of serum creatinine.

SUPPORT READING

Nguyen HT, Herndon CDA, Cooper C, et al. The Society for Fetal Urology consensus statement on the evaluation and management of antenatal hydronephrosis. J Pediatr Urol 2010; 6: 212–31

Hari P, Bagga A, Srivastava RN, on behalf of Indian Pediatric Nephrology Group. Consensus statement on management of Antenatally detected hydronephrosis. Indian Pediatr 2001; 38: 1244–51

Kitchens DM, Herndon CDA. Antenatal hydronephrosis. Curr Urol Rep 2009; 10: 126–33

6 Cystic Diseases

A renal cyst is an enclosed or communicating segment of nephron or duct that is dilated. Cystic kidney diseases are a clinically and genetically heterogeneous group of disorders that may present *in utero* or be clinically silent into adulthood.

Classification

A classification of cystic kidney diseases is shown in Table 6.1. An accurate diagnosis is important to determine the prognosis, treatment and, where appropriate, provide genetic counseling. *Multicystic kidneys* consist of unilateral involvement with multiple non-communicating cysts associated with dysplasia. *Polycystic kidneys* are genetically determined cystic lesions of either the autosomal dominant or autosomal recessive form. *Glomerulocystic kidneys* have glomerular cysts as a predominant finding. *Medullary sponge*

Table 6.1: Classification of renal cystic diseases

Multicystic dysplastic kidney

Polycystic kidney diseases (PKD)
  Autosomal recessive PKD
  Autosomal dominant PKD

Glomerulocystic kidney diseases (GCKD)
  Familial GCKD
  Hereditary GCKD (associated with polycystic kidneys)
  Syndromic nonhereditary GCKD
  Sporadic or acquired forms

Tubulointerstitial syndromes with cysts
  Nephronophthisis
  Medullary cystic diseases
  Bardet-Biedel syndrome

Renal cysts in hereditary syndromes (Table 6.2)

Miscellaneous cysts
  Simple cortical cysts
  Medullary sponge kidney
  Cystic nephroma, nephroblastoma, von Hippel–Lindau disease; renal cell carcinoma with cysts
  Acquired renal cystic disease

Table 6.2: Syndromic renal structural anomalies

	Renal abnormalities	Extrarenal abnormalities	Genetic locus; inheritance
Syndromes with cysts			
Bardet–Biedl	Renal dysplasia, cysts and calyceal malformations	Retinopathy, digit anomalies, obesity, diabetes mellitus, male hypogonadism	Multiple genes or loci; autosomal recessive (AR), digenic
Beckwith Wiedemann	Large dysplastic kidneys +/- cysts	Somatic overgrowth	*p57KIP2*
Meckel Gruber	Cystic renal dysplasia	Central nervous system & digital malformations	*MKS1* (17q23), *MKS3* (8q22.1); *RPGRIP1L*
Tuberous sclerosis	Angiomyolipomas, renal cell carcinomas, polycystic kidney disease	Neurocutaneous syndrome, hamartomas, angiofibromas, seizures, hypomelanotic macules, ash leaf spots, retinal phakomas	*TSC1* gene (hamartin) 9q34; *TSC2* gene (tuberin) 16p13.3; autosomal dominant (AD)
Renal cysts and diabetes	Cysts	Diabetes mellitus, hyperuricemia, uterine malformations	*HNF1β*
Situs inversus, nephronophthisis	Cystic renal malformations	Situs inversus	*Inversin*; AR
Zellweger	Cystic dysplastic kidneys	Dysmorphic features	Peroxisomal protein mutation; AR
Branchio-oto-renal	Renal agenesis and dysplasia	Deafness, branchial arch defects, e.g. neck fistulae	*EYA1*
Syndromes without cysts			
Campomelic dysplasia	Diverse malformations	Skeletal malformation	*SOX9*
CHARGE association	Urinary tract malformations, dysplasia	Coloboma, heart malformation, choanal atresia, mental retardation, genital and ear anomalies	Unknown
Di George	Renal agenesis, dysplasia, vesicoureteric reflux	Cardiac malformations, branchial arch defects	Microdeletion at 22q11
Fanconi anemia	Renal agenesis, ectopic or horseshoe kidney	Anemia, limb malformations	Genes of DNA repair pathways
Fraser	Renal agenesis and dysplasia	Digit and ocular eyelid malformations	*FRAS1* and *FREM*
Nail-patella	Renal agenesis, nephrotic syndrome	Dysplastic nails, joint contractures, absent/hypoplastic patellae, iliac wings	*LMX1B* mutation, *uroplakin IIIa* heterozygous mutation
Urofacial (Ochoa)	Obstructive bladder, dysplasia	Abnormal facial expression while smiling	*HPSE2* (10q); AR
VACTERL association	Multiple malformations	Vertebral, cardiac, tracheoesophageal, radial and other limb anomalies	Unknown mitochondrial gene
Kallmann	Renal agenesis	Hypogonadotrophic hypogonadism, anosmia	*Anosmin-1*
Klinefelter	Renal agenesis	Small, firm testis, gynecomastia, azoospermia, hypogonadism	47, XXY
MURCS association	Renal agenesis	Mullerian duct aplasia-hypoplasia, Renal malformation, Cervicothoracic Somite dysplasia	Undefined

HNF1β hepatocyte nuclear factor β

kidney is a sporadic, medullary cystic abnormality that is diagnosed radiologically.

Evaluation

History and Examination

Family history of cystic disease, chronic kidney disease and history of consanguinity is elicited. Clinical features including dysmorphic facial features, and location and morphology of cysts help in reaching a diagnosis. The patient is examined for cysts in the liver and pancreas. An effort is made to distinguish hereditary from non-hereditary forms, and isolated (non-syndromic) from conditions where renal cysts occur as part of a syndrome (Table 6.2).

Renal Imaging

Ultrasound is an appropriate first investigation. It is important to look at the kidney size and classify the cysts as unilateral or bilateral, solitary or multiple, communicating or non-communicating, and cortical or medullary. It is necessary to rule out hydronephrosis, which might be mislabelled as cysts. High resolution ultrasonography helps in increasing the sensitivity for detecting very small cysts. Presence of extrarenal cysts (liver, pancreas, spleen) and hepatic fibrosis should be looked for. It is also important to perform an ultrasound of the parents to look for renal cysts (especially if suspecting autosomal dominant PKD).

Patients with autosomal recessive PKD may show hyperechoic or "bright kidneys" on ultrasonography. Multiple conditions can mimic ARPKD, by having similar ultrasonographic features. This group includes many inherited and acquired diseases, often diagnosed during second or third trimester.

Differential diagnosis of bright kidneys includes: dysplasia, obstruction, nephrocalcinosis, Beckwith Wiedemann syndrome (Table 6.2), Meckel Gruber syndrome (Table 6.2), Perlman syndrome (renal hamartomas, nephroblastomatosis and fetal gigantism),

Simpson Golabi Behmel syndrome (X linked; dysplasia, overgrowth, craniofacial abnormalities), trisomy 13 (holoprosencephaly, polydactyly, ventricular septal defect).

Contrast enhanced computerized tomography (CT) shows a characteristic striate pattern of contrast excretion in autosomal recessive PKD. CT scan or magnetic resonance imaging (MRI) is useful to characterize renal cysts in other cases.

Autosomal Recessive Polycystic Kidney Disease (ARPKD)

The frequency varies between 1:20000 and 1:55000 live births. ARPKD begins *in utero* and is characterized by fusiform dilation of collecting tubules arranged radially from the medulla to the cortex. There is varying degree of non-obstructive renal ectasia, malformation of the biliary tract and hepatic fibrosis. Autosomal recessive PKD is caused by mutations in the *PKHD-1* gene that encodes fibrocystin or polyductin. Truncating mutations in *PKHD-1* are associated with a more severe phenotype.

Thirty percent patients die during the neonatal period, mainly due to pulmonary hypoplasia. Those who survive show renal damage, hepatic fibrosis, portal hypertension, cholangitis and esophageal varices. The chief causes of morbidity include end stage renal disease, portal hypertension with esophageal varices, hepatosplenomegaly and hypersplenism.

ARPKD has two presentations: *(i)* classic form in neonates and infants, and *(ii)* childhood form with hepatic fibrosis. The classic form presents in the neonatal period with severe respiratory impairment, Potters facies and pulmonary hypoplasia. Patients surviving the neonatal period may present during the first month and evolve to chronic renal failure in the first year of life. The childhood form presents between 6–12 months with renal and liver involvement, but the evolution to end stage renal disease is inevitable (Table 6.3).

Table 6.3: Features of autosomal recessive and dominant polycystic kidney disease (PKD)

	Autosomal recessive PKD	*Autosomal dominant PKD*
Presentation	Perinatal or neonatal period, respiratory distress or renal insufficiency Later childhood: renal insufficiency, portal hypertension	Onset in 3rd–5th decade, with hypertension, proteinuria and hematuria
Ultrasound	Symmetrically enlarged kidneys; increased echogenicity of renal parenchyma throughout cortex and medulla	Enlarged kidneys; cysts of different sizes in cortex and medulla; small at onset; sometimes large cysts in childhood
Involvement with cysts	Dilated collecting ducts and distal tubules	Cysts in all parts of the nephron
Associated pathology	Congenital hepatic fibrosis, hyperplastic biliary ducts and portal fibrosis (Caroli disease); pancreatic cysts (rare)	Liver, pancreatic cysts. Rarely, ductal plate malformation, congenital hepatic fibrosis, intracranial aneurysms
Risk for siblings	25%	50%
Parental ultrasound	Normal	One affected parent with ADPKD (unless parents are <30 years); rarely *de novo* mutation

The diagnosis of ARPKD may be suspected on ultrasonography as early as 17 weeks of gestation. In the postnatal stage, the kidneys are enlarged and echogenic bilaterally with poor corticomedullary differentiation. CECT scan showing radially arranged pattern of dilated collecting tubules extending from the medulla to the cortex is almost specific (Fig. 6.1).

Autosomal Dominant Polycystic Kidney Disease (ADPKD)

This condition manifests after the third or fourth decade of life, but may present in childhood. Its prevalence is 1:1000 live births. *ADPKD1*, with the mutation located on chromosome 16, represents 85% cases; *ADPKD2*, with the mutation on chromosome 4, accounts for 15% patients. While family history is present in 90%, 10% cases represent *de novo* mutations. The genes *ADPKD1* and *ADPKD2* encode polycystin 1 and polycystin 2, respectively. Polycystins are modular membrane proteins that regulate tubular and vascular development in the kidneys, liver, brain, and pancreas by assembling large signaling complexes and activate several pathways.

ADPKD presents with impaired ability to concentrate urine, progressive proteinuria or hematuria, flank pain, hypertension and urolithiasis (Table 6.3). Extrarenal features including cysts in liver, pancreas and spleen, subarachnoid hemorrhage, cerebral aneurysms and mitral valve prolapse are less common in children. Liver fibrosis is usually associated with ARPKD but can also be seen in ADPKD2.

Diagnosis

ADPKD should be suspected in any child with bilateral renal cysts. The presence of 3 or more cysts in cortex or medulla of both kidneys, family history of cysts, and presence of polycystic liver, valvar heart disease, pancreatic cysts and cerebral aneurysms are suggestive.

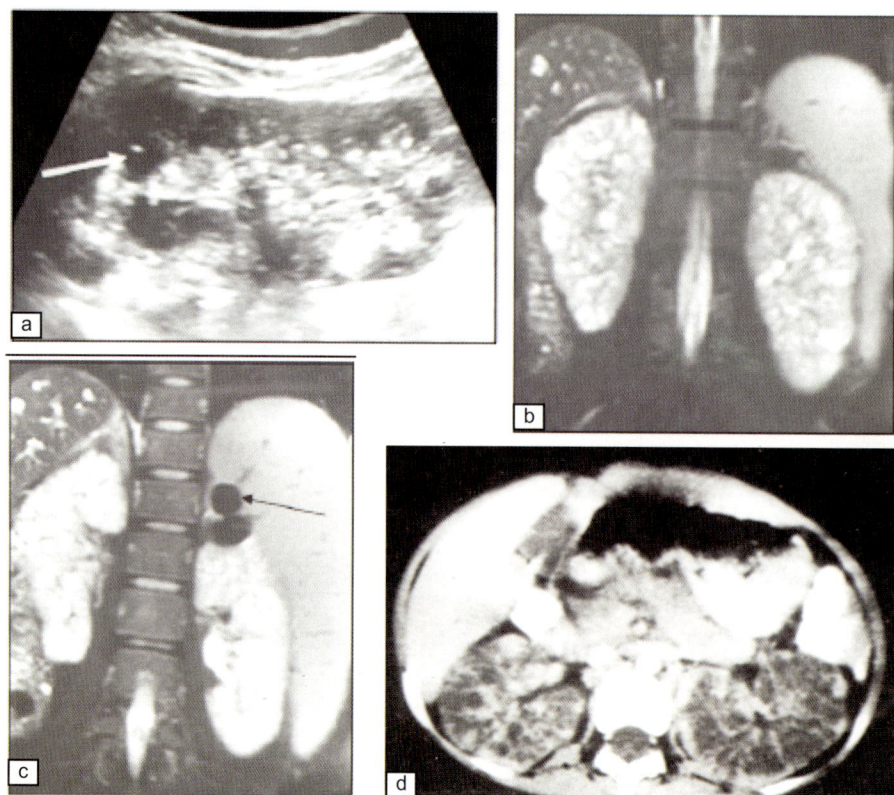

Fig. 6.1: Autosomal recessive polycystic kidney disease (ARPKD). (a) Ultrasonography shows bulky kidney, altered echogenicity with loss of corticomedullary differentiation and occasional visible cysts (arrow). (b) Coronal T2 weighted magnetic resonance image (MRI) of the abdomen shows multiple small cysts in bilateral kidneys. (c) Coronal T2W MRI of the same child shows gross splenomegaly and dilated splenic vein (arrow) secondary to portal hypertension. The child had congenital hepatic fibrosis. (d) Contrast enhanced computed tomography (CECT) showing numerous contrast filled linear channels extending across the entire width of both kidneys, giving the appearance of striate pattern, typical of ARPKD (*Courtesy* Dr. Arun K Gupta, AIIMS, New Delhi)

Ultrasonography may show few bilateral cysts in normal sized to enlarged kidneys (Fig 6 .2). Among at-risk individuals between 15 and 29 yr of age, at least two renal cysts (unilateral or bilateral) is sufficient; between 30 to 59 yr, at least two cysts in each kidney; and above 60 yr, at least four or more cysts in each kidney are required for the diagnosis.

If ultrasonography is equivocal, both CT scan and MRI (with or without contrast), are useful for reaching a diagnosis (Fig 6.2). Both these techniques can detect cysts of smaller size than ultrasonography. CT scan has a risk of radiation exposure and of contrast induced nephropathy. MRI allows detection of cysts 2-3 mm in diameter.

In the absence of family history, the diagnosis of ADPKD is challenging. In these cases, ADPKD can be due to a *de novo* mutation or, more likely, familial mild PKD, which often is otherwise missed. In the latter instance, ultrasound examination may demonstrate multiple renal cysts in one parent or grand-

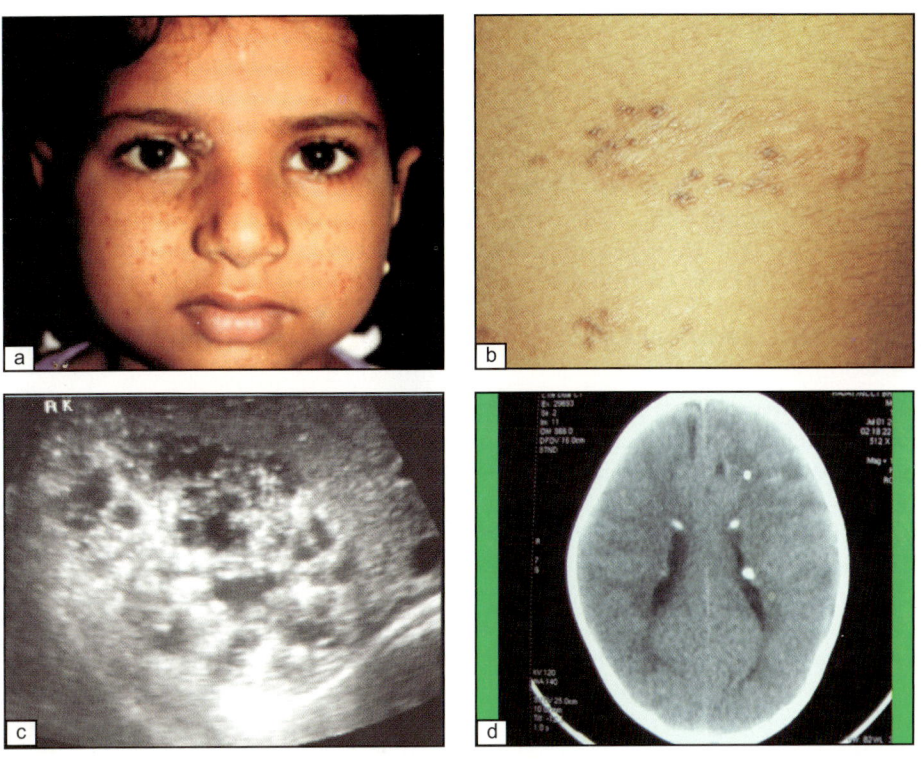

Fig. 6.2: Findings in a 9-yr-old girl with tuberous sclerosis and autosomal dominant polycystic kidney disease (ADPKD). (a) Adenoma sebaceum, appearing as tiny red nodules over the nose and cheeks. (b) Roughened, raised lesion with an orange-peel consistency located over the left lumbar region, characteristic of a shagreen patch. (c) Ultrasonography shows grossly disorganized architecture of the kidney with multiple irregular shaped cysts and foci of calcification. (d) Computed tomography of the brain showing calcified tubers in the periventricular area

parents (screened if parents are below 30-yr-old).

Molecular genetic testing may be indicated for the evaluation of at-risk individuals with equivocal imaging results, younger at-risk individuals while being evaluated as a living related kidney donor, and individuals with atypical or *de novo* renal cystic disease.

Management

Patients should be monitored frequently, with attention to diet and physical growth. Periodic screening should include evaluation for hypertension, proteinuria and creatinine. Blood pressure is maintained between 50th to 75th centile. Angiotensin converting enzyme inhibitors are preferred since they simultaneously reduce hyperfiltration induced injury and proteinuria. Reduction of cyst volume by surgical decompression or percutaneous aspiration is effective in relieving the pain.

Progression of renal disease is noted in third to fifth decade of life. Factors contributing to progression to ESRD include *PKD1* genotype, early age of presentation (<30 years), large cyst number in early childhood, presence of hypertension and hematuria before 35 years, heavy proteinuria and recurrent urinary infections.

The mammalian target of rapamycin (mTOR) is implicated in the pathogenesis of cysts. Two commercially available drugs, sirolimus and its derivative everolimus, can inhibit mTOR. It is possible that these agents may slow the kidney volume enlargement and renal function deterioration in a subset of patients. However, the therapeutic role of mTOR inhibitors in ADPKD is still uncertain.

Nephronophthisis Medullary Cystic Disease Complex

The nephronophthisis (NPHP) complex comprises a genetically heterogeneous group of cystic disorders, with autosomal recessive inheritance. Mutations have been detected at the locus 2q13 which has a group of genes, *NPHP1-9* encoding cytosolic proteins called nephrocystins. NPHP is the most frequent genetic cause of end stage renal disease up to the third decade of life. Medullary cystic kidney disease, inherited in an autosomal dominant manner, is indistinguishable histologically from NPHP. A discriminating feature is the different age at onset of symptoms and progression to renal failure. Because of clinical and morphological similarities, the term *nephronophthisis-medullary cystic disease complex* is used to describe these diseases.

Diagnosis

NPHP has a subtle onset; there is history of polyuria, polydipsia or secondary enuresis that begins around 3-5 yr of age. Symptoms of renal failure, such as fatigue, pruritus, nausea, vomiting, uremic gastritis, anemia and growth retardation may be present. There may be history of parental consanguinity. Extrarenal phenotypes include: (*i*) ocular (retinitis pigmentosa, colobomas, nystagmus), (*ii*) neurological (hypopituitarism, vermis agenesis), (*iii*) liver fibrosis, and (*iv*) skeletal dysplasia.

Mutations in the *NPHP2* gene, encoding inversin, cause the infantile form of NPHP, which presents with advanced renal function impairment developing before 5 years of age. Patients with Joubert syndrome (*NPHP1* mutation, *JBTS13*) have structural cerebellar and midbrain abnormalities, retinitis pigmentosa, conglenital hypotonia, and ocular motor apraxia or irregularities in breathing pattern in the neonatal period. Mutations at *NPHP3* (renal hepatic pancreatic dysplasia) and *NPHP2* are associated with congenital hepatic fibrosis. Patients with Jeune chondrodysplasia have renal disease with features consistent with NPHP.

Urinalysis shows a concentration defect (<300 mOsm/kg in morning urine). Renal function, complete blood counts and liver function tests are done. Renal ultrasound shows small kidneys with poor corticomedullary differentiation and corticomedullary cysts and, if present, liver fibrosis. The diagnosis of NPHP is confirmed on renal biopsy or mutation analysis (Fig. 6.3) (www.renalgenes.org). Molecular genetic analysis allows a definitive diagnosis, but is not readily available. An ophthalmological examination should be performed in all patients with NPHP to evaluate for retinal degeneration.

Glomerulocystic Kidney Disease (GCKD)

The presence of predominant glomerular cysts is seen in: non-syndromic GCKD,

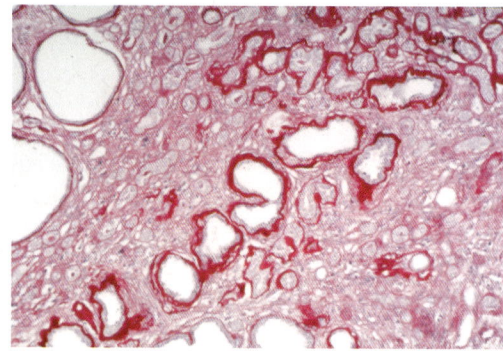

Fig. 6.3: Renal histology in a 12-yr-old girl with nephronophthisis. Light microscopy with periodic acid Schiff staining shows tubular atrophy, cystic dilatation of the tubules, peritubular and interstitial fibrosis

Cystic Diseases

dominantly inherited GCKD, and sporadic forms. It can be a feature of inherited syndromes (Table 6.2), e.g. tuberous sclerosis and trisomy 13, and also a manifestation of renal dysplasia. Early onset of renal failure is characteristic. Ultrasonography shows bilaterally increased kidney echogenicity and loss of cortical medullary differentiation. Cysts are small and subcortical.

Renal Cyst and Diabetes Syndrome

The main features are large hyperechoic fetal kidneys, renal hypodysplasia with cortical microcysts and diabetes mellitus (maturity onset disease of the young). Mutations are present in the hepatocyte nuclear factor 1β gene (*HNF 1β* or *TCF-2*). Other features include vaginal aplasia, rudimentary or bicornuate uterus; epididymal cysts, atresia of vas deferens and hypospadias; and hyperuricemia.

Syndromic Renal Cystic Diseases

A review of the clinical and radiological features may reveal an underlying disorder (Table 6.2). The presence of renal (e.g. multiple angiomyolipomas, renal cell carcinoma) or extrarenal clinical findings (e.g. facial and periungual fibromas, pancreatic cysts) that are atypical of ADPKD should raise the suspicion of inherited renal cystic syndromes. Tuberous sclerosis is characterized by varied skin lesions, seizures, and renal cysts with angiomyolipomas (Fig. 6.2).

The presence of retinal and central nervous system hemangioblastomas, renal cell carcinoma, pheochromocytoma, cystadenomas of the epididymis and pancreas suggests the diagnosis of von Hippel-Lindau syndrome.

Cystic dysplasia is a developmental disorder in which there is abnormal differentiation of renal parenchymal cells. The more characteristic morphology is the presence of primitive tubules lined with columnar epithelium, surrounded by rings of cartilage, fibromuscular and metaplastic nests. Many dysplastic kidneys have cysts and many cystic kidneys may show different degrees of dysplasia, termed as multicystic kidneys.

Simple cysts are rare in children. The prevalence of one or more simple renal cysts has been estimated to be less than 0.5% in individuals who are younger than 30 yr. They are usually unilateral, but may be multiple and bilateral. Ultrasonography shows cysts in the renal cortex, less than 1 cm in diameter.

Acquired renal cystic disease is common and observed in 7% patients with chronic kidney disease and in approximately 20% patients with end-stage renal disease. Despite presence of multiple renal cysts bilaterally with varying degree of renal insufficiency, the size of the kidneys is normal or small.

6

SUPPORT READING

Avni FE, Hall M. Renal cystic diseases in children: new concepts. Pediatr Radiol 2010; 40: 939–946

Avni FE, Garel L, Cassart M, *et al.* Perinatal assessment of hereditary cystic renal diseases: the contribution of sonography. Pediatr Radiol 2006; 36: 405–414

Guay-Woodford LM. Renal cystic diseases: diverse phenotypes converge on the cilium/centrosome complex. Pediatr Nephrol 2006; 21: 1369–76

7 Multicystic Dysplastic Kidney

Multicystic dysplastic kidney (MCDK) is the most common cystic renal malformation in children. Abnormal differentiation of the metanephros results in formation of MCDK, comprised of cartilage and unorganized tubules, which manifest grossly as multiple, variably sized cysts.

The reported incidence of MCDK varies between 1 in 2400 to 1 in 4300 live births, and is more common in boys. 20–50% of MCDK involute and are undetectable by ultrasound at 3–5 yr follow-up. The contralateral normal kidney generally shows compensatory hypertrophy (renal length greater than two standard deviations above the mean). MCDK are associated with contralateral renal abnormalities in 20–50% patients. Vesicoureteric reflux (VUR), pelviureteric junction (PUJ) obstruction and duplication of the collecting system are common.

Simple MCDK is unilateral dysplasia with a normal contralateral kidney, showing compensatory hypertrophy and no genitourinary anomalies. *Complex* MCDK implies either bilateral dysplasia or abnormalities of the contralateral kidney or genitourinary tract, detected on ultrasonography or on examination.

Complications

Vesicoureteric reflux and urinary tract infections: About 5–45% of children with MCDK have contralateral and/or ipsilateral VUR.

Although contralateral VUR is of low grade (I-II) in the majority, the risk is considerably more in patients showing anomalies of the contralateral kidney and urinary tract.

Hypertension: The risk of hypertension in patients with MCDK (5.4 per 1000 children) is no higher than that in the general population. Hypertension resolves with nephrectomy in 25–50% patients.

Wilms tumor: The risk of malignant transformation is negligible and does not warrant either nephrectomy or very close surveillance.

Chronic renal insufficiency: The risk of chronic renal insufficiency at 5–7 yr is 20–30% for patients with complex MCDK, and significantly lower for those with simple MCDK. Patients with a solitary functioning kidney of any etiology have an increased risk of proteinuria and renal insufficiency in adulthood.

Diagnosis and Management
Ultrasonography

While most cases of MCDK are now diagnosed in the antenatal period, some might be detected during evaluation for an abdominal mass.

If MCDK is suspected on an antenatal ultrasound the neonate should be screened postnatally to confirm the diagnosis and rule out significant contralateral abnormality.

On ultrasonography, MCDK is characterized by non-communicating cysts of variable sizes, lack of identifiable renal parenchyma and atretic proximal ureters (Fig. 7.1). The cysts in MCDK are multiple, thin-walled and distributed randomly throughout the kidney. Parenchymal tissue between the cysts is often hyperechogenic. The organ is enlarged with an irregular non-reniform outline.

The condition should be distinguished from severe hydronephrosis; the non-communicating cysts and absence of renal pelvis and proximal ureter help distinguish MCDK from

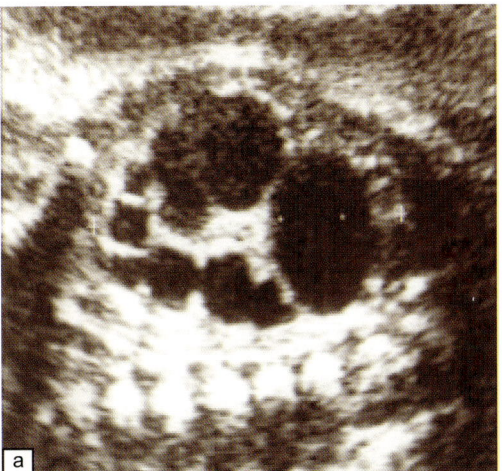

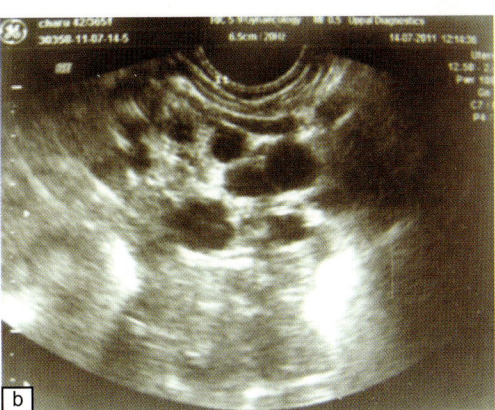

Fig. 7.1: Multicystic dysplastic kidney. Multiple, thin-walled and non-communicating cysts are seen to involve the left kidney on (a) antenatal ultrasonography, and (b) postnatal ultrasound at one month age

this entity. Other differentials include polycystic kidney diseases (dominant and recessive forms) and glomerulocystic disease. Unilateral involvement, the absence of renal arterial flow by Doppler, and variability in size of cysts distinguish MCDK from these diseases.

Nuclear Scintigraphy

A DMSA scan confirms non-function of the kidney with multicystic dysplasia. The demonstration of significant function in MCDK is exceedingly rare, and should suggest alternative diagnosis. DMSA scintigraphy, done between 8–12 weeks, also allows the evaluation of the contralateral kidney, especially for the presence of renal scars.

Micturating Cystourethrography (MCU)

In view of high risk of contralateral VUR, most patients with unilateral MCDK were previously advised to undergo radiocontrast imaging for detecting and grading reflux. The current approach is conservative, and MCU is advised only in patients with abnormalities of the contralateral kidney on ultrasonography, scarring on DMSA scan, or urinary tract infection.

Magnetic Resonance Urography

An MRU enables simultaneous evaluation of structure and function. Its limited availability, high cost and need for prolonged sedation preclude routine use in practice.

Follow up Evaluation

Patients with MCDK should be evaluated during immunization visits, and then annually. Physical examination at each visit includes anthropometry, blood pressure record and abdominal palpation for lump. Urine protein is evaluated annually; blood levels of creatinine are measured every 2-yr.

Follow up ultrasonography is required to monitor the involution of the affected kidney and for compensatory hypertrophy and

Structural Diseases

II

growth of the contralateral kidney. Ultrasounds are done every 4–6 months for the first year and yearly thereafter till involution or until 10-yr of age.

The indications of nephrectomy in patients with MCDK are limited and include: (*i*) presence of hypertension, (*ii*) suspected malignancy, or (*iii*) large cystic kidney (>6 cm diameter) that is palpable/fails to involute.

SUPPORT READING

Hains DS, Bates CM, Ingraham S, Schwaderer AL. Management and etiology of the unilateral multicystic dysplastic kidney: A review. Pediatr Nephrol 2009; 24: 233–41

Cambio AJ, Evans CP, Kurzrock EA. Non-surgical management of multicystic dysplastic kidney. BJU Int 2008; 101: 804–08

Woolf AS. Unilateral multicystic dysplastic kidney. Kidney Int 2006; 69: 190–93

8 Single Kidney

Single kidney or solitary functioning kidney may result from unilateral renal agenesis or unilateral nephrectomy. Unilateral renal agenesis is the condition of being born with non-ectopic, solitary functioning kidney, with failure of formation of the contralateral kidney. The incidence of unilateral renal agenesis is between 1 in 500 to 1000 live births. Unilateral nephrectomy may have been performed for significant renal disease or as a healthy donor for renal transplant; this entity is not discussed in this section.

Etiology

Renal agenesis results from either failure of the ureteric bud to arise, or its failure to engage with the renal mesenchyme.

Renal agenesis may occur as a part of syndromes involving mutations in genes that are expressed during differentiation of normal kidneys and ureters (*see* Table 6.2). Even without a syndromic association, renal agenesis may be familial, and inherited as a dominant trait with incomplete penetrance. Parents and siblings of infants born with solitary or dysgenetic kidneys(s) should therefore undergo ultrasonographic screening for renal anomalies.

Poorly controlled maternal diabetes mellitus, and therapy with inhibitors of renin angiotensin axis or high dose vitamin A during pregnancy may have a teratogenic effect on renal development.

Differential Diagnosis

On ultrasonography, an *empty renal fossa* might also be present in the following conditions:

1. Ectopic kidney, e.g. pelvic kidney or cross-fused ectopia
2. Renal hypodysplasia containing remnants of undifferentiated and metaplastic tissues
3. Renal atrophy secondary to renal artery stenosis or neonatal renal venous thrombosis
4. Involution of multicystic dysplastic kidney.

Evaluation for an ectopic kidney should include a careful ultrasound followed by radionuclide DMSA scintigraphy. Remnants of hypodysplasia, multicystic dysplastic kidney and atrophy may be detected on magnetic resonance imaging.

The solitary kidney may itself be abnormal due to variable degree of hypodysplasia or damage by antenatal or postnatal vesicoureteric reflux. Reported abnormalities include vesicoureteric reflux or obstruction, particularly at the pelviureteric junction.

Management

Physical examination: Anthropometry, dysmorphic features and hypertension.

Ultrasonography: Patients are evaluated for anomalies of the ipsilateral and contralateral renal tracts. Congenital single kidneys are usually larger due to compensatory hyper-trophy, and their size exceeds the upper normal age adjusted limits (Appendix 10). The contra-lateral kidney is considered abnormal if it is smaller than normal, or is echogenically bright.

^{99m}Tc Dimercaptosuccinic acid (DMSA) scan: Detects scarring secondary to significant reflux, and examines functional remnants of contralateral kidney and a kidney in ectopic location.

Micturating cystourethrography: This is advised in patients with pelvic or ureteric dilatation on ultrasonography, or those with renal scarring.

Diethylene triamine penta-acetic acid (DTPA) or LL-ethylene cysteine dimer (LLEC) scan: Pelvic or ureteric dilatation may be secondary to pelviureteric or vesicoureteric junction obstruction, detected by diuretic renography using DTPA or LLEC.

Screening of asymptomatic relatives: Asymp-tomatic first degree relatives should be scree-ned using ultrasound.

Follow up Evaluation

Blood pressure and urinary protein excretion should be checked every 6 months; blood levels of creatinine are estimated annually. Patients with renal dysfunction require more frequent evaluation according to the stage of chronic kidney disease. Treatment with angiotensin converting enzyme inhibitors is preferred in patients with hypertension and/or proteinuria.

Participation in Sports

The potential benefits from sports outweigh the small risk of catastrophic sports-related kidney injury. Usual physical activity and sports are not restricted in children with a solitary kidney. Activities most associated with serious renal trauma include bicycling, skiing, snowboarding and equestrian sports. Patients are generally advised to avoid contact sports, e.g. boxing, American football and ice hockey. Most experts recommend that no restrictions be placed on noncontact sports, and that clinical judgement should be used regarding placing any restrictions on contact or collision sports. Children should be encou-raged to engage in some form of physical activity, even if contact sports are ruled out.

Prognosis

Children with uncomplicated unilateral renal agenesis are expected to maintain glomerular function similar to that of two normal kidneys. However, it is likely that compensatory growth and hyperfiltration in the single kidney may lead to its injury on the long term. Potential consequences include glomerulosclerosis, hypertension, protei-nuria and even renal failure. The relative risk for gestational hypertension, pre-eclampsia or gestational proteinuria is increased twofold in pregnant women with unilateral renal agenesis compared to those with two normal kidneys. Adults with single kidneys also have a higher prevalence of hyper-tension and proteinuria.

SUPPORT READING

Zaffanello M, Brugnara M, Zuffante M, Franchini M, Fanos V. Are children with congenital solitary kidney at risk for lifelong complications? A lack of prediction demands caution. Int Urol Nephrol 2009; 41: 127–35

Woolf AS, Hillman KA. Unilateral renal agenesis and the congenital solitary functioning kidney: developmental, genetic and clinical perspec-tives. BJU Int 2007; 99: 17–21

Psooy K. Sports and the solitary kidney: what parents of a young child with a solitary kidney should know. Can Urol Assoc J 2009; 3: 67–68

Electrolyte Disorders and Tubular Diseases

9 Disorders of Sodium Balance

The normal blood levels of sodium vary between 135 and 145 mEq/L. Sodium, with urea and glucose, is the chief determinant, of extracellular fluid (ECF) osmolality. Urea and glucose, while contributing to the osmolality, diffuse freely across the cell wall and do not create a transcellular osmotic gradient. On the other hand, sodium is an effective solute and contributes to tonicity.

Sodium homeostasis is closely related to water homeostasis. Water balance is primarily maintained through monitoring the tonicity of the ECF (hypothalamic osmoreceptors) and secondarily by monitoring intravascular volume (volume receptors in great veins and right side of heart). An increase in tonicity is interpreted as a decrease in total body water, and *vice-versa*. In response, water is retained or lost until the serum sodium level returns to normal. However, if intravascular volume is severely depressed, the volume signal overrides the osmotic signal and water is retained irrespective of ECF osmolality. This phenomenon can lead to hyponatremia in volume depleted infants treated with hypotonic replacement fluids.

The blood brain barrier is composed of tight junctions between the capillary endothelial cells and astrocyte foot processes. Water flows freely across the blood-brain barrier, but solutes take hours to equilibrate. Because of the relative impermeability to solutes, changes in plasma osmolality create an osmotic gradient between plasma and central nervous system interstitial fluid.

Two mechanisms attenuate the change in brain volume resulting from osmotic gradients. The cerebral interstitial fluid is in communication with the cerebrospinal fluid (CSF). In the presence of hyponatremia, a portion of the excess water that enters the interstitial fluid goes into the CSF compartment and is absorbed by arachnoid granulations. The reverse occurs in hypernatremia.

Secondly, the brain cells adapt to changes in interstitial fluid osmolality by generating or extruding solutes. Brain potassium content increases within hours of hypernatremia. If hypernatremia persists for more than 24 hr, the brain generates an excess of low molecular weight organic solutes (sugar alcohols, methylamines and amino acids) that increase ICF osmolality (*idiogenic osmoles*), preventing dehydration of the brain cells. Similarly, in the first few hours following development of hyponatremia, potassium is lost from the cells, and this is followed by loss of low molecular weight organic solutes.

While the two mechanisms limit the change in brain volume, a rapid change in plasma osmolality can still lead to significant and symptomatic brain edema or dehydration. These adaptive mechanisms also have therapeutic implications. The osmotically compensated brain needs time to "uncompensate". If plasma osmolality rapidly returns to normal after the brain has adapted, cerebral dehydration will follow. A possible consequence of this dehydration is central pontine myelinolysis; similar lesions have been seen outside the pons. Rapid correction of persistent hyper- or hyponatremia should therefore be avoided.

HYPONATREMIA

Hyponatremia, defined as a serum sodium concentration less than 135 mEq/L, indicates an excess of body water relative to sodium. The development of hyponatremia is associated with abnormal water homeostasis. Though often asymptomatic, hyponatremia has the potential for causing severe neurological damage and death.

The sodium concentration, when determined by flame photometry, is factitiously reduced in patients with hyperproteinemia or hypertriglyceridemia. The error (*factitious hyponatremia*) is usually minor; an artifactual decrease in the sodium level by 1 mEq/L requires a 500 mg/dL increase in triglycerides or 4 g/dL increase in serum proteins. Instruments utilizing an ion selective electrode directly estimate sodium concentration in plasma water and are more accurate.

The presence of effective solutes other than sodium in the ECF can also lead to a reduction in serum sodium concentration. In the absence of insulin, as in diabetes, most tissues outside the CNS are impermeable to glucose; hence glucose behaves as an effective solute and preferentially increases ECF osmolality. Water is drawn from the intra-

cellular fluid (ICF) to the ECF and the sodium concentration is reduced because of dilution. For every 100 mg/dL increase in blood glucose level, the serum sodium concentration decreases by 1.5 mEq/L. Mannitol is another effective solute.

Causes

The causes of true hyponatremia are listed in Table 9.1. In most cases, history, physical examination and urinalysis enables assessment of the underlying etiology (Fig. 9.1).

Hyponatremic Dehydration

This is a common cause for hyponatremia in children. The diarrheal fluid is hypo-osmolar in relation to plasma, which tends to increase rather than decrease serum sodium. However, if volume depletion is significant, ADH secretion is stimulated and free water excretion by the kidneys is minimized. In this setting, replacement of diarrheal losses by hypo-osmolar fluids will lead to free water retention and hyponatremia. As long as volume depletion persists, water retention will continue in spite of low serum sodium. As the hypovolemia is corrected, the stimulus for ADH secretion is removed, the urine becomes dilute, a large volume of free water is excreted and the serum sodium concentration increase.

Water Intoxication (Oral, Rectal, Intravenous)

The ability of the kidneys to excrete free water is considerable, up to 20 L/day in adults. For hyponatremia to develop, the rate of water intake should exceed the rate of free water excretion, as might occur in near-drowning in fresh water.

Postsurgical Hyponatremia

Administration of hypotonic fluids following surgery can lead to hyponatremia and cerebral edema. Hypotonic solutions should not be used following surgery.

Table 9.1: Etiology of hyponatremia

Hypovolemic	Sodium and water are both lost; fluid loss is hypotonic in relation to plasma; losses may have been replaced by hypotonic fluid

Extrarenal	*Urine sodium concentration <20 mEq/L*

Gastrointestinal loss: diarrhea, vomiting, fistulas
Excessive sweating
Cystic fibrosis
Burns
Third-space losses: pancreatitis, peritonitis, abdominal surgery

Renal	*Urine sodium concentration >20 mEq/L*

Diuretics (thiazides, loop diuretics)
Osmotic diuresis
Mineralocorticoid deficiency
Pseudohypoaldosteronism
Renal tubular acidosis
Cerebral salt wasting

Euvolemic	*Urine sodium concentration >20 mEq/L*

Syndrome of inappropriate ADH secretion
Water intoxication
Post surgical hyponatremia
Hypothyroidism
Glucocorticoid deficiency

Hypervolemic

Edema forming states	*Urine sodium concentration <20 mEq/L*

Nephrotic syndrome
Hepatic cirrhosis
Congestive cardiac failure

Renal insufficiency	*Urine sodium concentration >20 mEq/L*

Acute renal failure
Chronic renal failure

Intranasal Desmopressin

Hyponatremia with seizures has been reported following the use of desmopressin acetate (DDAVP) for control of primary enuresis in children. Parents should be cautioned not to provide excess fluids to children receiving this drug.

Malnutrition

Hyponatremia is commonly observed in severely malnourished children, with or without concomitant dehydration. The low serum sodium level might be a compensatory response to the reduced intracellular osmolality resulting from potassium depletion. If intake of protein and salt is low, adequate solute might not be available to excrete a water load. The minimum urinary osmolality that the kidney can achieve is 50 mOsm/kg. In infants on low protein diet with high fluid intake, solute availability might be the limiting factor for water excretion.

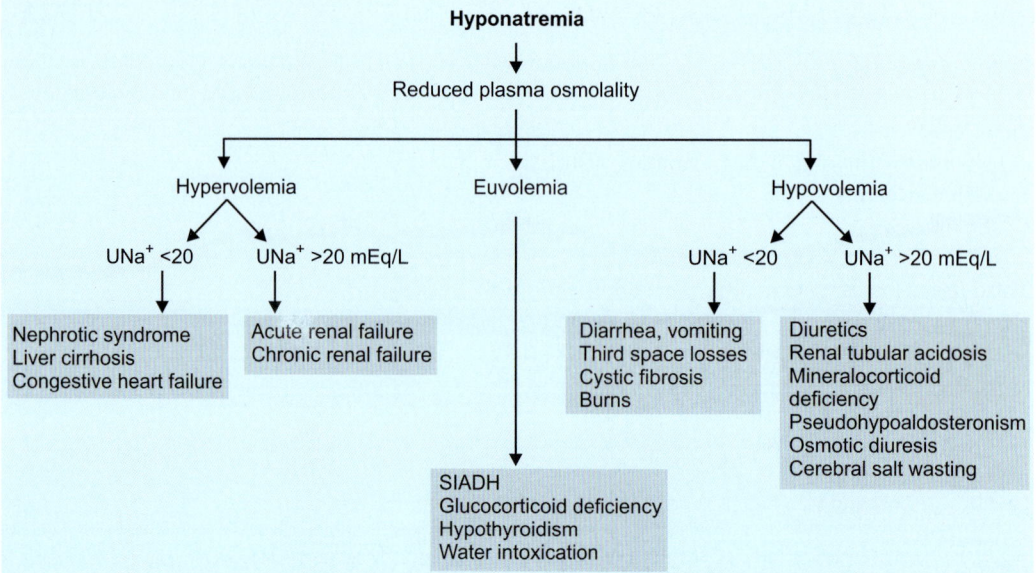

Fig. 9.1: Evaluation of hyponatremia. Patients with factitious and pseudohyponatremia show normal or increased plasma osmolality. A low urine sodium (UNa$^+$<20 mEq/L) suggests contracted effective blood volume and intact renal handling of sodium. Urine sodium >20 mEq/L implies either an intrinsic renal disorder or a natriuretic response to hypervolemia. SIADH syndrome of inappropriate antidiuretic hormone secretion

Syndrome of Inappropriate ADH Secretion (SIADH)

The diagnosis of SIADH requires the following:

1. Hyponatremia and low plasma osmolality
2. Urine that is not maximally dilute; but a urine osmolality less than plasma osmolality. A urine osmolality ~50 mOsm/kg is an appropriate response to hyponatremia. In SIADH, the urine osmolality is greater, but less than plasma osmolality.
3. Elevated urinary sodium concentration (>20 mEq/L), suggesting that the kidney is not actively conserving sodium, as it would if hyponatremia was a consequence of sodium deficiency. In patients with SIADH who are sodium restricted, the urinary sodium concentration can be <20 mEq/L

4. Absence of hypovolemia, or an edema-forming state (e.g. nephrotic syndrome, cardiac failure). This ensures that a non-osmotic stimulus is not responsible for ADH secretion
5. Normal renal, adrenal, pituitary and thyroid functions, since their hormones affect sodium and water balance

Disorders of the central nervous system are the most common cause of SIADH in children (Table 9.2). Patients with respiratory disorders show increased intrathoracic pressure and decreased venous return, resulting in apparent hypovolemia and ADH secretion.

Cerebral Salt Wasting

Patients with intracranial disease (brain injury, trauma, tumor or hematoma) might show depletion of ECF volume with renal salt wasting, polyuria and hyponatremia.

Table 9.2: Causes of the syndrome of inappropriate ADH secretion (SIADH)

Central nervous system

Meningitis	Brain abscess
Encephalitis	Head trauma
Guillain-Barre syndrome	Intracranial hemorrhage, thrombosis
Cerebral hypoxia	Acute intermittent porphyria
Craniopharyngioma	Pituitary surgery

Pulmonary, thoracic causes

Positive pressure ventilation	Bronchial asthma
Pneumothorax	Pulmonary tuberculosis
Pneumonia: viral, bacterial, fungal	

Medications

Carbamazepine, oxcarbazepine	Vincristine, vinblastine
Chlorpropamide	Morphine
Cyclophosphamide	Clofibrate

Malignancy

Hodgkin disease	Thymoma

Distinction of this disorder from SIADH can be difficult because both present with hyponatremia and relatively concentrated urine with natriuresis. The chief difference is their ECF volume status and urine output: cerebral salt wasting results in high urine output and hypovolemia, while patients with SIADH show normovolemia or mild hypervolemia. Random urine sodium concentrations are higher than 100 mEq/L in the former and lower in SIADH. Fluid restriction is useful in increasing blood sodium levels in SIADH.

Clinical Features

Mild hyponatremia is usually asymptomatic. Symptoms become common as the serum sodium level falls below 125 mEq/L. Hyponatremia is considered acute if it develops in less than 48-hr with a rate of decline in the serum sodium level >0.5 mEq/L/hr. Symptoms of acute hyponatremia include apathy, restlessness, altered sensorium and seizures.

Slowly developing (chronic) hyponatremia is asymptomatic or has subtle symptoms. These include anorexia, nausea, emesis, muscle weakness and cramps; irritability and changes in personality. At extremely low serum sodium, disturbances of gait, stupor and tremors are seen. Patients who develop central pontine myelinosis may have a biphasic course, with neurological improvement followed a few days later by deterioration. The initial symptoms are mutism, dysarthria, and lethargy; later features include spastic quadriparesis and pseudobulbar palsy.

Management

Symptomatic patients must be treated aggressively.

Symptomatic Hyponatremia

The goal of therapy in a patient with evidence of raised intracranial pressure is to raise the serum sodium level, but only as much as necessary to ensure that the patient shows normal respiration, is seizure-free and is alert.

Electrolyte Disorders and Tubular Diseases

III

The initial therapy consists of IV administration of 3% saline (0.5 mEq of sodium/ml) at a dosage of 4-6 mL/kg over 30–60 minutes. If clinical improvement is not seen, another 3–4 mL/kg is given. The infusion is stopped if child becomes asymptomatic or serum sodium is ~125 mEq/L. Persisting symptoms should raise suspicion of concomitant CNS hemorrhage or infection.

In patients with hypovolemia, resuscitation with saline takes precedence over correction of hyponatremia. Children who have severe hypovolemia and hyponatremia should receive one or more boluses of normal saline at 20–30 mL/kg. The potential for a rapid increase in the serum sodium level should be guarded against, especially in a setting of chronic hyponatremia.

Once the patient is asymptomatic, the remaining deficit is administered as normal saline. The total body sodium deficit in mEq/kg is estimated as follows:

$$Na^+ \text{ deficit (mEq)} = (130 - \text{serum } Na^+) \times 0.6 \times \text{body weight (kg)}$$

The rate of rise of the serum sodium level should not exceed 0.5 mEq/L/hr. The serum sodium level need not be corrected to normal in the acute phase; in the first two days, correction to ~130 mEq/L is advised. The rate of rise of sodium can be predicted as follows:

Rise of serum Na^+ per liter of fluid infused

$$= \frac{\text{Infusate } Na^+ - \text{Plasma } Na^+}{(0.6 \times \text{wt}) + 1}$$

The sodium content of 3% saline and isotonic saline is 513 and 154 mEq/L respectively. Serum sodium levels should be monitored frequently.

Asymptomatic Hyponatremia

Efforts to rapidly increase the serum sodium level are not necessary in patients with asymptomatic hyponatremia. Patients with hypovolemia and asymptomatic hyponatremia should receive normal saline for initial resuscitation, and subsequent maintenance and replacement therapy can be provided with half normal saline in 5% dextrose. The rate of increase in the serum sodium level should not exceed 0.5 mEq/L/hr.

If SIADH is suspected, the underlying cause should be investigated. Restricting intake of free water helps to increase the serum sodium level. If necessary, frusemide can be used to enhance free water loss.

In patients with hyponatremia secondary to malnutrition, liver disease, diuretic therapy and renal salt wasting, the management is guided by the underlying condition. Depending on the clinical situation, fluid restriction, diuretics, or isotonic saline may be used. Patients with cerebral salt wasting should receive enough fluids and sodium supplements. Therapy with fludrocortisone may be beneficial.

HYPERNATREMIA

Hypernatremia is defined as a serum sodium concentration exceeding 145 mEq/L. An elevation in the serum sodium level denotes a relative water deficiency in proportion to the total body sodium content. Increase in the sodium concentration, and therefore the tonicity, stimulate both ADH secretion and thirst. The latter is the chief protection against hypernatremia. Plasma sodium concentration >150 mEq/L is uncommon in an alert older child with a normal thirst mechanism and access to water.

A rapid increase in plasma osmolality causes a shift of water from cerebral interstitial fluid with cellular dehydration. Brain volume is decreased and there is vascular congestion. Subdural, subarachnoid and intraventricular hemorrhage and thrombosis of the venous sinuses may be seen in acute, severe hypernatremia.

Causes

Hypernatremia is often seen in infants with gastroenteritis and dehydration. It also occurs in infants or incapacitated older children who are maintained on a fixed fluid intake but have increased insensible losses from fever or tachypnea.

Hypernatremia is reported following accidental substitution of salt for sugar in oral rehydration solutions. In the hospital setting, hypernatremia is sometimes seen after cardiopulmonary resuscitation because of repeated use of IV sodium bicarbonate. Infants with diabetes insipidus with inadequate access to fluids will also develop hypernatremia. Other causes include hypothalamic disorders such as primary hypodipsia, reset osmostat or loss of osmoreceptor function. An approach to a child with hypernatremia is shown in Fig. 9.2.

Clinical Features

Since the ECF volume is relatively well preserved, clinical evaluation may underestimate the degree of dehydration. When the serum sodium level exceeds 160 mEq/L, patients show restlessness, irritability, lethargy, muscle twitching, hyperreflexia and spasticity. Coma, seizures and death may occur. Neurological symptoms may manifest as intracranial capillary and venous congestion with bleeding and venous thrombosis.

Management

The goals of therapy are to stabilize the intravascular volume and replace the relative water deficit. If there are signs of circulatory compromise, initial therapy should consist of rapid infusion of normal saline or Ringer lactate at 20–30 mL/kg; this can be repeated if necessary.

Once the patient is hemodynamically stable, therapy aims to repair the fluid and solute deficit and provide appropriate maintenance fluids. In order to reduce the risk of cerebral edema, the serum sodium levels should be reduced gradually, not exceeding a rate of 0.5 mEq/L/hr (about 10–12 mEq/L daily). The formula for predicting the rise in serum sodium depending on the sodium concentration of the fluid infused can be used to predict the drop in serum sodium as well.

The calculated fluid deficit is given over a period of 48 hr, so that the patient receives daily maintenance fluid and half the fluid deficit in the first 24 hr, followed by main-

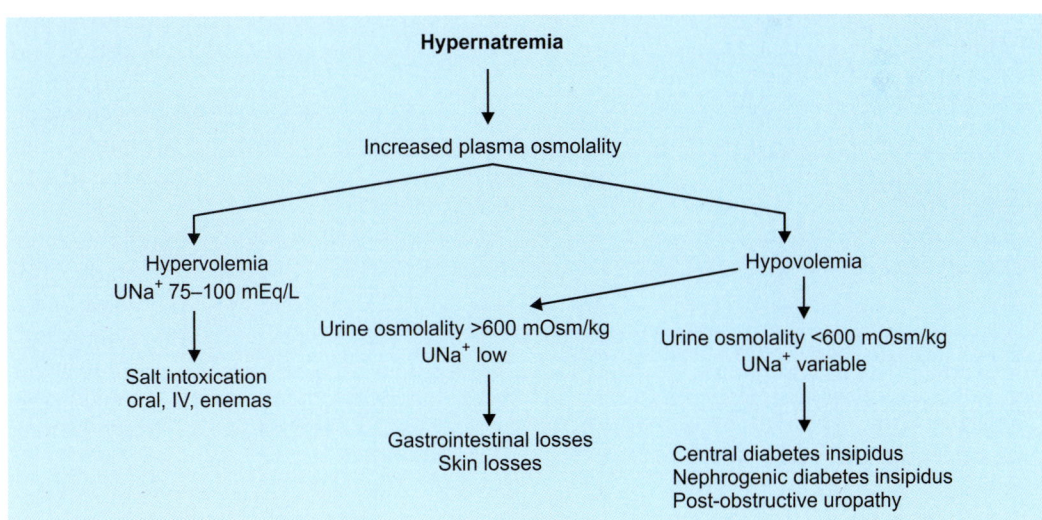

Fig. 9.2: Approach to hypernatremia. Assessment of volume status and urine osmolality allows determination of its underlying etiology. UNa$^+$ urine sodium concentration

tenance fluid and the other half of the deficit the following day. In most instances, this is achieved by providing hypotonic fluid such as N/4 or N/3 saline. Hypotonic infusates should however be given slowly and blood levels of sodium estimated every 4–6 hr, in order to avoid sudden reduction.

Hypocalcemia that occurs during treatment of hypernatremia is treated with calcium gluconate.

Patients who have hypernatremia secondary to excessive salt intake (oral, IV route), high levels of sodium (>180 mEq/L) and those who have renal insufficiency with volume overload may require peritoneal or hemodialysis.

SUPPORT READING

Androgue HJ, Madias NE. Hypernatremia. N Eng J Med 2000; 342: 1493–99

Androgue HJ, Madias NE. Hyponatremia. N Eng J Med 2000; 342: 1581–89

Barsoum N, Levine B: Current prescriptions for corrections of hypo- and hypernatremia: Are they too simple? Nephrol Dial Transplant 2002; 17: 1176–80

10 Hyperkalemia and Hypokalemia

HYPERKALEMIA

Hyperkalemia is defined as serum potassium level that exceeds 5.5 mEq/L. This disorder can be the result of decreased excretion as in renal failure, intracellular to extracellular shift in presence of acidosis, cellular breakdown, hypoaldosteronism and less commonly, increased potassium intake.

Spurious hyperkalemia refers to conditions in which the elevation in measured potassium is due to potassium movement out of the cells during or after the blood specimen has been drawn.

Evaluation

It is important to understand the etiology of hyperkalemia based on clinical features and investigations. A majority of patients with true hyperkalemia have renal failure (acute or chronic), or type 1 pseudohypoaldosteronism or take drugs that can cause hyperkalemia (Table 10.1). Measurement of blood level of creatinine, aldosterone and renin along with estimation of renal potassium excretion is required for a definitive diagnosis. The 24-hr urinary K^+ varies considerably but is usually <20 mEq/L in renal and >40 mEq/L in extra-renal causes.

ECG Changes

Mild hyperkalemia is usually asymptomatic and is detected on routine laboratory tests. In patients with severe hyperkalemia with serum potassium level >6.5 mEq/L, ECG changes are apparent and correlate with the degree of hyperkalemia (Fig. 1a). Cardiac toxicity is more evident if there is a rapid rise in the serum potassium level, if there are underlying cardiac problems and in individuals on digitalis therapy.

Transtubular Potassium Gradient

If renal function is normal, estimation of the transtubular gradient of potassium (TTKG) helps in assessing the renal response to hyperkalemia. Potassium is secreted in the late distal and cortical collecting tubules under the influence of aldosterone. TTKG is an important component in the evaluation of hyperkalemia and is calculated as follows:

$$TTKG = U_K \times P_{osm} / P_K \times U_{osm}$$

where,

U_K = urinary potassium concentration,
U_{osm} = urinary osmolality,
P_{osm} = plasma osmolality and
P_K = plasma potassium

While evaluating TTKG, it is important to ensure that the urinary sodium concentration is greater than 25 mEq/L so that insufficient sodium delivery is not limiting potassium secretion and the urine osmolality should exceed serum osmolality.

TTKG is a satisfactory indicator of aldosterone activity in normal children and in children with hypoaldosteronism and pseudo-hypoaldosteronism. Normally, the TTKG is less than 2.5 during hypokalemia and greater

Table 10.1: Causes of hyperkalemia

Spurious hyperkalemia

Hemolysis, leukocytosis, thrombocytosis

Decreased excretion

Acute and chronic renal failure
Renal tubular acidosis type IV

Transcellular shifts

β-adrenergic receptor antagonists, succinylcholine, digoxin intoxication
Metabolic acidosis
Hyperosmolality with insulin deficiency
Hyperkalemic periodic paralysis

Increased potassium intake or release from cells

Potassium ingestion or infusion
Nutritional and herbal supplements
Stored packed red blood cells, intravascular hemolysis
Rhabdomyolysis, severe exercise

Drugs

Potassium sparing diuretics
Trimethoprim, pentamidine
Nonsteroidal anti-inflammatory drugs
Angiotensin converting enzyme inhibitors (ACEI), angiotensin receptor blockers
Heparins (unfractionated and low-molecular-weight heparin)
Calcineurin inhibitors (e.g. cyclosporine, tacrolimus)

Mineralocorticoid deficiency, resistance

Normal plasma aldosterone

Sickle cell disease, systemic lupus erythematosus
Obstructive uropathy
Type 1 RTA (voltage defect)
ACEI, spironolactone, amiloride, trimethoprim

Low plasma aldosterone

Congenital adrenal hyperplasia, Addison disease
Chronic tubulointerstitial nephritis, diabetes mellitus

High plasma aldosterone

Pseudohypoaldosteronism types 1 and 2
Obstructive uropathy

than 7 during hyperkalemia. A high TTKG during hyperkalemia indicates an appropriate aldosterone effect. A value less than 5 suggests inadequate aldosterone effect. Estimation of the serum aldosterone level helps differentiate between hypoaldosteronism and renal resistance to aldosterone.

Management

Spurious hyperkalemia should be excluded. If the serum potassium level >6.5 mEq/L, or if ECG changes are present, therapeutic measures should be instituted immediately.

Emergencies

Recommended emergency interventions include:

1. *Intravenous calcium* directly antagonizes the effect of hyperkalemia on cell membranes. The onset of action is within 1–3 minutes and effect lasts for 30–45 minutes. Calcium gluconate (10%) is infused with cardiac monitoring at a dose of 100 mg/kg (1 mL/kg) over 3 to 5 minutes; the total dose should not exceed 10 ml.

2. *Intravenous insulin* lowers extracellular potassium levels by driving potassium into cells; concomitant administration of glucose prevents hypoglycemia. Insulin is given at a dose of 0.1 U/kg along with 0.5 g/kg (2 mL/kg) of 25% dextrose solution over 30 minutes. The dose may be repeated in 30 to 60 minutes, or as an infusion of 25% dextrose at 1–2 mL/kg/hr along with insulin 0.1 U/kg/hr. The onset of action is within 20–30 minutes and the effect lasts for 4–6 hr.

3. *Intravenous or nebulized β2-adrenergic agonists,* such as salbutamol (4-6 µg/kg/

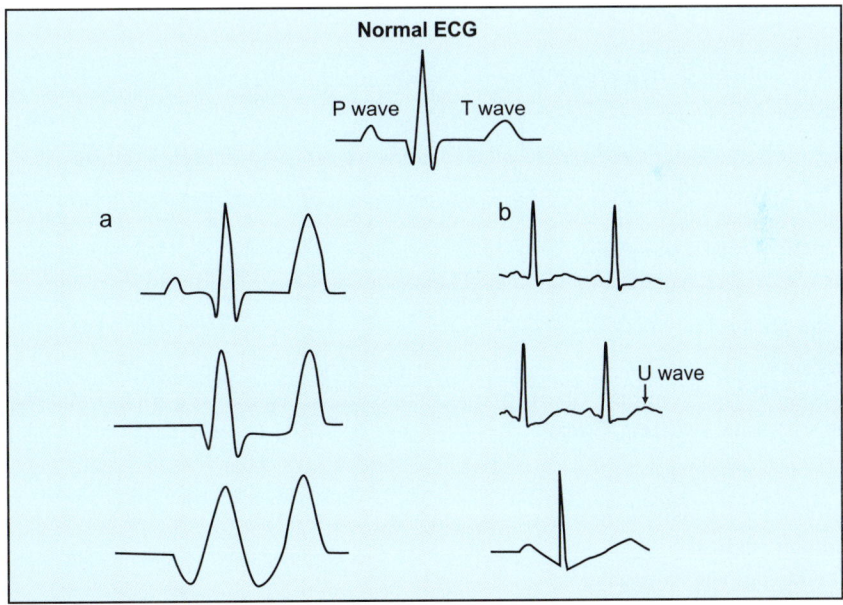

Fig. 10.1: ECG changes in (a) Hyperkalemia: The earliest change is peaking of the T-waves, which is followed by flattening of the P-waves, prolongation of PR interval, and widening of the QRS complex; terminal events include a sine-wave pattern with ventricular fibrillation and cardiac arrest. (b) Hypokalemia: Depression of ST segment is noted, followed by P wave widening, flattening of T waves, the appearance of U wave and fallacious QT prolongation

dose, max 5 mg) drive potassium into cells. The onset of action is within 20–30 minutes and the effect lasts for 4–6 hr.

4. *Intravenous sodium bicarbonate* results in release of hydrogen ions from cells and is accompanied by potassium movement into cells. It may be administered at a dosage of 1–2 mEq/kg over 5 to 10 minutes. Its onset of action is within 5–20 minutes and the effect lasts for 2 hr.

Other Measures

Restriction of dietary intake of potassium and discontinuation of drugs that may cause hyperkalemia is important. Increasing renal potassium excretion with the use of a loop diuretic, and less frequently a thiazide diuretic is useful. In addition, cation exchange resins (sodium polystyrene sulfonate 1 g/kg q8 hr) allow gastrointestinal potassium excretion. Finally, patients with end-stage renal disease and hyperkalemia require institution of dialysis.

HYPOKALEMIA

Hypokalemia is defined as serum potassium less than 3.5 mEq/L. It may be the consequence of true potassium depletion in the body or merely result from redistribution of potassium from the extracellular to intracellular compartment or expansion of "effective' circulating volume (Table 10.2). Spurious hypokalemia results when the cells take up potassium after blood has been drawn e.g. in patients with high leukocyte counts.

Mild hypokalemia (3–3.5 mEq/L) is usually asymptomatic. Values less than 3 mEq/L can result in generalized muscle weakness and cardiac conduction abnormalities (Fig. 10.1b). Chronic hypokalemia can result in impaired renal concentrating ability and polyuria.

Table 10.2: Causes of hypokalemia

Redistribution

Activation of β_2 adrenergic receptors: catecholamine excess, β-adrenergic agonists
Hormones: insulin, aldosterone
Metabolic alkalosis
Hypokalemic periodic paralysis
Expanded "effective" circulating volume: enhanced mineralocorticoid activity

Potassium depletion

Malnutrition
Gastrointestinal loss: vomiting, diarrhea, intestinal fistulas, laxative abuse, chloridiarrhea
Skin loss: excessive sweating, burns

Renal loss

Recovery from acute renal failure
Renal tubular acidosis
Bartter and Gitelman syndromes
Interstitial nephritis
Mineralocorticoid excess
Diabetic ketoacidosis
Use of loop, thiazide diuretics

Evaluation

Spurious hypokalemia is always without any EKG changes and can be avoided if plasma is rapidly separated from the cells or if the blood is stored at 4° C. Assessment of clinical features provides clues towards etiology (Table 10.2). Determination of blood pressure, blood pH, bicarbonate, electrolytes, urea, creatinine and urinary potassium concentration are useful (Fig. 10.2). Estimation of the fractional excretion of potassium (FEK) helps determine renal potassium handling:

$$FEK = \frac{\text{urine } K^+ \times \text{serum creatinine} \times 100}{\text{serum } K^+ \times \text{urine creatinine}}$$

It is important to differentiate hypokalemia due to renal versus non-renal losses. FEK of <6% indicates appropriate renal response. A random urine potassium/creatinine (K⁺/Cr) ratio can be used when a 24-hour urine collection is difficult. Urinary K^+ >15 mEq/ g of creatinine in a spot sample suggests renal losses.

Hypokalemia associated with high blood pressure and metabolic alkalosis

High blood pressure with hypokalemia suggests mineralocorticoid excess, primary aldosteronism (hyperplasia or adenoma), apparent mineralocorticoid excess, Liddle

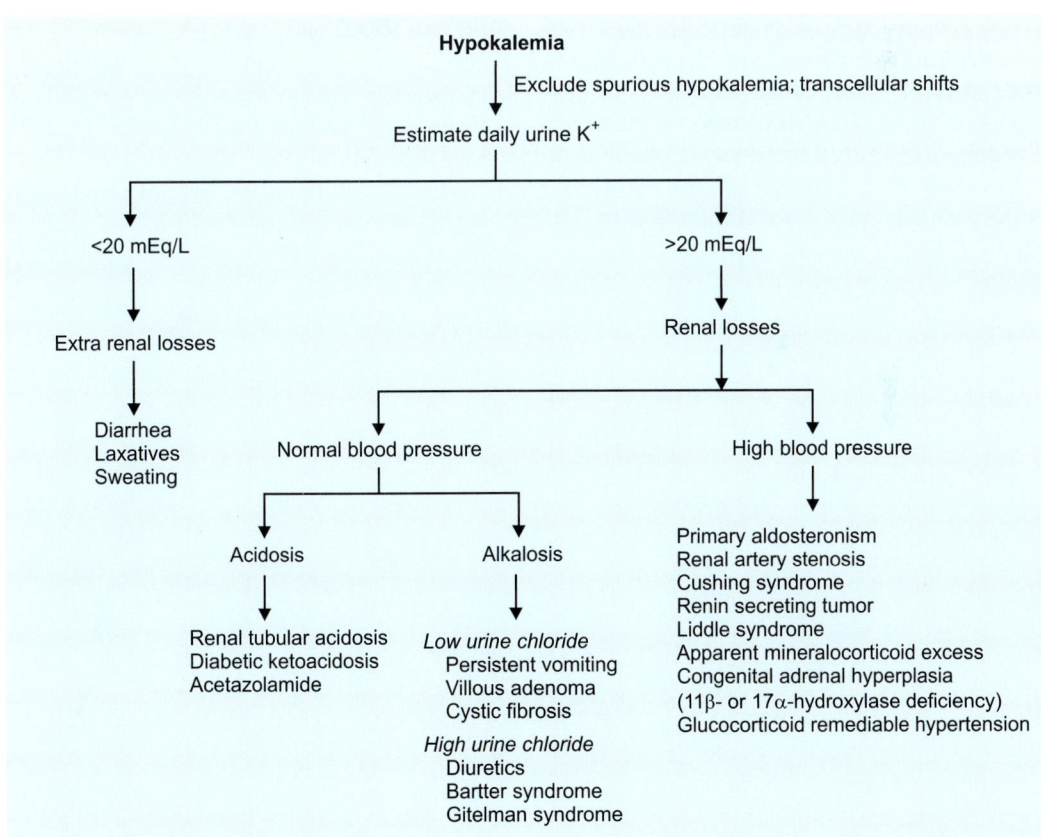

Fig. 10.2: Evaluation of hypokalemia based on urine concentration of potassium and presence of acidosis or alkalosis.

syndrome, congenital adrenal hyperplasia due to 11β-hydroxylase or 17α-hydroxylase deficiency, Cushing disease, exogenous mineralocorticoids and licorice ingestion.

The evaluation of hypokalemic metabolic alkalosis is discussed in Chapter 12.

Management

In most cases, oral replacement with potassium chloride (1–4 mEq/kg body weight daily in divided doses; syrup Potklor 15 mL = 20 mEq K^+) is effective in correcting hypokalemia. An alkaline salt such as potassium citrate is appropriate if there is accompanying acidosis. Oral potassium phosphate is useful with concomitant phosphorus deficiency.

Intravenous supplementation is necessary in patients with severe hypokalemia (<2.5 mEq/L), and those with ECG abnormalities or muscle weakness. Potassium chloride (0.5–1 mEq/kg/dose) is given as an infusion over 1–2 hr. The IV infusion rate should usually not exceed 1 mEq/kg/hr. The maximum concentration at which potassium can be administered safely is 40 mEq/L for peripheral lines and 150–200 mEq/L through a central line. Higher concentrations in peripheral lines lead to local discomfort, venous spasm and sclerosis. Potassium supplementation should be limited if hypokalemia is considered secondary to redistribution of potassium stores.

Magnesium deficiency should be suspected and treated if there is lack of response to potassium supplements. Potassium sparing diuretics such as spironolactone, triamterene or amiloride should be used cautiously with supplemental potassium because of the risk of hyperkalemia.

SUPPORT READING

Groeneveld J, Sijpkens Y, Lin S, Davids M, Halperin M. An approach to the patient with severe hypokalemia: the potassium quiz. Q J Med 2005; 98: 305–16

Raserger A Soleimani M. Hypokalemia and hyperkalemia. Postgrad Med J 2001; 77: 759–64

11 Renal Tubular Acidosis

Renal tubular acidosis (RTA) is a group of transport defects secondary to reduced proximal tubular reabsorption of bicarbonate (HCO_3^-), the distal secretion of protons (hydrogen ion, H^+) or both, resulting in impaired capacity for net acid excretion and persistent hyperchloremic metabolic acidosis.

Based on pathophysiology, RTA has been classified into three types: type 1 (distal) RTA; type 2 (proximal) RTA; and type 4 RTA. The above conditions are either secondary to other causes or primary, with or without known genetic defects.

Pathophysiology

The primary defect in *proximal RTA* is reduced renal threshold for HCO_3^-, resulting in bicarbonaturia (Fig. 11.1). Proximal RTA may represent isolated or generalized proximal tubular dysfunction, the latter (Fanconi syndrome) being characterized by tubular proteinuria and aminoaciduria and variable degrees of bicarbonaturia, phosphaturia, electrolyte wasting and glucosuria.

Distal RTA is characterized by metabolic acidosis secondary to decreased secretion of H^+ ions. Patients with distal RTA are unable to excrete ammonium (NH_4^+) ions in amounts adequate to keep pace with a normal rate of acid production. In hypokalemic distal RTA (classic RTA or type 1 RTA), urine pH cannot reach maximal acidity (i.e. remains >5.3) despite acidemia, indicating low H^+ concentration in the collecting duct. This condition is secondary to either a secretory (rate) defect or a gradient (permeability) defect. In the former, the rate of secretion of H^+ is low for the degree of acidosis. The defect in secretory distal RTA may be secondary to defective function of H^+ ATPase, H^+/K^+ ATPase, or the Cl^-/HCO_3^- exchanger (Fig. 11.2). Patients with the gradient (permeability) defect show normal secretory capacity of H^+ but an increased backleak resulting in dissipation of the pH gradient.

In distal RTA, the titrable acidity and NH_4^+ secretion are low. Hypokalemia is attributed to its increased losses in the tubular lumen, and urinary Na^+ loss and volume contraction leading to aldosterone stimulation that further increases tubular K^+ secretion and decreases proximal resorption.

Incomplete distal RTA is a variant or milder form of classic distal RTA, in which there is defective tubular H^+ secretion but plasma HCO_3^- levels are normal. Daily net acid excretion is maintained by enhanced ammoniagenesis. Hypercalciuria and hypocitraturia are present, and there is a risk for nephrolithiasis and nephrocalcinosis.

Distal RTA associated with hyperkalemia may occur due either to a voltage-defect or rate-defect due to aldosterone deficiency or resistance. The voltage-defect is uncommon and is caused by an insufficient negative intratubular potential at the level of cortical collecting duct, which results in reduced secretion of H^+ and K^+, with decreased

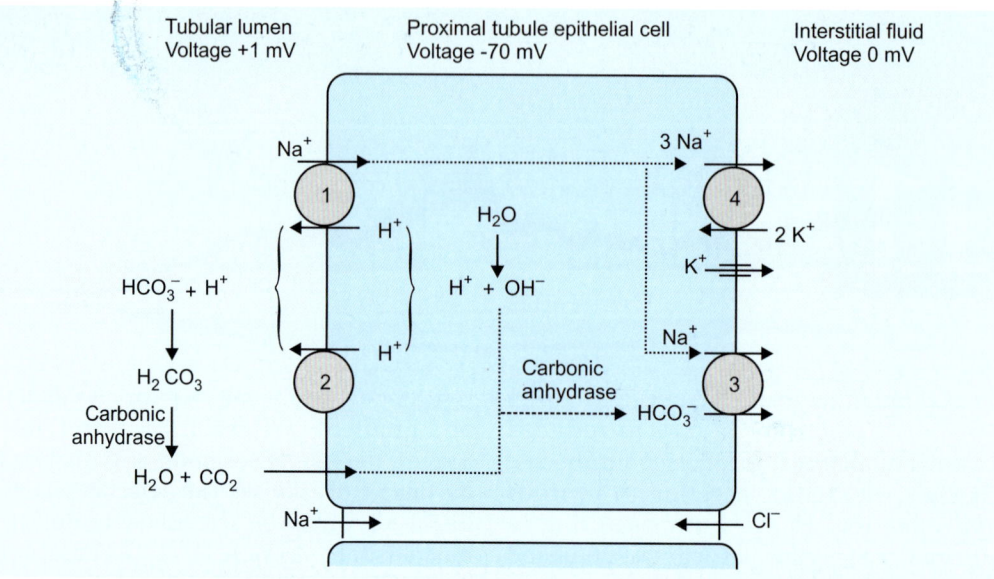

Fig. 11.1: Bicarbonate absorption in the proximal tubule. Protons (H^+) are secreted into the lumen through the actions of the Na^+/H^+ antiporter (1) and the H^+ ATPase (2). Secreted H^+ combines with HCO_3^- to form H_2CO_3, which, under the action of luminal membrane carbonic anhydrase dissociates to H_2O and CO_2. The CO_2 travels across the membrane into the cell where it combines with OH^- to generate HCO_3^-. The HCO_3^- and Na^+ cross the basolateral membrane using the Na^+/HCO_3^- symporter (3). Na^+ also exits the cell via the Na^+/K^+ ATPase (4). Electrogenic H^+ secretion generates a small lumen positive voltage, which creates current flow across the paracellular pathway.

trapping and excretion of NH_4^+ and hyperkalemia.

Hyperkalemia with distal RTA might also be due to aldosterone resistance or deficiency (*type 4 RTA*). Aldosterone increases Na^+ absorption and results in a negative intratubular potential. It also increases luminal membrane permeability to K^+ and stimulates basolateral $Na^+/K^+/$ATPase, causing increased urinary K^+ losses. Since aldosterone also directly stimulates the proton pump, aldosterone deficiency or resistance is expected to cause hyperkalemia and acidosis. Another factor in decreasing net H^+ excretion, in these patients, is reduced ammoniagenesis due to hyperkalemia.

In type 4 RTA, maximally acidic urine (<5.3) can be formed, indicating the ability to establish a maximal H^+ gradient. However, the rate of ammonium excretion is low.

Clinical Features

Clinical features of RTA include growth retardation, failure to thrive, polyuria, polydipsia, preference for savory foods and refractory rickets. Children with proximal RTA present with stunted growth. Rickets and/or osteomalacia may be associated, and suggest the presence of Fanconi syndrome. Nephrocalcinosis and urolithiasis are not seen. Symptoms related to hypokalemia (weakness, paralysis) are uncommon. Proximal RTA is either a primary (isolated) defect or a part of Fanconi syndrome, due e.g. to cystinosis, galactosemia, Lowe syndrome, fructose intolerance or Wilson disease (Table 11.1).

Features in distal RTA include impaired growth, polyuria, nephrocalcinosis, nephrolithiasis and symptoms of hypokalemia.

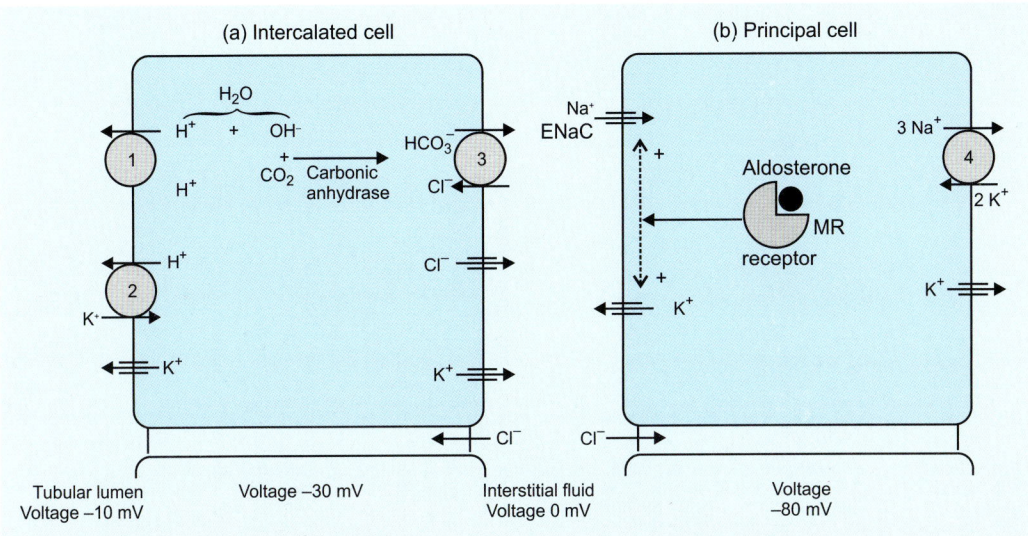

Fig. 11.2: Mechanism of distal acidification and potassium excretion. (a) The intercalated cells of the cortical collecting ducts secrete H^+ through the H^+ ATPase (1) and H^+/K^+ ATPase (2), independent of Na^+ transport. The hydroxyl (OH^-) ions generated in the cell through H^+ secretion exit the cell by the HCO_3^-/Cl^- exchanger (3). The secreted H^+ is buffered by luminal ammonia forming NH_4^+ and phosphate (titrable acids), to prevent a drop in luminal pH that would prevent further H^+ secretion. (b) Principal cells mediate sodium (Na^+) absorption and potassium (K^+) transport. The apical membrane contains an amiloride sensitive Na^+ channel (epithelial sodium channel, ENaC); Na^+ exits basolaterally *via* Na^+/K^+ ATPase (4). Sodium transport creates a lumen negative transepithelial potential that increases the rate of H^+ secretion by intercalated cells. Aldosterone binds to the mineralocorticoid (MR) receptor and enhances Na^+ absorption and H^+ and K^+ secretion

Progression of nephrocalcinosis might lead to chronic renal failure. In children, distal RTA is almost always a primary entity, and rarely secondary to systemic lupus erythematosus or Sjogren syndrome (Table 11.2). Some patients have sensorineural deafness, which is present from birth or manifests later.

Type 4 RTA is associated with hypoaldosteronism or resistance to the action of aldosterone. Nephrocalcinosis and urolithiasis are absent and bone lesions are rare. Older children may develop RTA due to advanced tubulointerstitial diseases leading to mineralocorticoid resistance, drugs or mineralocorticoid deficiency.

Pseudohypoaldosteronism (PHA) type 1 may involve only the kidney (autosomal dominant form) or, in the generalized (auto-somal recessive) disorder, affect sweat glands, salivary glands and colon. Both forms show elevated levels of renin and aldosterone but the autosomal dominant form of PHA type 1 is less severe. PHA type 1 should be considered in the differential diagnoses in neonates and infants presenting with salt loss, hypotension, hyperkalemia and metabolic acidosis. Treatment consists of oral sodium chloride supplementation that leads to expansion of ECF and increased delivery of sodium to the distal nephron resulting in increased excretion of potassium.

Patients with PHA type 2 (Gordon syndrome) have hypertension, acidosis and hyperkalemia with low levels of renin. Therapy with thiazides corrects these abnormalities (Table 12.3).

Table 11.1: Inherited forms of renal tubular acidosis (RTA)

Type of RTA	Inheritance	Non renal manifestation	Defective protein and gene
Type 1 (distal)	Dominant	None	Anion exchanger 1 (AE1); *SCL4A1*
	Recessive	Hemolytic anemia	AE1; *SCL4A1*
	Recessive	Early hearing loss	B1 subunit of H+-ATPase; *ATP6V1B1*
	Recessive	Normal hearing/delayed hearing loss	A4 subunit of H+-ATPase; *ATP6V0A4*
Type 2 (proximal)			
Isolated	Recessive	Ocular abnormalities (band keratopathy, cataracts, glaucoma)	Sodium bicarbonate cotransporter 1 (NBC1); *SCL4A4*
		Defective dental enamel	
		Intellectual impairment	
		Basal ganglia calcification	
Multiple tubular dysfunction (Fanconi syndrome)	Recessive, dominant	None	Not known
	X-linked	Dent's disease	Renal chloride channel; *CLCN5*
	Syndromic*	Cystinosis	Cystinosin; *CTNS*
		Tyrosinemia type 1	Fumarylacetoacetate hydrolase; *FAH*
		Fanconi Bickel	Glucose transporter GLUT2; *GLUT2/SLC2A2*
		Wilson disease	ATPase, Cu2+-transporting polypeptide; *ATP7B*
		Galactosemia	Galactose-1-phosphate uridylyltransferase; *GALT*
		Hereditary fructose intolerance	Fructose-1-phosphate aldolase; *ALDOB*
		Lowe syndrome	Phosphatidylinositol 4,5-bisphosphate 5-phosphatase; *OCRL1*
		Glycogen storage disease type I	Glucose-6-phosphatase-alpha; *G6Pα*
		Mitochondrial disorders	Multiple defects described
Type 3 (combined)	Recessive	Osteopetrosis; blindness, deafness	Carbonic anhydrase type II (CAII); *CA2*
Type 4 (hyperkalemic)	Recessive	Congenital adrenal hyperplasia	21 hydroxylase, *CYP21*; aldosterone synthase, *CYP11B2*
	Dominant	Pseudohypoaldosteronism (PHA) type 1	Mineralocorticoid receptor (MR) (*NR3C2*)
	Recessive	Pseudohypoaldosteronism (PHA) type 1	Epithelial sodium channel (ENaC); *SCNN1B*
	Recessive	PHA type 2, Gordon syndrome	WNK1 or WNK4; *PHA2B, PHA2C*

* Syndromic forms of Fanconi syndrome are inherited in autosomal recessive pattern, except for Lowe syndrome with X linked recessive inheritance

Table 11.2: Causes of acquired renal tubular acidosis

	Etiology
Type I (distal)	Systemic lupus erythematosus
	Sjögren syndrome, sickle cell anemia
	Obstructive uropathy; reflux nephropathy
	Nephrocalcinosis
	Amphotericin B toxicity
Type II (proximal)	*Isolated*
	Carbonic anhydrase inhibitors (acetazolamide)
	Fanconi syndrome
	Vitamin D dependent rickets
	Primary hyperparathyroidism
	Sjögren syndrome
	Paroxysmal nocturnal hemoglobinuria
	Acute tubulointerstitial nephritis with uveitis
	Drugs: ifosfamide, valproate, aminoglycosides, cisplatin
	Heavy metals & toxins: lead, cadmium, mercury, toluene
Type IV (hyperkalemic)	
Aldosterone deficiency without renal disease	*Aldosterone resistance*
Addison disease	Post transplantation
Isolated aldosterone deficiency	Drugs: amiloride, spironolactone, ACE inhibitors,
Adrenal tuberculosis; necrosis	heparin, NSAIDs, calcineurin inhibitors
Aldosterone deficiency in renal insufficiency	
Obstructive uropathy	
Interstitial nephritis	
Nephrocalcinosis	

EVALUATION

Metabolic acidosis may result from extrarenal processes, which result in either increased endogenous acid synthesis (e.g. ketoacidosis) or enhanced bicarbonate losses. Intestinal and pancreatic secretions and bile have considerable quantities of HCO_3^-, therefore conditions like diarrhea, removal of pancreatic or intestinal secretions or bile by tube drainage or fistula leads to loss of HCO_3^- and metabolic acidosis. Hyperchloremic metabolic acidosis may also result from ureterosigmoidostomy due to presence in the colon of an anion exchange pump that absorbs luminal Cl^- (of urinary origin) and exchanges it for HCO_3^-, and due to colonic absorption of NH_4^+ (of urinary origin), which releases H^+ when metabolized in the liver. Cholestyramine also cause metabolic acidosis by acting as anion exchange resins, where colonic luminal HCO_3^- is absorbed in exchange for Cl^- released by the resin.

Since all types of RTA are associated with hyperchloremic normal anion gap metabolic acidosis, the initial step is to determine the plasma anion gap (Fig. 11.3). Further evaluation of metabolic acidosis is detailed in steps below and in Fig. 11.4.

Step 1. Determine plasma anion gap

Plasma anion gap is calculated as follows:

Anion gap = $Na^+ - (Cl^- + HCO_3^-)$

The normal plasma anion gap is 8–12 mEq/L. Assessment of the anion gap facilitates distinction between RTA and diarrhea on one hand, and diabetic ketoacidosis, lactic acidosis due to shock or poor peripheral perfusion,

Electrolyte Disorders and Tubular Diseases

III

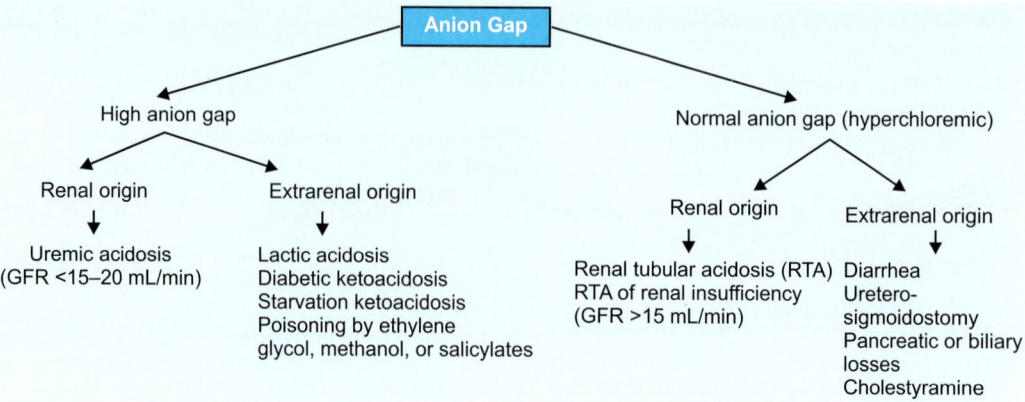

Fig. 11.3: Differential diagnosis of the causes of metabolic acidosis. GFR glomerular filtration rate

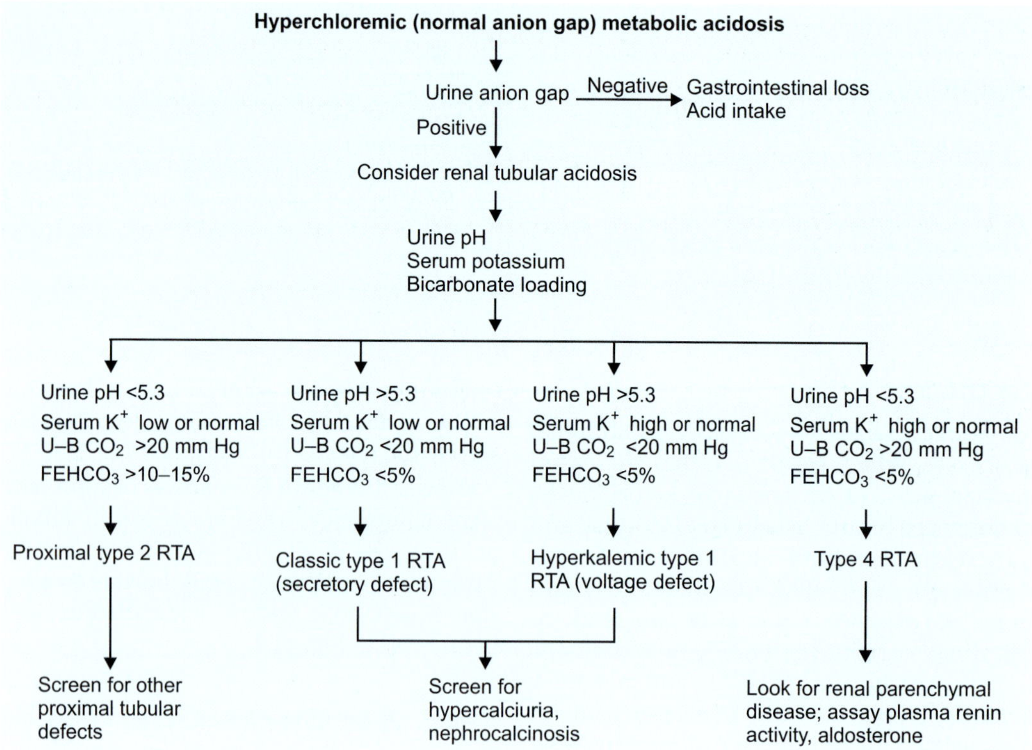

Hyperchloremic (normal anion gap) metabolic acidosis

↓

Urine anion gap ——Negative——→ Gastrointestinal loss
Acid intake

Positive ↓

Consider renal tubular acidosis

↓

Urine pH
Serum potassium
Bicarbonate loading

↓

Urine pH <5.3	Urine pH >5.3	Urine pH >5.3	Urine pH <5.3
Serum K$^+$ low or normal	Serum K$^+$ low or normal	Serum K$^+$ high or normal	Serum K$^+$ high or normal
U–B CO$_2$ >20 mm Hg	U–B CO$_2$ <20 mm Hg	U–B CO$_2$ <20 mm Hg	U–B CO$_2$ >20 mm Hg
FEHCO$_3$ >10–15%	FEHCO$_3$ <5%	FEHCO$_3$ <5%	FEHCO$_3$ <5%
↓	↓	↓	↓
Proximal type 2 RTA	Classic type 1 RTA (secretory defect)	Hyperkalemic type 1 RTA (voltage defect)	Type 4 RTA
↓	↓		↓
Screen for other proximal tubular defects	Screen for hypercalciuria, nephrocalcinosis		Look for renal parenchymal disease; assay plasma renin activity, aldosterone

Fig. 11.4: Evaluation of a patient with renal tubular acidosis. RTA renal tubular acidosis, U-B CO$_2$ urine to blood PCO$_2$ gradient, FEHCO$_3$ fractional excretion of HCO$_3^-$

some inborn errors of metabolism, poisoning and uremia on the other. While advanced renal failure with GFR <15 mL/min/1.73 m^2 results in metabolic acidosis with elevated anion gap, normal anion gap (hyperchloremic) acidosis is not infrequent at GFR 20–50 mL/min, especially in patients with tubulo-interstitial diseases.

Step 2. Estimate urine anion gap (UAG)

Having established the presence of metabolic acidosis with a normal plasma anion gap, the next step is to distinguish renal (RTA) from extrarenal causes. The UAG (or urine net charge) is useful for estimating NH_4^+ excretion in patients with hyperchloremic metabolic acidosis. While metabolic acidosis due to extrarenal HCO_3^- losses (diarrhea) is associated with high urinary NH_4^+ excretion, the excretion is low in patients with RTA. Since the sum of charges on cations and anions is equal:

$Na^+ + K^+ + NH_4^+ +$ unmeasured cations

$= Cl^- +$ unmeasured anions

The difference between urinary unmeasured anions (sulfates, phosphates, organic anions) and cations (calcium, magnesium) is relatively constant (about 80 mEq/L), thus:

$$Na^+ + K^+ + NH_4^+ = Cl^- + 80$$

The UAG or urine net charge is the difference between the sum of urinary Na^+ and K^+ and Cl^-. Hence, the UAG gives an approximate estimate of urinary NH_4^+ excretion.

$$NH_4^+ = 80 - UAG$$

Under normal circumstances, the UAG is positive due to the presence of dissolved anions. Metabolic acidosis with normal mechanism of renal acidification causes the UAG to become negative due to an increase in the NH_4^+ synthesis and excretion with the Cl^- ion. Thus in patients with hyperchloremic metabolic acidosis with preserved mechanism of renal acidification a negative UAG implies adequately increased NH_4^+ excretion. A positive UAG indicates inappropriately low renal NH_4^+ excretion, as in RTA.

Step 3. Determine urine pH

Urine pH is useful for assessing the integrity of distal urinary acidification. In the presence of systemic acidosis, the urine pH is normally <5.3. Presence of urine pH >5.3 during metabolic acidosis suggests defective distal secretion of H^+. It should be noted that urine pH measures the concentration of free H^+. However, this constitutes <1% of H^+ ions

secreted during systemic acidosis, since most protons are excreted as NH_4^+ or as titrable acidity. Urine pH values <5.3 are seen in subjects with proximal RTA during systemic acidosis and low filtered load (plasma HCO_3^- <15 mEq/L), or in patients with selective aldosterone deficiency (type 4 RTA).

The pH is measured electrometrically on fresh voided specimen. The use of dipstick is not recommended. Urine kept standing might get contaminated or infected with urea-splitting organisms, resulting in high urine pH.

If systemic acidosis is absent, an oral ammonium chloride (0.1 mg/kg) or calcium chloride (2 mEq/kg) load might be given, followed by the measurement of blood and urine pH every hr for the next 2–8 hr. If the plasma total CO_2 content falls by 3–5 mEq/L and capillary pH <7.35, the urine pH should fall to <5.3. Another protocol involves giving the same dose of the agent daily for 3–5 days, followed by measurement of pH. The test is done rarely, since ammonium chloride is unpalatable and associated with vomiting.

The ability of the distal tubule to secrete H^+ ions can also be determined by the frusemide or the frusemide-fludrocortisone test (page 63). The test is useful in evaluation of hypercalciuria detected during evaluation of nephrolithiaisis (Chapter 14). Urine pH following administration of these agents should normally result in urine pH <5.3.

Caveats in Assessment of Urine pH

The urine pH should be estimated in conjunction with urinary NH_4^+ content. Firstly, low urine pH does not always suggest an intact acidification mechanism, if excretion of NH_4^+ is low, as in proximal RTA. Secondly, patients with chronic metabolic acidosis (e.g. after chronic diarrhea) show increased ammoniagenesis that consumes most distally secreted H^+ ions, resulting in enhanced urine NH_4^+ excretion. *The urine pH in this instance may therefore be high despite appropriate H^+ excretion.* Finally, urine pH should be inter-

Table 11.3: Investigations to differentiate types of renal tubular acidosis (RTA)

	Proximal RTA	*Distal RTA*		*Type 4 RTA*
		Classic	*Hyperkalemic*	
Plasma K^+	Normal/low	Normal/low	High	High
Urine pH	<5.5	>5.5	>5.5	<5.5
Urine anion gap	Positive	Positive	Positive	Positive
Urine NH_4^+	Low	Low	Low	Low
Fractional HCO_3^- excretion	>10–15%	<5%	<5%	>5–10%
U-B PCO_2 mm Hg	>20	<20	</>20	>20
Urine calcium	Normal	High	High	Normal/low
Other tubular defects	Often present	Absent	Absent	Absent
Nephrocalcinosis	Absent	Present	Present	Absent
Bone disease	Common	Often present	Uncommon	Absent

U-B PCO_2 urine to blood PCO_2 gradient

preted in relation to urine Na^+ levels. When urine Na^+ level is <5–10 mEq/L, distal H^+ secretion is negligible. Thus, in patients with low urinary Na^+ concentration (e.g. acute diarrhea with dehydration), the presence of a high urine pH does not imply defective urinary acidification.

Step 4. Bicarbonate loading test

Sodium bicarbonate is given as half-strength IV infusion (0.5 mEq/mL) at the rate of 3 mL/minute through a peripheral vein, while measuring urine pH in timed samples 30–60 minutes apart. The urine should be collected under mineral oil. A steady state is achieved after 3–4 hr of the infusion, and the test is terminated when consecutive samples show urine pH >7.5. The medication may also be given orally (2–4 mEq/kg/d for 3 days) with the aim to achieve urine pH >7.5 and normal plasma HCO_3^-. Measurement of fractional excretion of HCO_3^- and urine to blood CO_2 gradient allows characterization of RTA (Fig. 11.4).

Urine to Blood CO_2 Gradient

In alkaline urine, such as after a load of sodium bicarbonate, urine PCO_2 increases because of distal H^+ secretion and is considered a sensitive indicator of distal acidification. The secreted H^+ in the distal tubule reacts with luminal HCO_3^- to form carbonic acid, which dehydrates slowly in the medu-

llary collecting duct to form CO_2 that is trapped in the renal tubule.

If urine pH is >7.5 and plasma HCO_3^- concentration is normal, the urine PCO_2 exceeds 70 mm Hg and the urine to blood PCO_2 gradient is greater than 20 mm Hg in normal individuals. Patients with decreased rates of tubular H^+ secretion (classical type 1 RTA) show subnormal values, with urine PCO_2 less than 50 mm Hg and U-B PCO_2 <10 mm Hg. Normal results are obtained in those with back leak and voltage defects and in type 4 RTA.

Fractional Excretion of Bicarbonate ($FEHCO_3$)

The fractional excretion, calculated after alkalization, is an index of proximal tubular handling of HCO_3^-. The proximal tubule normally reabsorbs almost all filtered HCO_3^-. $FEHCO_3$ (%)

$$= \frac{\text{urine bicarbonate} \times \text{plasma creatinine}}{\text{plasma bicarbonate} \times \text{urine creatinine}} \times 100$$

When serum HCO_3^- is normal (>22 mEq/L), a value >15% indicates proximal RTA. Levels are in the normal range (<5%) in classic distal RTA. In hyperkalemic distal RTA, the $FEHCO_3$ varies from 5–10%.

Step 5. Additional Investigations

Table 11.3 summarizes the assessment that allows the distinction of various types of RTA from each other. Some additional tests may be required, depending on the type of RTA.

Tests for Phosphate Handling

The plasma phosphate level indicates proximal tubular function. The fractional excretion of phosphate determined on a timed (6-hr, 12-hr or 24-hr) urine specimen, is useful for detecting phosphate wasting, as in Fanconi syndrome. Normally 5–12% of the filtered phosphate is excreted and the tubular reabsorption is 88–95%.

Fractional excretion of phosphate =

$$\frac{\text{urine phosphate} \times \text{plasma creatinine}}{\text{plasma phosphate} \times \text{urine creatinine}} \times 100$$

Tubular reabsorption
= 100 – fractional excretion

Tubular reabsorption of phosphate depends on plasma phosphate and GFR and is not an optimum index of tubular phosphate handling, especially in patients with hypophosphatemia. The *tubular maximum for phosphate,* corrected for GFR (TmP/GFR), is independent of plasma phosphate and renal functions for assessment of phosphate handling. TmP/GFR (Bijvoet index) represents the concentration above which most phosphate is excreted and below which most is reabsorbed. This can be calculated from the plasma phosphate and TRP, using a commonly available nomogram. The normal value is 2.8–4.4 mg/dL, with lower values for older children (Appendix 9).

Transtubular Potassium Gradient (TTKG)

While spot and 24-hr urinary excretion of K^+ are useful for evaluating patients with hypokalemia, their role in evaluating hyperkalemia is limited. In patients with hyperkalemia and normal glomerular function, the TTKG provides an accurate estimate of aldosterone effect on late distal and cortical collecting tubules.

The secretion of K^+ in the cortical and outer medullary collecting ducts chiefly accounts for its excretion in the urine, that is influenced by aldosterone, plasma K^+ and anion composition of the luminal fluid. Negligible amounts of K^+ are secreted or reabsorbed distal to these sites. The final urinary K^+ concentration then depends on water reabsorption in the medullary collecting ducts, which results in a rise in urinary K^+. The TTKG is determined as follows:

$$\text{TTKG} = \frac{\text{urine } K^+ \times \text{plasma osmolality}}{\text{plasma } K^+ \times \text{urine osmolality}}$$

The TTKG is an index of K^+ gradient in the distal tubular lumen and interstitial blood capillaries. The ratio of urine to plasma osmolality allows for correction of the final urinary K^+ concentration for the water reabsorbed in the medullary collecting duct. TTKG in normal persons varies within the range of 6-12. Hypokalemia from extrarenal causes results in renal K^+ conservation and a TTKG <2. A higher value suggests renal K^+ losses, as in hyperaldosteronism. During hyperkalemia, the expected TTKG is >10. An inappropriately low TTKG (<8) suggests hypoaldosteronism or tubular resistance to aldosterone. Administration of fludrocortisone enables TTKG to rise to >7 in patients with hypoaldosteronism, but not in those with aldosterone resistance.

Fludrocortisone Frusemide Test

This is a sensitive test for assessing distal urinary acidification.

Principle: Administration of frusemide increases the delivery of sodium ions to the distal tubules. In normal individuals, these ions are resorbed in exchange for H^+ ions resulting in acidic urine. The avidity of sodium resorption and change in urine pH are greater if the individual is sodium depleted or following administration of a mineralocorticoid (e.g. fludrocortisone).

Procedure: Following an overnight fast, the early morning urine pH is recorded. Frusemide 1–2 mg/kg (maximum 40 mg) and fludrocortisone 0.025 mg/kg (tablet 0.1 mg; maximum 1 mg) are administered orally. Fluid intake is allowed *ad lib.* Urine is collected every hour for next 6 hours

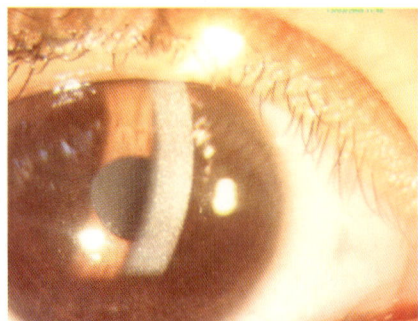

Fig. 11.5: Slit lamp examination of the cornea in a 4-year-old girl with cystinosis: Diffuse crystal deposition is noted

and the urine pH measured with a pH meter. In patients with hypokalemia (<3.5 mEq/L), oral potassium supplements should be given for 3–4 days before the test.

Interpretation: A normal response is lowering of urine pH to <5.3 by 4 hours. This rules out a defect in distal urinary acidification. Frequent urine pH measurements are necessary to avoid misinterpretation.

In patients with hypokalemic distal RTA, the urine pH does not fall but the urine K$^+$ excretion increases since the function of principal cells is intact. Patients with H$^+$ ATPase pump defect limited to the medulla show a relatively normal increase in both H$^+$ and K$^+$ secretion because cortical tubule function is stimulated appropriately by a rise in luminal electronegativity. Patients with primary defect in cortical Na$^+$ reabsorption (voltage defect) have baseline hyperkalemia; following frusemide they show no increase in H$^+$ or K$^+$ excretion, since luminal electronegativity is not enhanced. A normal response is observed in patients with type 4 RTA, hypoaldosteronism (where voltage sensitive activity is retained), reversible voltage dependent defects and proximal RTA.

Genetic Studies

Mutations have been identified in the genes encoding transporters involved in pathogenesis of RTA (Table 11.1). Identification of these mutations provides insight into the pathogenesis.

Proximal RTA

The diagnosis of proximal RTA requires evaluation of other proximal tubular functions. Apart from assessment of phosphate excretion, evaluation for aminoaciduria, glucosuria, low

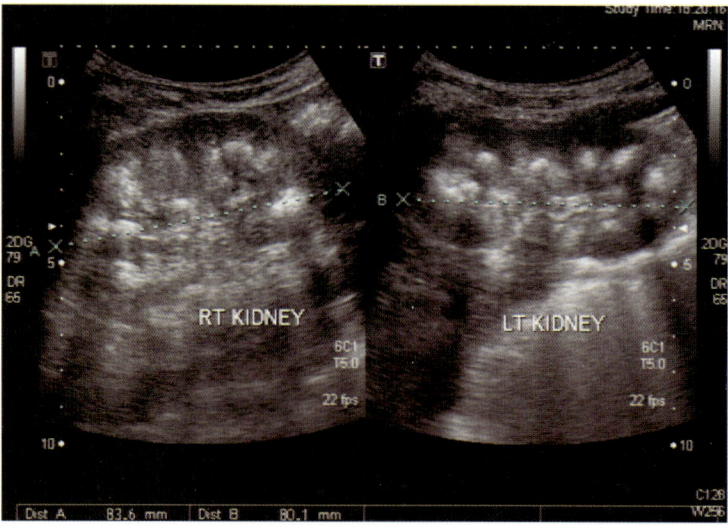

Fig.11.6: Medullary nephrocalcinosis. Ultrasonography in a 3-yr-old boy with distal renal tubular acidosis shows hyperechoic medulla

molecular weight proteinuria, calcium excretion and for rickets is important. Disorders that are associated with proximal RTA and Fanconi syndrome should be screened for, including cystinosis (Fig. 11.5), Lowe syndrome, galactosemia and Wilson disease.

Distal RTA

Additional work-up for evaluation of distal RTA includes ultrasonography for nephrocalcinosis (Fig. 11.6) and renal calculi, and measurement of urinary calcium and citrate excretion.

Hypercalciuria and hyperphosphaturia occur due to the release of calcium phosphate from bone in order to buffer excess H^+ during acidosis, and the direct effects of acidosis on tubular reabsorption of these ions. Hypocitraturia results from citrate utilization in proximal tubular cells, and due to the high luminal pH favoring conversion of citrate^{3-} to the readily resorbable citrate^{2-}. Hypercalciuria, hypocitraturia and high urine pH contribute to occurrence of calcium phosphate renal stones. Hypercalciuria is suspected when the value of urinary calcium to creatinine ratio is above age related norms, and confirmed by 24-hr excretion exceeding 4 mg/kg/day.

All patients with idiopathic distal RTA should undergo a hearing evaluation. Type 1 RTA in older children may also be associated with systemic lupus, osteopetrosis, Sjogren syndrome or chronic hepatitis.

Type 4 RTA

In children, aldosterone unresponsiveness is more common than aldosterone deficiency, and is commonly associated with obstructive uropathy. Diagnostic work-up should thus include investigations for underlying nephropathy, ultrasound to identify structural abnormalities and renal function tests for parenchymal dysfunction. TTKG is useful in diagnosing type 4 RTA, and when done before and after a mineralocorticoid challenge helps distinguish between deficiency and resistance to aldosterone. Measurement of plasma renin activity and aldosterone levels are necessary.

TREATMENT

The principles of management include ensuring adequate nutrition, and fluid and electrolyte intake. Acidosis is corrected by administration of alkali supplements (Polycitra, Shohl solution; Appendix 6)

Distal RTA: The requirement of alkali in patients with distal RTA is 2–3 mEq/kg/day, which can be increased until bicarbonate levels are normal. Alkali requirements decrease after the age of 5-yr. With correction of acidosis, renal potassium losses are reduced; however some patients require prolonged potassium supplements. Early treatment results in higher growth velocity, and reduction of hypercalciuria and increase in urinary citrate excretion, thus preventing nephrocalcinosis. Urinary calcium excretion should be monitored and if hypercalciuria persists, administration of thiazides is necessary.

Proximal RTA: The correction of acidosis requires administration of 5–20 mEq/kg/d of alkali supplements. This is usually given as a combination of sodium and potassium citrate, with restriction of dietary sodium. Supplements of phosphate (Appendix 6) are necessary in patients with the Fanconi syndrome. Small doses of vitamin D are often required to enable healing of rickets.

SUPPORT READING

Soriano JR. Renal tubular acidosis, the clinical entity. J Am SocNephrol 2002; 13: 2160–70

Bagga A, Bajpai A, Menon S. Approach to renal tubular disorders. Indian J Pediatr 2005; 72: 771–76

Bagga A, Sinha A. Evaluation of renal tubular acidosis. Indian J Pediatr 2007; 74: 679–86

Sayer JA, Pearce SHS. Diagnosis and clinical biochemistry of inherited tubulopathies. Ann Clin Biochem 2001; 38: 459–70

Walsh SB, Shirley DG, Wrong OM, Unwin R. Urinary acidification assessed by simultaneous furosemide and fludrocortisone treatment: an alternative to ammonium chloride. Kidney International 2007; 71: 1310–16

12 Metabolic Alkalosis

Patients with metabolic alkalosis have a high blood pH (>7.45) and high serum bicarbonate [HCO_3^-] (normal 22–26 mEq/L). Most conditions with metabolic alkalosis also have hypokalemia (serum K^+ <3.5 mEq/L). Patients present with increased neuromuscular irritability such as tetany or exaggerated reflexes. In addition, symptoms and signs of hypokalemia may be present. Metabolic alkalosis is not innocuous; in severe cases, arrhythmias and seizures may occur, leading to death.

Etiology

Conditions presenting with metabolic alkalosis are listed in Table 12.1; common causes include use of diuretics and persistent vomiting.

Excess base may be produced in the body by loss of chloride from the extracellular fluid (ECF) compartment in excess of Na^+ and K^+ ('unaccompanied' chloride depletion or deficiency) but 'accompanied' by H^+ or NH_4^+, which is equivalent to the gain of HCO_3^-. Such

Table 12.1: Differential diagnosis of metabolic alkalosis

Chloride responsive (urinary chloride <15 mEq/L)

Diuretics (loop or thiazide)
Gastric losses (vomiting; nasogastric suction)
Chloride losing diarrhea
Chloride deficient formula
Cystic fibrosis
Post-hypercapnia

Chloride resistant (urinary chloride >20 mEq/L)

Normal blood pressure	*High blood pressure*
Gitelman syndrome	Cushing syndrome
Bartter syndrome	Steroid administration
Administration of alkali	Renovascular disease; renin secreting tumor
	Adrenal hyperplasia, adenoma or carcinoma
	Glucocorticoid remediable aldosteronism
	11β-hydroxysteroid dehydrogenase deficiency
	17α-hydroxylase deficiency
	11β-hydroxylase deficiency
	Liddle syndrome

Metabolic Alkalosis

patients have a contracted effective circulating volume and normal to low blood pressure. In an attempt to conserve the ECF, there is a reduction in glomerular filtration rate (GFR), all the filtered HCO_3^- is reabsorbed proximally, and the renin angiotensin aldosterone system is activated, which promotes hypokalemia and maintains the metabolic alkalosis. The urine chloride is low, except in case of current diuretic use; once the diuretic effect has worn off, the urinary chloride level is low (<15 mEq/L) due to appropriate renal chloride retention in response to volume depletion. Since the alkalosis is driven by chloride losses, this is responsive to administration of chloride orally or intravenously (chloride responsive).

In another situation, metabolic alkalosis is the result of retention of HCO_3^- within the ECF to accompany the major cation Na^+. This is usually the result of avid resorption of HCO_3^- due to altered mineralocorticoid action or avid distal sodium resorption.

Rarely, it may occur with excessive intake (e.g. ingestion of milk and the antacid calcium carbonate) in a setting of reduced GFR. These patients have an expanded ECF volume, high blood pressure and low or high urine chloride. The alkalosis in these patients does not respond to chloride administration (chloride resistant).

Evaluation

History is important to rule out an apparent cause for alkalosis, such as vomiting, nasogastric suction, administration of diuretics, bicarbonate, licorice or steroids, and history suggesting cystic fibrosis or significant respiratory illness (Fig. 12.1). Patients are examined for presence of dehydration/hypovolemia or hypertension. Failure to thrive and triangular facies suggests Bartter syndrome.

1. Serum electrolytes and venous blood gas: to confirm metabolic alkalosis and hypokalemia

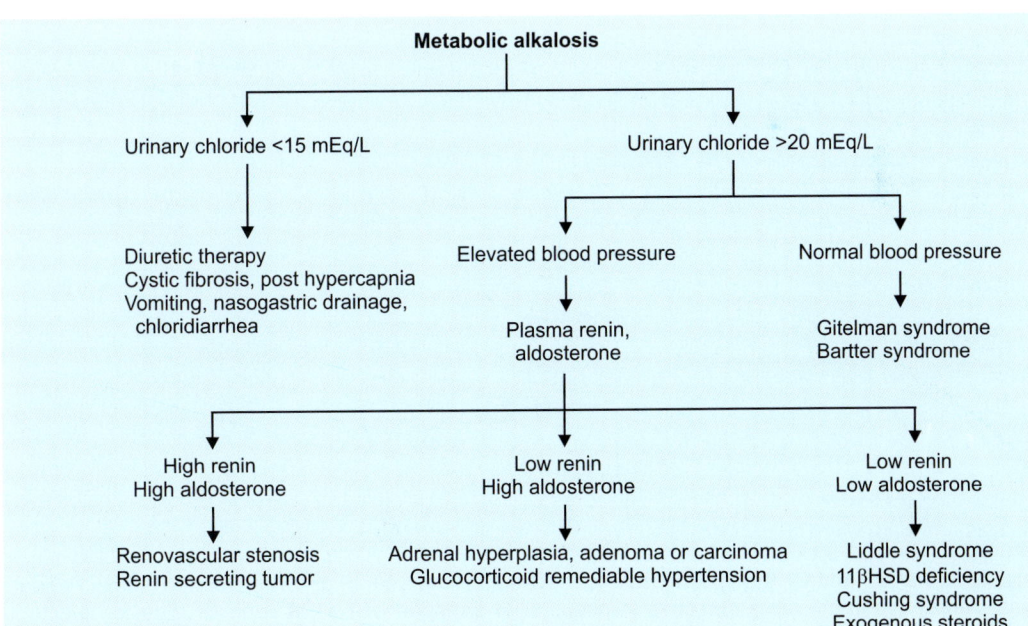

Fig. 12.1: Evaluation in a patient with metabolic alkalosis. 11βHSD 11β hydroxysteroid dehydrogenase

2. Urine electrolytes (chloride, sodium, potassium)
3. Plasma renin activity and aldosterone, in patients with hypertension

Figure 12.1 provides a plan for evaluation of patients with metabolic alkalosis and hypokalemia.

Metabolic Alkalosis with Urinary Chloride Wasting

Patients with tubulopathies such as Bartter and Gitelman syndrome should be differentiated from non renal causes of chloride loss such as vomiting, dietary deficiency and cystic fibrosis. Further characterization of the underlying defect is essentially based on molecular testing, but differences in presentation may help characterize the defect. These are summarized in Fig. 12.2 and Table 12.2.

In Bartter syndrome, tubular losses of K$^+$, Na$^+$, Cl$^-$ and water lead to volume contraction that in turn causes secondary hyperaldosteronism. Hypokalemia stimulates prostaglandin synthesis, leading to hyperreninemia and hyperaldosteronism. Several subtypes of Bartter syndrome are recognized. Table 12.2 lists these subtypes and other conditions with similar biochemical features.

Metabolic Alkalosis with Hypertension

Rare monogenic disorders present with hypertension, mild metabolic alkalosis and hypokalemia. Table 12.3 provides a summary of diagnostic evaluation and management of these causes. In all cases, hypertension is caused by an upregulation of Na$^+$ resorption in the distal nephron, causing an expansion of the extracellular volume. On the basis of site of defect, these disorders can be characterized into two groups. In the first group, mutations involve Na$^+$ transport in the distal convoluted tubule (DCT) cell and the principal cell of the collecting duct, e.g. Liddle syndrome (activating mutation of epithelial sodium channel, ENaC) and syndrome of apparent mineralocorticoid excess (inactivating mutation in the gene encoding glucocorticoid-metabolizing 11β-hydroxysteroid dehydrogenase type 2).

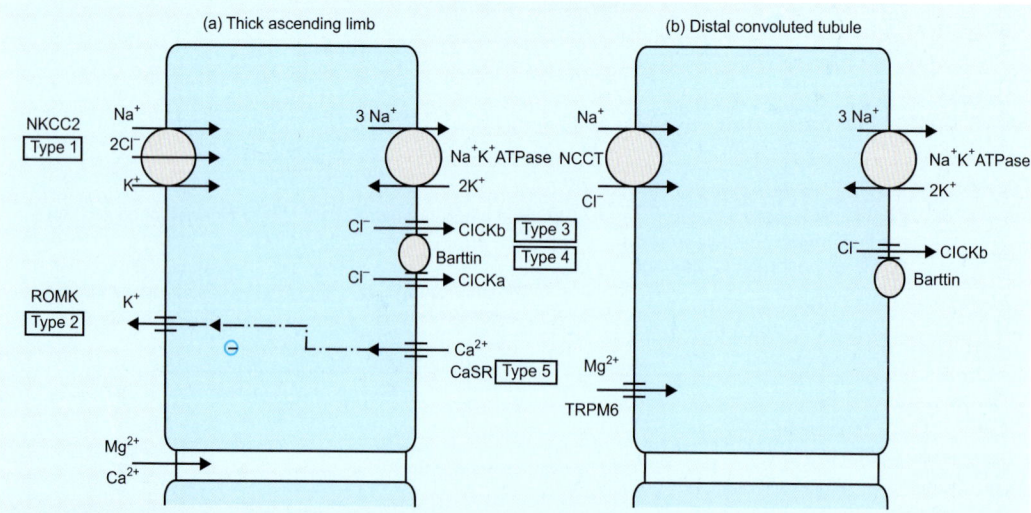

Fig. 12.2: Na$^+$, K$^+$ and Cl$^-$ transport in (a) thick ascending limb and (b) distal convoluted tubule. Patients with Bartter syndrome have defective transepithelial transport of Na$^+$, K$^+$ and Cl$^-$ due to defects in transport of these ions in the thick ascending limb. Bartter types 1 to 5 are caused by defects in individual channels, as detailed in Table 12.2 (b) Gitelman syndrome is caused by defective transport of Na$^+$ and Cl$^-$ in the distal convoluted tubule by the thiazide (NCCT) channel

Table 12.2: Diseases presenting with hypochloremic metabolic alkalosis with hypokalemia, and normal or low blood pressure

Disorder	Protein	Location	Gene; location	Presentation
Bartter syndromes (BS)				
Type 1, antenatal BS, aBS	Sodium potassium chloride cotransporter-2 (NKCC2)	Luminal thick ascending limb (TAL)	*SLC12A1*; 15q15–q21.1	Antenatal; polyhydramnios, prematurity, failure to thrive, nephrocalcinosis
Type 2, aBS	Potassium channel ROMK1	Luminal TAL, cortical collecting duct	*KCNJ1*; 11q24	Antenatal; polyhydramnios, prematurity, failure to thrive, nephrocalcinosis; hyperkalemia may occur
Type 3, classic BS (cBS)	Chloride channel, kidney, b (CLCKb)	Basolateral TAL, distal collecting duct (DCT)	*CLCNKB*; 1p36	Growth retardation, hypercalciuria; no nephrocalcinosis, normal serum magnesium
Type 4, aBS with sensorineural deafness	Barttin (beta subunit of CLCKa, CLCKb)	Basolateral TAL and DCT	*BSND CLCNKA-CLCNKB*	Antenatal; polyhydramnios, prematurity, sensorineural deafness
Bartter syndrome	Calcium sensing receptor (activation)	TAL	*CaSR*; 3q 13.3–q21	Hypercalciuria, nephrocalcinosis, hypomagnesemia
Gitelman syndrome				
Gitelman syndrome	Thiazide sensitive sodium chloride cotransporter	DCT	*SLC12A3*; 16q12.3	Hypocalciuria, hypomagnesemia, chondrocalcinosis (see Table 12. 4)

All conditions are inherited in an autosomol recessive manner, except Bartter syndrome due to mutation in the calcium sensing receptor, which is autosomal dominant

12

Table 12.3: Differential diagnosis of monogenic low renin hypertension

Disorder	Defect, inheritance	Diagnosis	Additional features	Treatment
Metabolic alkalosis and hypokalemia				
Liddle syndrome	Activating mutation of epithelial sodium channel (ENaC); autosomal dominant (AD)	Low plasma aldosterone; genetic testing	Most common type; variable hypokalemia and alkalosis	Low-salt diet; amiloride or triamterene
Apparent mineralocorticoid excess	11β-hydroxysteroid dehydrogenase type 2; autosomal recessive (AR)	Low plasma aldosterone; increased ratio of urinary tetrahydrocortisol (THF) and 5αTHF to tetrahydrocortisone	Variable polyuria, low birth weight, failure to thrive, hypercalciuria and nephrocalcinosis	Low-salt diet; eplerenone or spironolactone ± amiloride or thiazide
Glucocorticoid remediable aldosteronism	Hybrid gene between ACTH-responsive promoter and aldosterone synthase; AD	High aldosterone to PRA ratio*; increased urinary 18-oxocortisol; screening for hybrid gene	Increased risk of cerebral aneurysms	Low dose glucocorticoids
Congenital adrenal hyperplasia	11β hydroxylase or 17α hydroxylase; AR	Low plasma aldosterone; specific plasma or urine steroid profiles	Genital ambiguity	Eplerenone or spironolactone
Metabolic acidosis and hyperkalemia				
Gordon syndrome (pseudohypoaldosteronism type II)	Kinases WNK1 (activating mutation) or WNK4 (loss of function); AD	High aldosterone to PRA ratio*	Hyperkalemia, acidosis and failure to thrive may precede hypertension; hypercalciuria	Low salt diet; thiazide diuretic

*Ratio of aldosterone (in ng/dL) to plasma renin activity (PRA, ng/mL/hr) >30

Metabolic Alkalosis

Table 12.4: Magnesium wasting diseases

Disorder	Protein	Location	Gene, locus	Inheritance	Features
Gitelman syndrome	Thiazide sensitive sodium chloride cotransporter	DCT	SLC12A3, 16q 12.3	AR	Hypokalemic metabolic alkalosis, hypocalciuria, chondrocalcinosis
Familial hypomagnesemia, hypercalciuria, nephrocalcinosis (FHHNC)	Paracellin-1 (claudin-16), tight junction protein	TAL	CLDN16, 3q28	AR	Nephrocalcinosis, hyperuricemia, neonatal seizures, sensorineural deafness, progressive renal failure
Familial hypomagnesemia, hypercalciuria, nephrocalcinosis and severe ocular involvement	Claudin-19, tight junction protein	TAL	CLDN19, 1p34	AR	Severe myopia, nystagmus or macular coloboma in addition to symptoms described for FHHNC
Familial hypomagnesemia with hypocalciuria	Transient receptor potential cation channel, subfamily M (TRPM6)	DCT	TRPM6, 9q22	AR	Secondary hypocalcemia; calcinosis (myocardial, kidneys, cerebral arteries)
Isolated dominant hypomagnesemia	γ subunit of the sodium potassium ATPase	DCT	FXYD, 11q23	AD	Hypocalciuria
Isolated recessive hypomagnesemia	Not known	Not known	Not known	AR	Seizures, neurodevelopmental defects; normal calcium excretion
Hypomagnesemia/metabolic syndrome (mitochondrial hypomagnesemia)	Mitochondrial-coded tRNA (isoleucine)	DCT	(mt) tRNA (Ile)	Maternal	Hypercholesterolemia, hypertension
Autosomal dominant hypoparathyroidism	Calcium magnesium sensing receptor (CaSR)	TAL, DCT	Activating mutation of CASR; 3q13	AD	Onset in childhood; seizures or carpopedal spasms; hypocalcemia and low PTH; Bartter like phenotype

DCT distal convoluted tubule; TAL thick ascending limb; AR autosomal recessive; AD autosomal dominant

Patients with Gordon syndrome have mutations in regulatory kinases (WNK 1 or 4) and present with hypertension with *hyperkalemia* and *metabolic acidosis*.

In the second group are disorders with abnormal adrenal steroid production, causing an inappropriate stimulation of the mineralocorticoid receptor in the distal nephron. These include abnormal aldosterone production in glucocorticoid-remediable aldosteronism (GRA) and familial hyperaldosteronism type I and II, abnormal cortisol production (in familial glucocorticoid resistance), or other steroid metabolites in congenital adrenal hyperplasia with 11β or 17α hydroxylase deficiency.

Plasma renin activity and aldosterone are satisfactory screening tools that allow distinction between these conditions (Fig. 12.1, Table 12.3).

Treatment

Treatment of chloride responsive states includes management of the underlying problem, volume repletion, and oral or intravenous supplementation of potassium and sodium chloride. If essential, a potassium sparing diuretic should be used. Use of proton pump inhibitor minimizes gastric acid loss in patients with continuous gastric drainage.

For patients with metabolic alkalosis that does not respond to normal saline, the source of aldosterone or glucocorticoid should be removed. Treatment with spironolactone or amiloride may be useful. The management of Bartter syndrome includes fluid replacement and supplements of potassium chloride (1–3 mEq/kg/day). Administration of indomethacin (2–3 mg/kg/day) or ibuprofen (30 mg/kg/day) decrease the elevated prostaglandins and ameliorate fever and polyuria. Side effects of indomethacin include vomiting, abdominal pain, peptic ulcer and renal toxicity. Potassium sparing diuretics and angiotensin converting enzyme inhibitors have been used to aid potassium retention. Hypomagnesemia requires magnesium supplementation (see below). Specific medications for monogenic forms of hypertension are listed in Table 12.3.

Disorders of Magnesium Wasting

The clinical features of hypomagnesemia (normal levels 1.7 to 2.2 mg/dL) include muscle weakness or cramps, arrhythmia, vertigo, ataxia, seizure or altered mental status. Patients receiving long term therapy with thiazide diuretics show normal or low blood pressure, hypokalemic metabolic alkalosis hypomagnesemia and hypocalciuria.

Investigations include estimation of blood levels of creatinine, electrolytes, pH, bicarbonate, calcium and phosphate. Urine is examined for excretion of calcium, and for fractional excretion of magnesium. Important causes of hypomagnesemia are shown in Table 12.4.

Management

Oral supplementation (magnesium gluconate, oxide or hydroxide) is sufficient to correct hypomagnesemia when serum level is >1 mg/dL and the patient is asymptomatic. Parenteral administration of magnesium is necessary for symptomatic patients or those with blood level <1.0 mg/dL. This can be given as magnesium sulfate 25–50 mg/dose (maximum 2 g) by IM injection or slow IV infusion every 6-hr for 3–4 doses. Hypomagnesemia is often accompanied by hypokalemia and hypocalcemia that require treatment.

SUPPORT READING

Chadha V, Alon US. Hereditary renal tubular disorders. Semin Nephrol 2009; 29: 399–411

Vehaskari VM. Heritable forms of hypertension. Pediatr Nephrol 2009; 24: 1929–37

Electrolyte Disorders and Tubular Diseases

III

13 Polyuria

Polyuria is defined as urine output exceeding 6 mL/kg/hour or 2 L/m² in children, and 3L/day in adults. Actual polyuria is uncommon; more often, a history of frequency or nocturia is not associated with an increase in urine output.

Etiology

The causes of polyuria can be summarized on the basis of underlying defect. Common causes are listed in Table 13.1.

Polyuria is also a feature of some structural renal disorders including juvenile nephronophthisis, renal dysplasia secondary to reflux nephropathy or obstructive uropathy, and chronic tubulointerstitial nephritis. Recognition of these conditions is important since patients with these disorders show progressive kidney disease.

Some important entities presenting with polyuria are described briefly.

Primary (Psychogenic) Polydipsia: This condition is characterized by a primary increase in water intake. Daytime polydipsia and polyuria are noted. The disorder is uncommon in children, most often seen in anxious adolescents, in patients with psychiatric illnesses, or those prescribed anticholi-

---

Table 13.1: Causes of polyuria

Water diuresis: Abnormally increased excretion of water
Diabetes insipidus
    Central (deficiency of vasopressin)
    Nephrogenic (insensitivity to vasopressin)
Excessive water intake: psychogenic polydipsia; iatrogenic

Solute or osmotic diuresis: Abnormally increased excretion of solute
Renal sodium wasting: loop diuretics; Bartter syndrome
Exogenous sodium chloride or bicarbonate loading
Glucose: diabetic ketoacidosis, exogenous loading
Diuretic phase of acute tubular necrosis
Post-obstructive diuresis
Mannitol or glycerol administration
Urea: hypercatabolic state, post rhabdomyolysis

Miscellaneous
Juvenile nephronophthisis
Chronic tubulointerstitial nephritis
Renal dysplasia: associated with obstructive uropathy; reflux nephropathy

---

nergic agents or phenothiazines leading to a dry mouth.

Central Diabetes Insipidus (DI): A deficiency in secretion of antidiuretic hormone (ADH) may be idiopathic or secondary to a hypothalamic lesion that affects the thirst center, e.g. malignancy, head trauma, pituitary surgery, hypoxic or ischemic encephalopathy or granulomatous disease (Langerhans cell histiocytosis, tuberculosis, sarcoidosis). Familial cases have been described with an autosomal dominant mode of inheritance.

Nephrogenic Diabetes Insipidus (NDI): This rare condition is characterized by tubular unresponsiveness to ADH. The disease is usually inherited, in an X-linked recessive pattern (90% cases) with mutations in the gene for the arginine vasopressin V2 receptor (*AVPR2*; Xp28), or in an autosomal recessive or autosomal dominant manner with mutations in the gene encoding aquaporin 2 (chromosome 12q). NDI may be acquired, as with obstructive uropathy, analgesic nephropathy, sickle cell disease, chronic pyelonephritis, hypercalcemia, hypokalemia, amyloidosis, sarcoidosis, and with use of lithium and tetracyclines.

Clinical Features

Infants may present with irritability, failure to thrive, recurrent episodes of dehydration and fever. Constipation is common. Repeated episodes of hypernatremia and dehydration, with or without cerebral edema due to rapid rehydration, result in neurological abnormalities with psychomotor retardation and intracranial calcification, sequelae of hemorrhage and necrosis. Many patients show attention deficit, hyperactivity and restlessness. Rarely, seizures are noted during therapy, particularly if correction of dehydration is rapid.

Evaluation

It is important to confirm polyuria and/or polydipsia by asking the parent to maintain a record of the child's daily fluid intake and output, noting both the timing and quantity. In infants, the confirmation of polyuria may require hospitalization and/or catheterization.

History of nocturia and primary or secondary enuresis suggest an organic basis. Pointers to specific etiology include (*i*) absence of nocturnal voiding (psychogenic polydipsia); (*ii*) history of injury to the central nervous system, e.g. meningoencephalitis, head trauma, birth asphyxia (central diabetes insipidus); (*iii*) recent surgery for bladder outlet obstruction (postobstructive diuresis); and (*iv*) use of drugs such as diuretics or lithium. An assessment of the extracellular fluid volume (hydration) is an important component of physical examination. Important investigations include:

1. Blood electrolytes, pH, bicarbonate
2. Blood sugar, calcium, urea, creatinine
3. Ultrasound kidneys, bladder
4. Urinary osmolality, electrolytes, sugar, ketones
5. Water deprivation test
6. Pitressin challenge

A practical approach to evaluation of polyuria is based on urine osmolality. In "pure" water diuresis, the urine osmolality [Uosm] is typically <150 mOsm/kg, in "pure" solute diuresis it is higher at 300–500 mOsm/kg, while in "mixed" water-solute diuresis it ranges between 150 and 300 mOsm/kg.

Contraction of the extracellular fluid volume leads to dehydration in conditions with persistent water or solute diuresis if the intake of solute and water is insufficient. While hypernatremia is a hallmark of water diuresis, it is also noted with solute diuresis if water intake is insufficient.

Hypokalemia may be present in patients with solute diuresis. During dehydration, the blood urea and creatinine levels may be raised, but return to normal with adequate hydration.

Water Deprivation Test

Indications

The test helps differentiate between diabetes insipidus and psychogenic polydipsia. An early morning urine specific gravity >1015 or urine osmolality >400–600 mOsm/kg (>750 mOsm/kg is normal) rules out an organic concentrating defect. Water deprivation testing is indicated where diabetes insipidus is suspected.

Pre-requisites

1. Baseline plasma sodium is normal (<145 mEq/L)
2. Concurrent urine osmolality <300 mOsm/kg on *ad lib* fluid and food intake
3. Normal plasma potassium and calcium
4. Normal blood sugar; no glucosuria
5. Normal renal functions

Procedure

Heparinized blood (*not* serum or EDTA plasma) is used for estimation of plasma sodium and osmolality. Plasma sodium can be used to calculate osmolality in case the latter cannot be measured:

Plasma osmolality = 2 × plasma sodium

The patient is called fasting in the morning for a daycare admission. An early morning urine volume, osmolality, pH and sodium are recorded, to confirm the need for the test. The child is weighed to the nearest 0.1 kg; blood pressure and pulse rate are recorded. The patient is placed recumbent and a large bore intravenous cannula is placed; a sample is drawn for sodium and osmolality.

During the water deprivation test, the child is asked to stay semi-recumbent (except when standing to void). Urine and blood tests are repeated every hour or with each spontaneous void. Complete water deprivation is continued till *any one* of the following end-points is achieved:

1. Plasma sodium >145 mEq/L or osmolality >295 mOsm/kg

2. Urine osmolality >750 mOsm/kg
3. Weight loss of 5%
4. Plateau urine osmolality (<30 mOsm/kg/hr increase for 3 consecutive hr)

The period of water deprivation should not exceed 4 hours in infants and 7–8 hours in older children. The test should be terminated if any of the following are noted: an increased body temperature, tachycardia, or orthostatic hypotension (≥10 mm Hg decrease in systolic blood pressure upon standing and ≥10 beats/minute increase in heart rate upon standing), loss of body weight by >5% or presence of dehydration (dry skin and mucous membranes, decreased skin turgor).

If the serum sodium concentration is <145 mEq/L or the plasma osmolality is <295 mOsm/kg, consider infusion of hypertonic saline (3% saline at a rate of 0.1 ml/kg/minute for 1–2 hours) in order to reach the endpoints discussed above.

Interpretation

Figure 13.1 illustrates the response to water deprivation and pitressin administration in

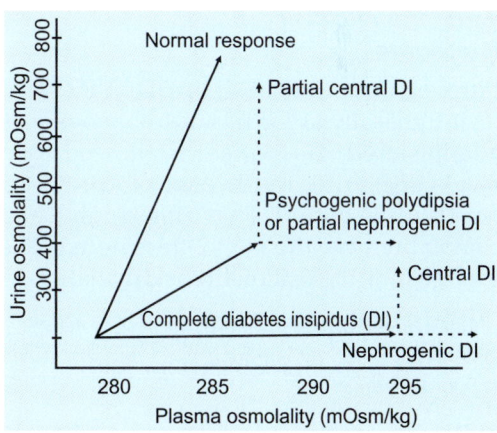

Fig. 13.1: Interpretation of the water deprivation test. Solid lines depict changes in urine and plasma osmolality in responses to water deprivation and interrupted lines indicate the response following administration of desmopressin/pitressin

various conditions. Patterns of response are characterized as follows:

1. *Plasma sodium >145 mEq/L or plasma osmolality >295 mOsm/kg and urine osmolality <300 mOsm/kg:* Strongly indicative of complete forms of diabetes insipidus. The type of DI should be characterized further by response to pitressin or DDAVP.

2. *Urine osmolality ≥300 mOsm/kg before plasma sodium >145 mEq/L (or osmolality >295 mOsm/kg):* Rules out complete forms of diabetes insipidus. This set of results suggests either partial forms of DI or psychogenic polydipsia

3. *Urine osmolality >750 mOsm/kg:* Suggests normal evaluation; no further testing is required.

Response to Pitressin

Indication

The test is indicated if the results of water deprivation test show either of the following:

1. Plasma sodium >145 *mEq/L*, osmolality >295 *mOsm/kg*; and urine osmolality <300 *mOsm/kg*
2. Urine osmolality 300–750 mOsm/kg

Procedure

Pitressin (5 units IV/IM) or DDAVP (10–20 µg intranasally or 1–3 µg subcutaneously) is administered. The patient is allowed light meals and drink fluids equal to previous hour's urine output. The urine volume and osmolality over the next 2-hr is noted. The change in urine osmolality is calculated.

Patients with plasma sodium >145 mEq/L, osmolality >295 mOsm/kg and urine osmolality <300 mOsm/kg

Rise in urine osmolality to >150% of baseline suggests complete central DI, while no change (<110% of baseline) suggests complete nephrogenic DI. Patients with responses in between these values (rise in urine osmolality 110–150%) may have a partial form of either central or nephrogenic DI. These patients require repeat testing 5–7 days after administration of subcutaneous pitressin (2 units) or DDAVP (10 µg).

Patients with plasma sodium >145 mEq/L, osmolality >295 mOsm/kg and urine osmolality 300–750 mOsm/kg

Rise in urine osmolality to >150% of baseline suggests complete central DI; while no change (<110% of baseline) suggests psychogenic polydipsia. Partial central or nephrogenic DI, or psychogenic polydipsia should be suspected in patients with change in urine osmolality by 110–150%. The presence of a hyperintense signal of posterior pituitary on MRI suggests psychogenic polydipsia or nephrogenic diabetes insipidus. However, such patients require further evaluation with repeat water deprivation following administration of subcutaneous pitressin.

Low Dose Pitressin Challenge

After water restriction, once urine osmolality of 300–750 mOsm/kg is reached, pitressin (2 units) or DDAVP (10 µg) is administered. No change in osmolality (<110%), in presence of a hyperintense signal of posterior pituitary on cranial MRI, suggests nephrogenic DI. A change in osmolality by 110–150% with the hyperintense signal being absent, suggests partial central DI. In cases with equivocal response, a therapeutic trial is required.

Therapeutic Trial

Pitressin (5 units IV) or DDAVP (10–20 µg nasally) is administered daily for 4–7 days. The volume status, thirst response and plasma sodium are assessed daily. Patients with partial nephrogenic DI do not respond, and continue to be symptomatic with polyuria and hypernatremia. Patients with partial forms of central DI respond completely, with normalization of urine output and serum sodium. In psychogenic polydipsia, response is often delayed; rarely, patients may develop hyponatremia.

Treatment

An adequate intake of water is necessary to compensate for the urinary losses, in both central and nephrogenic DI. Patients with central DI respond favorably to daily therapy with DDAVP (10–20 µg intranasal).

Restriction of dietary sodium to 1 mEq/kg/day reduces the osmolar load in patients with nephrogenic DI. Administration of hydrochlorothiazide (2 to 4 mg/kg/day), with or without amiloride (0.3 mg/kg/day) is useful in reducing urine output. These diuretics act at different sites to increase sodium excretion resulting in reduced extracellular sodium content and an increase in proximal tubular reabsorption of sodium and water. Indomethacin (2 mg/kg/day) has also been found to reduce urine volume.

SUPPORT READING

Bichet DG. Nephrogenic diabetes insipidus. Adv Chronic Kidney Dis 2006; 13: 96–104

Makaryus AN, Mcfarlane SI. Diabetes insipidus: diagnosis and treatment of a complex disease. Cleve Clin J Med 2066; 73: 65–71

14 Nephrolithiasis and Nephrocalcinosis

Nephrolithiasis is a common condition in patients attending pediatric nephrology services. An underlying metabolic cause is detected in 50–75% patients. Nephrocalcinosis is relatively uncommon, and an underlying metabolic disorder is usually detected.

Children have a high risk of recurrent urolithiasis; the annual risk of new stone formation is >5% in those diagnosed with a single stone. Stones may cause endstage renal disease in patients with staghorn calculi, repeated obstruction and recurrent urinary tract infections. Similarly, progressive nephrocalcinosis results in renal failure. Specific and intensive evaluation is required for every child with renal stones and/or nephrocalcinosis.

Table 14.1 provides a summary of stone types, their characteristics and association with diseases. Nephrocalcinosis is classified according to location as cortical, medullary or diffuse. Medullary nephrocalcinosis is graded according to the degree of echogenicity as mild (grade I), moderate (grade II) and severe (grade III).

Etiology

Common metabolic abnormalities underlying nephrolithiasis or nephrocalcinosis include idiopathic hypercalciuria, distal renal tubular acidosis, cystinuria and hyperoxaluria (Table 14.2). *Hypercalciuria* is the most common abnormality. Some patients with hypercalciuria may have an incomplete form of distal renal tubular acidosis that is only revealed when the acidification mechanism is stressed, as during the frusemide fludrocortisone test (Chapter 11). Patients with Dent's disease show proximal tubular dysfunction (low-molecular-weight proteinuria, glucosuria, aminoaciduria and phosphaturia). Familial hypomagnesemia with hypercalciuria and nephrocalcinosis (FHHNC) is characterized by urinary wasting of magnesium and calcium, nephrolithiasis, nephrocalcinosis and muscle weakness. Patients with Bartter syndrome may have nephrocalcinosis with hypercalciuria, but do not develop stones, possibly because of polyuria and dilute urine. Most uric acid stones are formed in acidic urine in patients with impaired renal ammoniagenesis; abnormalities of the purine or pyrimidine pathway are rare.

Stones often develop in context of a structural abnormality of urinary tract. Common causes include obstruction (pelviureteric junction obstruction, posterior urethral valves), medullary sponge kidney, autosomal dominant polycystic kidney disease and horseshoe kidney. Urinary tract infection, particularly with urease producing organisms like *Proteus, Staphylococcus* and *Pseudomonas* spp. favor precipitation of magnesium ammonium phosphate and calcium phosphate, and aggravate the structural abnormality.

Common etiologies for medullary nephrocalcinosis include idiopathic hypercalciuria,

78

Table 14.1: Characteristics of kidney stones

	Frequency	Shape of crystals	Urine pH favoring growth	Associations
Calcium oxalate	40–80%	Dihydrate: bipyramidal Monohydrate: dumb bell	–	Primary hyperoxaluria; enteric hyperoxaluria
Calcium phosphate	1–25%	Wedges	>7	Hyperparathyroidism; renal tubular acidosis; nephrocalcinosis
Uric acid	2–10%	Rhomboid; rosettes; barrels	5	Gout; sometimes form staghorn
Triple phosphate (magnesium ammonium phosphate)	10–25%	Rectangle; coffin lids	8	Infection with urease producing organisms; staghorn calculi
Cystine	1–10%	Hexagon	5	Cystinuria

Table 14.2: Metabolic abnormalities underlying nephrolithiasis or nephrocalcinosis

Hypercalciuria with hypercalcemia	*Hyperoxaluria*
Vitamin D overdose	Primary hyperoxaluria, type I
Primary hyperparathyroidism	Primary hyperoxaluria, type II
Production of PTH related peptide (malignancy, sarcoidosis)	
Hypercalciuria with normal serum calcium	*Abnormal purine, pyrimidine metabolism*
Idiopathic hypercalciuria	Lesch Nyhan syndrome*
Familial hypophosphatemia with hypercalciuria	Partial HPRT deficiency*^
Dent's disease*	Glycogenosis type 1a, type 1b APRT deficiency^
Bartter syndrome	Xanthinuria
Autosomal dominant hypocalcemic with hypercalciuria	
Familial hypomagnesemia, hypercalciuria & nephrocalcinosis	
Lowe syndrome*	
Frusemide use	
Hypocitric aciduria and hypercalciuria	*Miscellaneous*
Distal renal tubular acidosis	Cystinuria
	Melamine toxicity#

*X linked recessive inheritance

^Patients with adenine phosphoribosyltransferase (APRT) deficiency form dihydroxyadenine stones and those with hypoxanthine-guanine phosphoribosyl transferase deficiency (HPRT) have uric acid stones

#Contamination of melamine in powdered infant formulae results in crystals that contain melamine with cyanuric acid

hyperoxaluria, distal renal tubular acidosis and use of diuretics in preterm neonates; uncommonly, this is secondary to Bartter syndrome, Dent's disease, primary hyperparathyroidism or FHHNC. Cortical nephrocalcinosis is secondary to renal injury, as seen in acute cortical necrosis, chronic glomerulonephritis and chronic graft rejection.

Clinical Evaluation

History is taken for passage of stones or gravel, dysuria, flank or abdominal pain, hematuria, enuresis, frequent voiding or urinary retention; family history of urolithiasis; history of recurrent urinary tract infections; intake of vitamin D, mineral supplements, frusemide, salicylates or steroids.

The presence of polyuria, thirst, failure to thrive, muscle cramps and rickets suggest renal tubular acidosis. Patients with Crohn disease, cystic fibrosis, and post bowel resection may have enteric hyperoxaluria.

Nephrocalcinosis is mostly asymptomatic. Unless picked up incidentally on an imaging study, diagnosis is delayed until presentation with tubular dysfunction manifest as polyuria, poor growth, rickets or uremia (Fig. 14.1).

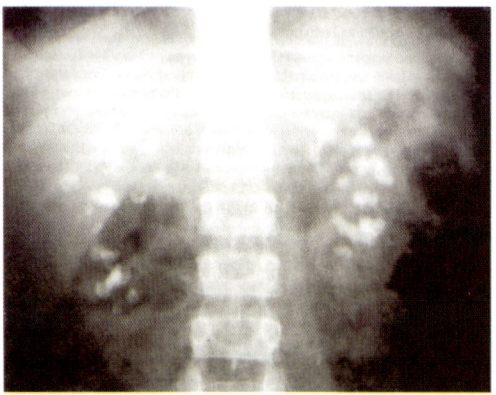

Fig. 14.1: Plain X ray abdomen in a 6-yr-old girl evaluated for failure to thrive and abdominal pain. Bilateral nephrocalcinosis is noted

Diagnosis

Ultrasonography is satisfactory for detection of urolithiasis because of high diagnostic yield, easy availability, avoidance of ionizing radiation and detection of hydronephrosis (Fig. 14.2). Helic*al non-contrast computed tomography* (NCCT) is less observer dependent, and provides equivalent diagnosis of hydronephrosis, accurate estimation of stone size and greater sensitivity, allowing diagnosis of small calculi. NCCT is the imaging modality of choice in patients with renal colic. *Plain radiographs* are rarely required.

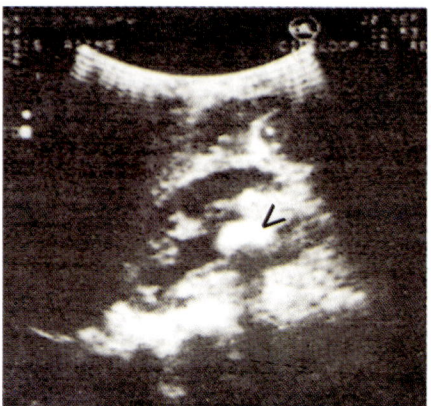

Fig. 14.2: Ultrasound of the kidney showing single echogenic calculus (arrowhead) with acoustic shadowing and hydronephrosis

Imaging of the urinary tract to screen for stasis or obstruction is an essential component of evaluation. *Contrast studies* such as intravenous pyelography (IVP), CT urography, and rarely, retrograde ureteroscopy or pyelography, are indicated if suspecting *(i)* obstruction, *(ii)* radiolucent or low density stones, or *(iii)* an anatomical abnormality of the urinary tract (such as a duplicated collecting system). Ureteral stones are better detected and localized using NCCT than IVP; however, IVP may still be favored in young children in order to avoid sedation and to reduce exposure to ionizing radiation.

The appearance of a stone on radiological imaging varies according to the composition.

While calcium oxalate and calcium phosphate stones are most dense, struvite and cystine stones have intermediate density. Uric acid and xanthine stones have a low density on CT and are radiolucent on plain radiographs. Stones composed of indinavir, ceftriaxone, sulfadiazine or matrix have variable density. Small stones of any composition are difficult to appreciate by radiographs.

High resolution ultrasonography is an optimal technique for the diagnosis and monitoring of nephrocalcinosis (Fig. 14.3). The procedure is more sensitive than NCCT (96% vs. 64%), but less specific (85% vs. 96%) (Fig.14.4). Over-

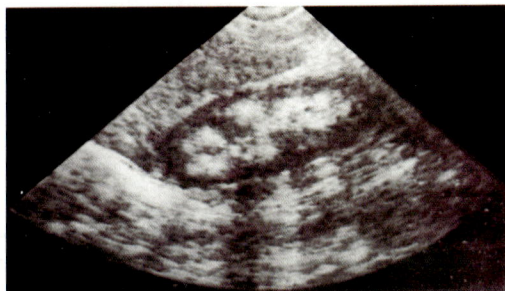

Fig. 14.3: Ultrasound of the kidney shows nephrocalcinosis and focal areas of increased echogenicity in the medullary pyramids

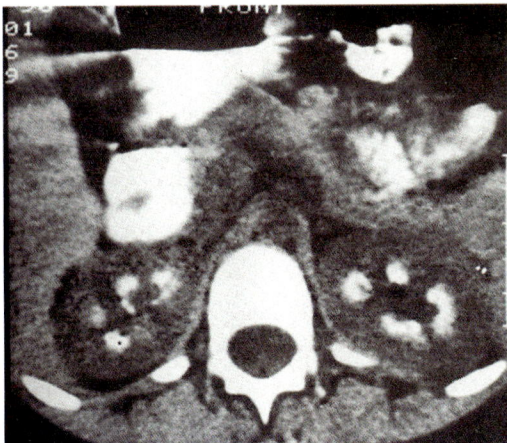

Fig. 14.4: Nephrocalcinosis is noted on plain CT film of the abdomen. Note the multiple calcific densities in medullary pyramids on both sides

diagnosis is common, particularly in early neonatal period when the physiologically increased echogenicity or deposits of Tamm Horsfall protein are mistaken for medullary nephrocalcinosis. The evaluation should be repeated after few weeks.

Other conditions that might result in increased echogenicity of both kidneys include: autosomal recessive polycystic kidney disease, renal parenchymal infection with cytomegalovirus or candida in neonates, and medullary sponge kidney in older children.

Metabolic Evaluation

This is required in all patients with urolithiasis and/or nephrocalcinosis (Table 14.3). Repeated evaluations are essential before an underlying cause can be excluded.

Timed urine collections (24-hr or 12-hr) are preferred for estimation of excretion of solutes. Completeness of each collection is confirmed with measurement of urinary creatinine level. Where such collection is impractical, the first or second morning void is used. Metabolic evaluation should be avoided for 2–4 weeks following extracorporeal shock wave lithotripsy. For urinary oxalate determination, the urine is collected in a container containing hydrochloric acid (0.1 N) in order to avoid precipitation of oxalate and conversion of ascorbate to oxalate.

Table 14.4 gives values for normal excretion of solutes in the urine. Important causes of hypercalciuria including hypomagnesemia, abnormalities of the thyroid hormone and partial forms of distal renal tubular acidosis should be ruled out before hypercalciuria is labeled idiopathic. The latter requires testing with the fludrocortisone frusemide test (Chapter 11).

Idiopathic Calculi

Even after extensive evaluation there remain patients in whom an etiology is not found. Excretion of calcium, oxalate and uric acid is

Electrolyte Disorders and Tubular Diseases

III

Table 14.3: Evaluation in a patient with nephrolithiasis and nephrocalcinosis

Step 1

Blood: Calcium, phosphorus, creatinine, uric acid, pH, bicarbonate

Urinalysis

    pH (in fresh urine by pH meter)

    Microscopy for crystals, casts

    Measurement of solutes in urine: calcium, oxalate, uric acid, protein, creatinine

    Culture

Stone analysis

Step 2

Hypercalcemia	*Hypercalciuria with normal serum calcium*	*Normal urinary calcium*
Blood PTH	*Blood*	Nitroprusside test
25-hydroxyvitamin D	pH, bicarbonate	Aminoacidogram
Evaluate for sarcoidosis	Magnesium	Urine oxalate excretion
	Thyroxine, thyroid stimulating hormone	Urine cystine excretion
	Urine	
	Fasting urine pH	
	Glucosuria	
	Aminoacidogram	
	Protein; β2 microglobulin	
	Tubular reabsorption of phosphate	
	Frusemide fludrocortisone test	

Table 14.4: Normal values for excretion of important solutes

Constituent	*24 hr excretion*	*Solute/creatinine ratio*
Calcium	<4 mg /kg /day	0–6 month: <0.8 mg/mg 6–12 month: <0.6 mg/mg 1–2 yr: <0.4 mg/mg >2 yr: <0.2 mg/mg
Oxalate	<40 mg /1.73 m^2 <2 mg/kg/day	<1 yr: 0.15–0.26 mmol/mg 1–5 yr: 0.11–0.12 mmol/mg >5 yr: 0.006–0.15 mmol/mg
Uric acid	<35 mg/kg/day 750–800 mg/1.73 m^2	
Citrate	<320 mg/1.73 m^2	<300 mg/g of creatinine
Cystine	30–50 mg/1.73 m^2	<75 mg/g of creatinine
Protein	<100 mg/m^2/day	<0.2 mg/mg
Creatinine	*Children:* 15–20 mg/ kg/day *Newborn:* 8–10 mg/kg/day	

normal. The results of stone analysis are important in such cases.

Management

Patients with renal stones should be advised to increase fluid intake (>2-2.5 L/1.73 m^2) and decrease animal protein and salt intake. Long-term therapy with potassium citrate (2 mEq/kg/day) results in decreased stone formation; citrate binds to urinary calcium forming a soluble complex and reducing precipitation of calcium with other anions. Compliance is ensured by regularly measuring the urine pH. There is limited data on the efficacy and long-term safety of therapy with magnesium and phosphate supplements in patients with recurrent stones.

Idiopathic Hypercalciuria

The treatment of idiopathic hypercalciuria consists of ensuring a high fluid intake and avoiding periods of dehydration. Since dietary sodium loading increases urinary calcium excretion, moderate salt restriction is recommended. A high-protein diet (animal protein) should be avoided. Recommended dietary allowances for protein and calcium should be provided. Administration of potassium citrate (1.5–2 mEq/kg/day) results in reduction of calcium excretion and increase of urinary citrate and potassium.

Long acting thiazide diuretics (hydrochlorthiazide, 1–2 mg/kg/day) increase calcium resorption in the distal convoluted tubule, thereby reducing its excretion. Patients receiving thiazide diuretics should be monitored for hypokalemia and, if necessary, supplemented with potassium or a potassium sparing diuretic (e.g. amiloride). Therapy with thiazides may adversely affect lipid metabolism and lead to hyperuricemia.

Primary Hyperoxaluria

Supportive measures consist of reduction of oxalate from the diet (spinach, peanuts, cocoa), and ensuring a large fluid intake and

administration of pyridoxine (3–5 mg/kg). Most patients with primary hyperoxaluria and end stage renal disease require combined liver-kidney transplantation to correct the metabolic defect and restore kidney function. Otherwise, there is high risk of recurrence of oxalosis in the allograft.

Cystinuria

Management comprises of adequate fluid intake, urinary alkalization (pH 7.5–8) and restriction of dietary methionine (moderate restriction of meat, fish, eggs, soy, wheat). Effective medications cleave the disulfide bond of cystine to form cysteine, a soluble homodimer. Sulfhydryl agents such as penicillamine (20–40 mg/kg/d, starting at 7.5 mg/kg in two doses) or α-mercaptoproprionyl-glycine (tiopronin, 20–40 mg/kg/d, starting at 15 mg/kg in two doses) are recommended. Treatment is titrated to achieve urine cystine <300 mg/day. Side effects, more common with the former, include rash, arthralgia, pemphigus, thrombocytopenia, polymyositis and proteinuria. Captopril (1–2 mg/kg/d) is a useful adjunct to therapy.

Surgical Treatment

Therapy depends on the site, size and composition of the stone, and anatomy of the urinary tract. Ureteric stones below 5 mm are likely to pass spontaneously and do not require specific therapy.

Small stones (less than 20 mm diameter) are treated by *extracorporeal shock wave lithotripsy* (ESWL), in which shock waves are focused at the stone, resulting in its fragmentation. Calculi composed of uric acid and calcium oxalate disintegrate easily, but cystine and calcium phosphate, that are comparatively harder do not. ESWL is suitable for radiopaque stones in the renal pelvis and upper ureter, but has lower success rates for stones in the lower renal calyces. Passing stone fragments can cause renal colic; other complications include hematuria, perirenal hema-

Electrolyte Disorders and Tubular Diseases

III

toma and local bruising. ESWL is a safe procedure with no long term influence on renal growth or function.

Percutaneous nephrolithotomy (PCNL) is preferred in patients with stones that are large (>20 mm) or in the lower pole, or having relative contraindications to ESWL (bleeding diathesis, oliguric renal failure, urinary tract obstruction). Stone fragmentation is achieved using pneumatic lithoclast, ultrasound or laser probes; the fragments are collected through special wire baskets or graspers, inserted through the working channel of the instrument.

The availability of small ureteroscopic endoscopes (4.5–5F) has enabled the application of *ureterorenoscopy* in children. This procedure is ideally suited for calculi in the mid and distal ureter.

Open surgery is preferred for removing stones that are large (e.g. staghorn calculi) or associated with anatomical abnormalities (pelviureteric junction obstruction, obstructive megaureter).

SUPPORT READING

Tanaka ST, Pope IV JC. Pediatric stone disease. Current Urology Reports 2009, 10: 138–43

Nicoletta JA, Lande MB, Medical evaluation and treatment of urolithiasis. Pediatr Clin N Am 2006; 53: 479–91

Hoppe B, Kemper MJ. Diagnostic examination of the child with urolithiasis or nephrocalcinosis. Pediatr Nephrol 2010; 25: 403–13

15 Rickets

Rickets results from a lack of adequate mineralization of growing bones. The diagnosis is based on the constellation of clinical findings, radiological features and blood biochemistry. While nutritional rickets is the chief etiology in India and developing countries, there is resurgence of the condition in developed countries. The evaluation and management of patients with nutritional and refractory rickets are discussed.

Vitamin D Metabolism

Both ergocalciferol (vitamin D_2), synthesized in the skin, and cholecalciferol (vitamin D_3), available from animal sources, are converted by hepatic microsomes to 25-hydroxycholecalciferol [25(OH) D_3, calcidiol]. Calcidiol is the chief form of vitamin D in circulation, and its plasma concentration is the best indicator of vitamin D status. 25(OH) vitamin D_3 is hydroxylated by 1α hydroxylase in the proximal renal tubular cells to form 1, 25 (OH)$_2$ D_3 (calcitriol). Calcitriol is the most potent vitamin D metabolite, but has a very short half life, and its plasma level is only 0.1% of the level of 25(OH) D_3. The chief functions of calcitriol are to increase the intestinal absorption of calcium and phosphate, decrease urinary calcium losses and increase bone resorption of calcium to maintain normal concentrations of extracellular calcium. The activity of 1α hydroxylase is regulated by extracellular concentrations of ionized calcium, inorganic phosphate, parathormone (PTH), and fibroblast growth factor (FGF)-23. When serum calcium levels are normal, feedback inhibition leads to decreased synthesis of 1, 25 (OH)$_2$ D_3 and increase in conversion of 25(OH) vitamin D to inactive metabolites.

A sodium-phosphate cotransporter (NPT2) is responsible for phosphate reabsorption in the proximal tubule. Several hormones including PTH, insulin like growth factor-1 and FGF-23 regulate this transport system. FGF-23, a circulating peptide secreted by the bone, is an important regulator of phosphate and vitamin D homeostasis. It acts by binding with high affinity to its receptor in the kidney in the presence of Klotho, a membrane bound protein, to impair phosphate reabsorption and inhibit synthesis of 1, 25(OH)$_2$ vitamin D_3 (Fig. 15.1). The former action is mediated by decrease in expression of renal NPT2a in proximal renal tubular cells, and the latter through suppression of 25-(OH) D-1α hydroxylase (Cyp27b1) gene expression and stimulation of 24-hydroxylase (Cyp24) expression. High levels of FGF-23 may independently inhibit PTH release. Additionally, 1,25 (OH)$_2$ D_3 upregulates expression of the FGF-23 and Klotho genes, providing a negative feedback loop for serum vitamin D.

Evaluation

Patients with non-nutritional rickets have often received multiple courses of oral or intramuscular vitamin D. History may provide

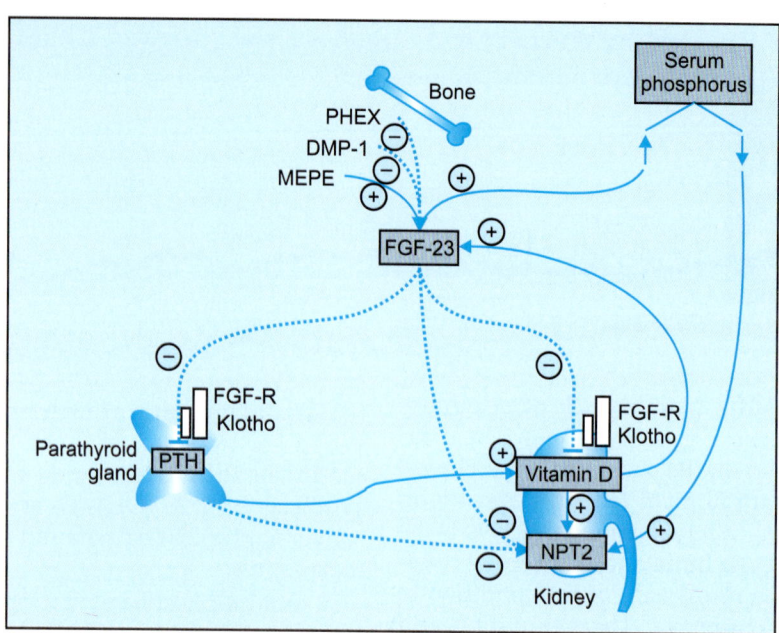

Fig. 15.1: The endocrine axis between bone, kidney and parathyroid. The expression of fibroblast growth factor-23 (FGF-23) is increased in osteocytes in response to elevated serum phosphorus and binding of 1,25-dihydroxyvitamin D_3. FGF-23 acts through binding to the Klotho-FGF receptor (FGF-R) complex. In the kidney, FGF-23 suppresses the synthesis of active vitamin D through downregulation of 1 α-hydroxylase, and upregulation of 24 hydroxylase. It suppresses renal tubular excretion of phosphorus through Na^+-dependent Pi cotransporter type 2 (NPT2). FGF-23 also suppresses the production and secretion of parathyroid hormone (PTH). Production of FGF-23 by osteocytes is regulated by the PHosphate regulating gene with homologies to Endopeptidases on the X-chromosome (PHEX), matrix extracellular phosphoprotein (MEPE) and dentin matrix protein 1 (DMP1). Mutations in the FGF-23 gene that affect normal degradation of the peptide are responsible for the autosomal dominant form of hypophosphatemic rickets, while the X linked dominant and autosomal recessive forms are caused by mutations in the *PHEX* and *DMP-1* genes, respectively

clues to etiology, such as polyuria, polydipsia or failure to thrive (renal tubular acidosis), diarrhea or liver disease (malabsorption), and use of anticonvulsants or glucocorticoids (accelerated metabolism of vitamin D). Maternal short stature suggests the X-linked dominant form of hypophosphatemic rickets. Onset in early infancy, and delayed motor milestones suggest vitamin D dependent rickets. A history of tetany, seizures and fractures is elicited in children with vitamin D dependent rickets type II.

Signs of rickets in infancy include craniotabes, large head, wide open fontanelle, caput quadratum, wrist widening and rachitic rosary. Older children show bony deformities, including bowing or knock knees (genu varum, genu valgum) and double malleoli. Hypotonia is seen in nutritional rickets and in vitamin D dependence. The latter may also have delayed dentition, enamel hypoplasia, ectodermal defects (oligodontia, epidermal cysts) and alopecia, and show positive Trousseau or Chvostek signs. Predominant involvement of lower limbs with a waddling gait and stunting suggests X-linked hypophosphatemic rickets or metaphyseal dysplasia. Children with X-linked hypophosphatemic rickets may have dental abscesses and pulp abnormalities and deformities of the skull and maxillofacial region.

NUTRITIONAL RICKETS

The vitamin D content of breast milk in vitamin D sufficient mothers is 15–50 IU/L. With an average consumption of 750 mL/day, exclusively breastfed infants without sun exposure would have intake of 11–38 IU/day of vitamin D, much below the recommended allowance of 200 IU/day. Most food items rich in vitamin D (oily fish, egg yolks, organ meats) are consumed occasionally. Fully clothed infants require 2-hr of sun exposure per week to maintain vitamin D levels >25 nmol/L (>10 ng/mL); requirements are higher in dark skinned persons. Calcium deficiency contributes to and might increase the severity of rickets. Nutritional rickets is common in the Indian subcontinent where dairy products are not fortified.

Initial Evaluation

Rickets is confirmed on wrist or knee X-ray. Loss of demarcation between the meta-physis and growth plate and loss of the provisional zone of calcification are the earliest signs of rickets. This is followed by osteopenia and widening of the growth plate; later changes include metaphyseal widening, splaying, cupping and fraying (Fig. 15.2).

Laboratory findings include hypophosphatemia, variable hypocalcemia, and increased levels of alkaline phosphatase and parathormone. If available, the diagnosis should be confirmed with levels of 25 hydroxy-vitamin D. Deficient patients have levels <15 ng/mL; <5 ng/mL indicates severe deficiency. Children showing vitamin D levels between 20–100 ng/mL are considered vitamin D replete.

Management

Various regimes for administration of vitamin D are listed in Table 15.1. The choice of the regimen depends on physician and parental preference, but should take into account issues of compliance. Children with nutritional rickets also require dietary supplements of calcium.

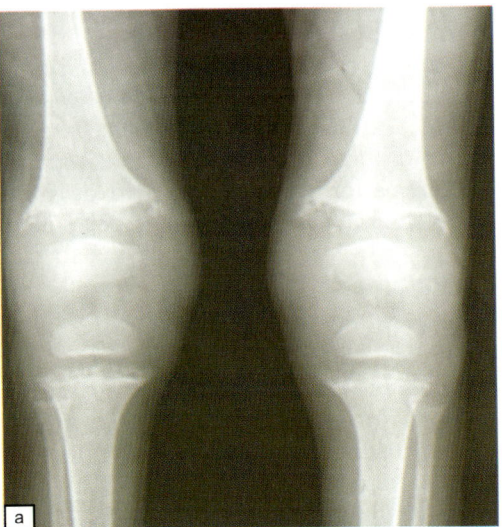
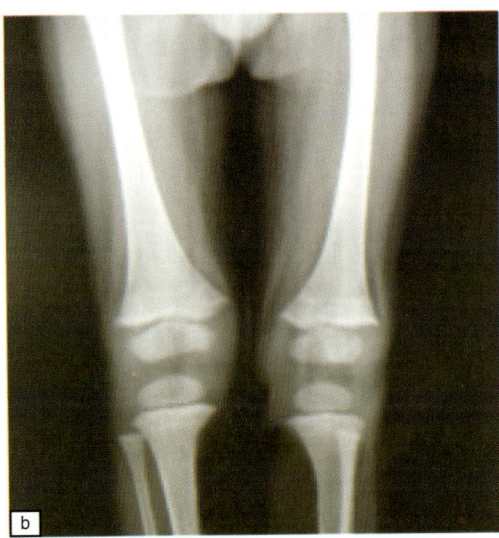

a

b

Fig. 15.2: Radiograph of both knees in a 4-year-old boy showing (a) widening, flaring and irregularity of the metaphyseal ends of long bones; (b) healing of rickets at 12 weeks, following a single dose of oral vitamin D (600000 IU)

Table 15.1: Therapy of nutritional rickets

Vitamin D (vitamin D₃; cholecalciferol)
Initially any of the following

Double of recommended allowance: 800 IU (20 μg) daily for 3–4 months
Pharmacologic doses: 1000–10000 IU (25–125 μg) daily for 8–12 weeks
Stoss therapy: 100000–600000 IU (2.5–15 mg) over 1–5 days; *or* 60000 IU (1.5 mg) every week for
6–8 weeks or daily for 10 doses

Subsequently

400–800 IU (10–20 μg) vitamin D per day
Calcium 30–75 mg/kg/day of elemental calcium in 2–3 divided doses for 2–4 weeks (start at the
higher end of the dose range, and taper to a lower dose)

Response to Therapy

Blood levels of calcium, phosphorus and alkaline phosphatase are obtained 1 month after initiating therapy. With *stoss* therapy, the first sign of biochemical response is an increase in blood levels of phosphate that occurs in 1–2 weeks. Levels of alkaline phosphatase rise in the short term, as bone formation increases. There is an initial increase in blood levels of 1, 25 dihydroxy-vitamin D; later alkaline phosphatase declines, and 25-hydroxyvitamin D levels normalize. Complete radiologic healing may take months, but changes are evident in 1–2 weeks.

A repeat X-ray to examine for line of healing should be done at 3–4 weeks. In case radiological response is absent, the dose of vitamin D is repeated and evaluation for refractory rickets should begin simultaneously.

REFRACTORY RICKETS

The term refers to patients who fail to show evidence of radiological healing and normalization of biochemical abnormalities, despite therapy with two large doses of vitamin D. The causes of refractory rickets are divided into two main groups according to the predominant metabolic abnormality: abnormal vitamin D metabolism or defective renal tubular phosphate handling (Table 15.2). The former group of conditions is characterized by low blood levels of calcium and phosphate,

aminoaciduria and high PTH. The latter show hypophosphatemia, and normal blood levels of calcium and PTH. Rickets in patients with distal renal tubular acidosis is attributed to impaired renal hydroxylation of calcidiol and a negative calcium balance secondary to persistent metabolic acidosis.

Evaluation

Work-up includes *(i)* estimation of blood levels of calcium, phosphorous, alkaline phosphatase, creatinine, pH, electrolytes, bicarbonate, 25 hydroxyvitamin D and parathormone; *(ii)* urinalysis, *(iii)* estimation of timed excretion of calcium, phosphate, protein and creatinine, and *(iv)* ultrasonography of kidneys and urinary tract. Based on results of these investigations, more specific tests are performed for a definitive diagnosis. Figure 15.3 gives an approach to evaluation.

Management

The therapy of rickets is tailored to the underlying cause. Management of mineral bone disease associated with chronic kidney disease (MBD-CKD) relies on control of hyperphosphatemia (dietary restriction, use of oral phosphate binders), and therapy with active vitamin D analogs and calcium supplements (*see* Chapter 34). Children with deformities might require corrective osteotomy after rickets has healed.

Rickets

Table 15.2: Causes of refractory rickets

Type	Cause	Gene; inheritance	Additional features
Calcipenic rickets			
Vitamin D dependent rickets, type 1	Deficiency of 1α-hydroxylase	CYP27B1; autosomal recessive (AR)	Onset in infancy; hypocalcemia, tetany, seizures, delayed dentition, enamel hypoplasia
Vitamin D dependent rickets, type 2	Mutation of the vitamin D receptor (VDR)	VDR (12q); AR	Onset in infancy; severe hypocalcemia, tetany, severe rickets; alopecia, ectodermal defects (oligodontia, epidermal cysts)
Hypophosphatemic rickets			
X-linked dominant	Inadequate proteolysis of FGF-23	PHEX (Xp22.1); XD	Short stature, lower limb deformities; dental abnormalities (pulp deformities, abscess); normal blood and urinary calcium; low tubular maximum for phosphate ($TmPO_4$/GFR); normal PTH; low levels of $1,25(OH)_2$ D; no aminoaciduria
Autosomal dominant (AD)	Mutant FGF-23 resistant to proteolysis	FGF-23; AD	
Autosomal recessive (AR)	Mutant DMP1 inhibits FGF-23 action	DMP1; AR	
Hypophosphatemia with hypercalciuria	Loss of function of NPT2	SLC34A3 (NPT2c) or SLC34A1 (NPT2a); AR	Increased $1,25(OH)_2$ D; hypercalciuria. Use of vitamin D analogs not necessary
Dent disease	Loss of function of voltage gated chloride channel	CLCN5 or OCRL1; X-linked	β-2 microglobulinuria, phosphaturia, hypercalciuria, nephrolithiasis, nephrocalcinosis
Fanconi syndrome	Proximal tubular dysfunction	AR; also secondary forms (chapter 11)	Metabolic acidosis, hypophosphatemia, failure to thrive; glucosuria, aminoaciduria, low molecular weight proteinuria
Distal renal tubular acidosis			
	Acidosis, negative calcium balance, impaired 1α-hydroxylation	AR or AD; secondary forms	Metabolic acidosis, failure to thrive; hypercalciuria, hypokalemia

FGF-23 fibroblast growth factor 23; PHEX phosphate regulating gene with homologies to endopeptidases on the X chromosome; DMP-1 dentin matrix protein 1; NPT sodium phosphate cotransporter

15

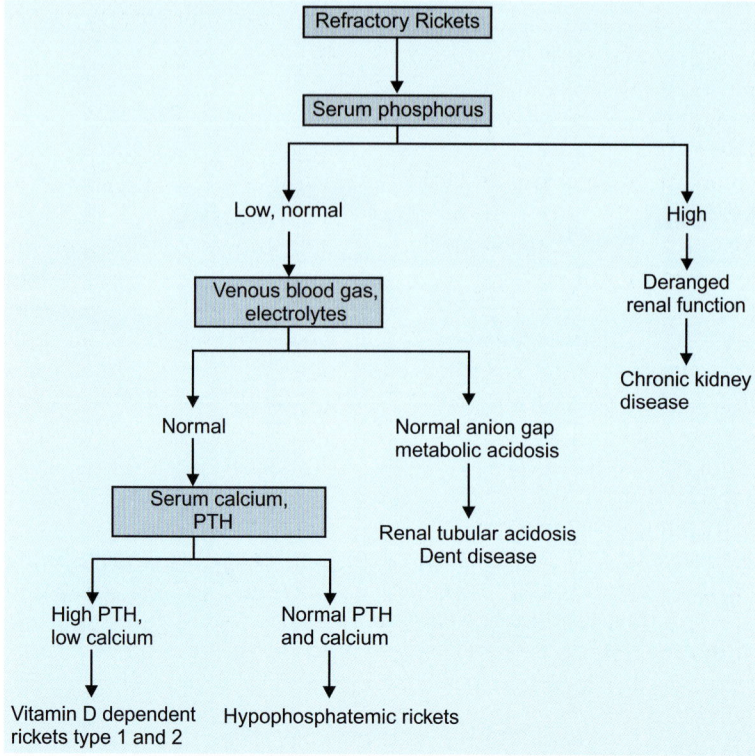

Fig.15.3: Biochemical evaluation of a patient with refractory rickets. The evaluation of renal tubular acidosis is detailed in chapter 11. Patients with vitamin D dependent rickets type 2 show severe manifestations, alopecia and elevated levels of parathormone (PTH) and 1,25 dihydroxyvitamin D. Patients with clinical features of rickets but with normal serum biochemistry should be evaluated for metaphyseal dysplasia

Patients with proximal renal tubular acidosis (RTA) show hyperchloremic metabolic acidosis and hypophosphatemia. The rickets responds satisfactorily to correction of acidosis (oral bicarbonate at 4–6 mEq/kg/d in 3–4 divided doses; Polycitra solution, see Appendix 6 and supplements of oral phosphate. Patients with secondary causes for proximal RTA, require specific therapy apart from the use of alkali and phosphate supplements, e.g. cysteamine for cystinosis. Vitamin D may be used in small supplements if required, and if not contraindicated by hypercalciuria. Patients with distal RTA do not require phosphate supplements. In these patients, treatment with

bicarbonate or citrate supplements (2–4 mEq/kg/d; Shohl's or Polycitra K, see Appendix 6 results in correction of metabolic acidosis, healing of rickets and reduction of hypercalciuria.

Patients with hypophosphatemic rickets (familial hypophosphatemic rickets, proximal RTA, Dent disease) require supplements of phosphate to compensate for its urinary losses. Supplementation is given at a dose of 30–50 mg/kg/day (1–3 g per day) in 4–5 divided doses in the form of neutral phosphate (1 g sodium acid phosphate and 3.66 g dibasic sodium phosphate in 60 mL water provides 1 g of inorganic phosphorus) or acid phosphate (Joulie solution) (each ml provides 30 mg phosphorus). The dose may be increased to 100 mg/kg/day, to ensure normalization of blood phosphorus levels (3–3.2 mg/dL), while watching for adverse effects (diarrhea, abdominal pain).

Since conversion to calcitriol (1,25 dihydroxyvitamin D) is impaired in patients with X-linked hypophosphatemic rickets, small doses of calcitriol (25–50 ng/kg/day; 0.25–0.5 µg daily) are necessary in addition to phosphate supplements. Patients are monitored by regular blood levels of calcium and phosphate, and for hypercalciuria and nephrocalcinosis. The presence of elevated levels of PTH suggests excessive treatment with phosphate, inadequate treatment with vitamin D analogs or concomitant vitamin D deficiency. Not all patients require therapy with calcitriol. Patients with hereditary hypophosphatemic rickets with hypercalciuria (HHRH) show healing of rickets following phosphate supplements alone.

Patients with vitamin D dependent rickets (VDDR) type 1 are treated with physiological doses of calcidiol or calcitriol (1–2 µg daily), and supplements of calcium and phosphate. With appropriate therapy radiological healing occurs within 6–8 weeks. Patients with VDDR type 2 require high doses of calcitriol (0.05 µg/kg/d, increased up to 0.2 µg/kg/d) and supplements of calcium and phosphate. The response to treatment is variable. Some patients benefit from long-term administration of high dose calcium infusions, followed by oral calcium supplements.

Response to Therapy

Monitoring requires regular assessment of symptoms, measurement of height and record of bony deformities. Blood levels of calcium, phosphorus and alkaline phosphatase levels should be estimated every 3–6 months. Patients on vitamin D or calcium supplementation should be evaluated for hypercalciuria, using timed urinary samples or the spot calcium to creatinine ratio. Therapy with vitamin D analogs should be withheld or its dose reduced in patients showing hypercalcemia or hypercalciuria. Radiological features of rickets should be evaluated at 3–6 months and then annually. An abdominal ultrasound is useful before beginning therapy to evaluate and follow up for nephrocalcinosis.

SUPPORT READING

Misra M, Pacaud D, Petryk A, et al; Drug and Therapeutics Committee of the Lawson Wilkins Pediatric Endocrine Society. Vitamin D deficiency in children and its management: review of current knowledge and recommendations. Pediatrics 2008; 122: 398–417

Allgrove J. A practical approach to rickets. Endocr Dev 2009; 16: 115–32

Pettifor JM. What's new in hypophosphataemic rickets? Eur J Pediatr 2008; 167: 493–99

Kuro-O M. Overview of the FGF23-Klotho axis. Pediatr Nephrol 2010; 25: 583–90

Malloy PJ, Feldman D. Genetic disorders and defects in vitamin D action. Endocrinol Metab Clin North Am 2010; 39: 333–46

Nephrotic Syndrome

16 Steroid Sensitive Nephrotic Syndrome

Nephrotic syndrome is characterized by heavy proteinuria, hypoalbuminemia (serum albumin <2.5 g/dL), hyperlipidemia (serum cholesterol >200 mg/dL) and edema. The large majority (>90%) is primary (idiopathic); a secondary cause, e.g. amyloidosis, systemic lupus, Henoch Schonlein purpura is seen rarely.

In most (>80%) children with idiopathic nephrotic syndrome, the disease is *sensitive* to therapy with oral corticosteroids. The prognosis in these cases is favorable. The disease course is variable; while a few children have no relapses or a single relapse, others show multiple relapses that occur either infre- quently or frequently (Table 16.1). A small proportion of children may develop resistance to steroids after a period of steroid responsive- ness (late steroid resistance).

Evaluation at Onset

Evaluation of a patient with suspected nephrotic syndrome includes history and physical examination, with attention to secondary etiology, prior therapies, edema, blood pressure, anthropometry and evidence of infections. Heavy or 'nephrotic range' proteinuria is defined as 3-4+ (300–2000 mg/ dL) urine protein by dipstick or boiling test on early morning urine for 3 consecutive days,

---

Table 16.1: Important definitions to clarify course of nephrotic syndrome

Remission: Urine albumin nil or trace (or proteinuria <4 mg/m^2/hr) for 3 consecutive early morning specimens

Relapse: Urine albumin 3-4+ (or proteinuria >40 mg/m^2/hr) for 3 consecutive early morning specimens, having been in remission previously

Frequent relapses: Two or more relapses in initial six months, or four or more relapses in any twelve months

Steroid dependence: Two consecutive relapses while on alternate day steroids or within 14 days of its discontinuation

Steroid resistance: Absence of remission despite therapy with daily prednisolone at a dose of 2 mg/ kg per day for 4 weeks

spot urine protein/creatinine ratio >2 mg/ mg, or urine protein excretion >40 mg/m^2/hr. A precise assessment of proteinuria is not necessary for the diagnosis. Relevant investigations are listed in Table 16.2.

Indications for Renal Biopsy

Most children with idiopathic nephrotic syndrome do not require a renal biopsy. Renal biopsy may be indicated at the onset of nephrotic syndrome in situations where a cause other than minimal change nephrotic syndrome is considered likely, such as: *(i)* age at onset <1 yr or >16 yr; *(ii)* gross hematuria, persistent microscopic hematuria or low serum C3; *(iii)* renal failure, not attributable to hypovolemia; *(iv)* suspected secondary causes; and *(v)* sustained severe hypertension.

A renal biopsy is considered later if *(i)* diagnosis of steroid resistance is made; or *(ii)* therapy with calcineurin inhibitors is planned.

Management of the Initial Episode

Adequacy of treatment of the initial episode, both in terms of dose and duration of corticosteroids, is an important determinant of the long term course.

Agents: Only prednisolone and prednisone are of proven benefit in the treatment of proteinuria. Other agents such as deflazacort, methylprednisolone, dexamethasone, beta-methasone, triamcinolone or hydrocortisone should not be used for this purpose. Prednisolone is administered after meals to reduce its gastrointestinal side effects; concomitant administration of antacids is not required, unless there is gastrointestinal intolerance.

Dose and duration: Prednisolone is given at a dose of 2 mg/kg per day (maximum 60 mg) in single or divided doses for 6 weeks, followed by 1.5 mg/kg (maximum 40 mg) as a single morning dose on alternate days for the next 6 weeks. Therapy with corticosteroids is then stopped.

Prolongation of initial steroid therapy for *12 weeks or longer* is associated with significantly reduced risk for subsequent relapses. Some experts suggest that therapy with corticosteroids should not be stopped abruptly, but tapered over the next 8–12 weeks. However, this benefit must be viewed recognizing the increased risk of steroid adverse effects with prolonged therapy.

Based on available evidence and opinion, and while awaiting results of ongoing prospective studies, *therapy with oral steroids is recommended for 12 weeks.*

Failure to achieve remission of proteinuria despite treatment with daily prednisolone for 4 weeks is labeled as *steroid resistant* nephrotic syndrome. The management of these patients is discussed in Chapter 17.

Table 16.2: Investigations at the first episode of nephrotic syndrome

Essential

Urinalysis: proteinuria, red cells, casts
Blood levels of urea, creatinine, albumin, cholesterol
Complete blood counts
Tuberculin test

If required (indication)

C3 and antistreptolysin O (gross or persistent microscopic hematuria)
Chest X-ray (positive tuberculin test; history of contact with tuberculosis)
Hepatitis B surface antigen (recent jaundice, raised levels of transaminases)
Antinuclear antibodies (systemic lupus erythematosus)
Urine culture (urinary tract infection)

Therapy for Relapse

Prednisolone is given at a dose of 2 mg/kg/day (single or divided doses) until urine protein is nil or trace for three consecutive days *(remission)*, and subsequently as a single morning dose of 1.5 mg/kg on alternate days for 4 weeks, and then discontinued. Treatment for a relapse usually lasts for 5 to 6 weeks.

Relapses are often triggered by minor infections. Symptomatic therapy of infectious illness often results in remission of 1+/2+ proteinuria. However, persistence of 3+/4+ proteinuria with infections requires the aforementioned therapy for relapse.

In case the patient is not in remission despite two weeks treatment with daily prednisolone, the treatment is extended for 2 more weeks. Patients not showing remission despite 4 weeks' treatment with daily prednisolone are labelled as *steroid resistant* nephrotic syndrome, and are referred for evaluation. The subsequent management of a patient with steroid sensitive nephrotic syndrome depends on the course of the illness, as is described below.

Infrequent Relapses

Patients suffering from three or fewer relapses a year should receive treatment for each disease relapse as described above, i.e. prednisolone at 2 mg/kg/day (single or divided doses) until remission, followed by the same agent given in a single morning dose of 1.5 mg/kg on alternate days for 4 weeks. Therapy is then discontinued.

Frequent Relapses and Steroid Dependence

Patients with frequent relapses or steroid dependent nephrotic syndrome require prolonged treatment in order to maintain disease remission. The strategies to maintain remission in such patients are as follows:

Long term, alternate day steroids

Following treatment of a relapse, prednisolone is gradually tapered to maintain the patient in remission on alternate day dose of 0.3–0.7 mg/kg, which is given for 9-18 months. This strategy is effective in maintaining remission in a proportion of patients.

Relapses may often be precipitated following minor infections. *Increasing the frequency of administration of prednisolone from alternate day to daily during minor infections might prevent infection precipitated relapses.*

Steroid Sparing Agents

The addition of an alternative agent is recommended if: *(i)* the prednisolone threshold required for maintaining remission is higher than 0.5–0.7 mg/kg on alternate days, or *(ii)* features of corticosteroid toxicity (growth failure, hypertension and cataract) appear. The agents used, usually in successive order, are listed below and in Fig. 16.1.

Levamisole

Dose and duration: 2–2.5 mg/kg on alternate days for 12–24 months.

Adverse effects: Rare; flu-like symptoms, neutropenia, hepatotoxicity, convulsions and skin rash.

Monitoring: Monitor total and differential leukocyte count every 3–4 months.

Concomitant steroid therapy: The dose of prednisolone is decreased every 2–4 weeks to 0.25–0.5 mg/kg on alternate days. While therapy with prednisolone may be discontinued in a proportion of cases, many patients continue to require a small dose of prednisolone, given on alternate days.

Cyclophosphamide

This agent is preferred in patients with: *(i)* significant steroid toxicity, *(ii)* severe relapses with episodes of hypovolemia, life threatening infections or thrombosis, and *(iii)* poor compliance or difficult follow up.

Dose and duration: 2–2.5 mg/kg/day for 8–12 weeks.

Adverse effects: Leukopenia, alopecia, nausea, vomiting and hemorrhagic cystitis; long-term

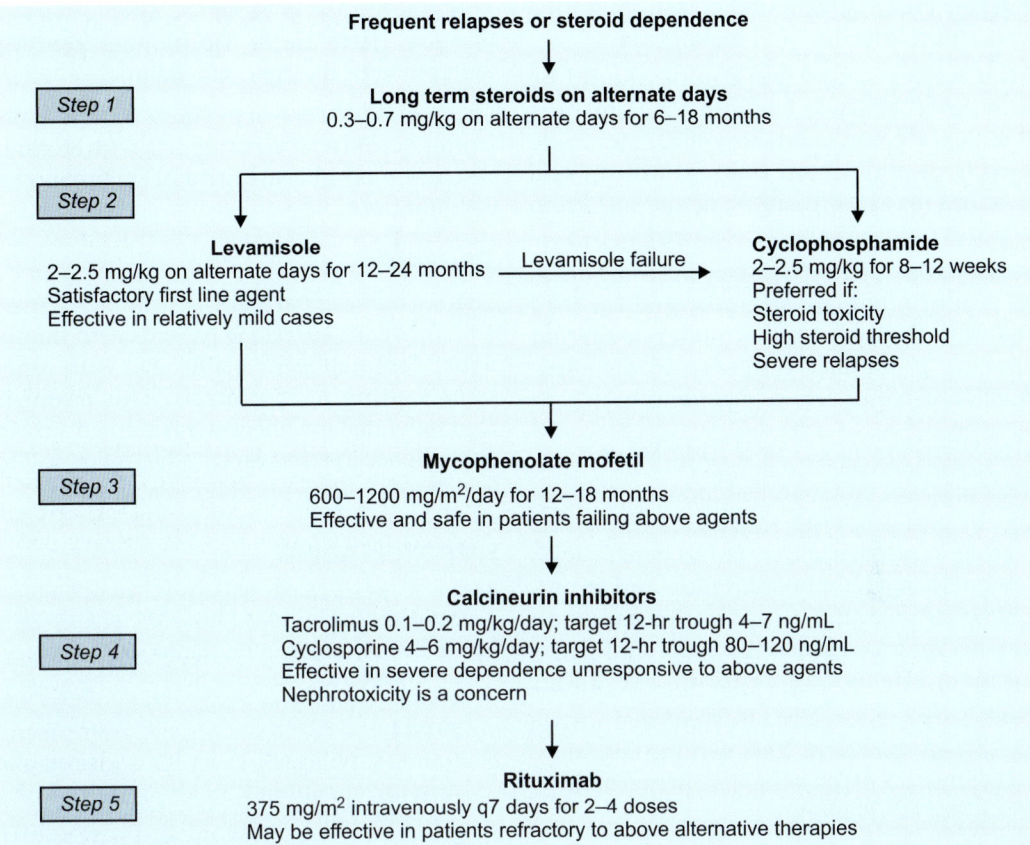

Frequent relapses or steroid dependence

Step 1 — **Long term steroids on alternate days**
0.3–0.7 mg/kg on alternate days for 6–18 months

Step 2

Levamisole
2–2.5 mg/kg on alternate days for 12–24 months — Levamisole failure →
Satisfactory first line agent
Effective in relatively mild cases

Cyclophosphamide
2–2.5 mg/kg for 8–12 weeks
Preferred if:
Steroid toxicity
High steroid threshold
Severe relapses

Step 3 — **Mycophenolate mofetil**
600–1200 mg/m^2/day for 12–18 months
Effective and safe in patients failing above agents

Step 4 — **Calcineurin inhibitors**
Tacrolimus 0.1–0.2 mg/kg/day; target 12-hr trough 4–7 ng/mL
Cyclosporine 4–6 mg/kg/day; target 12-hr trough 80–120 ng/mL
Effective in severe dependence unresponsive to above agents
Nephrotoxicity is a concern

Step 5 — **Rituximab**
375 mg/m^2 intravenously q7 days for 2–4 doses
May be effective in patients refractory to above alternative therapies

Fig. 16.1: Alternative agents in steroid sensitive nephrotic syndrome. Therapy with cyclophosphamide and calcineurin inhibitors is preferred in children with severe relapses (hypovolemia; life-threatening infections) and/or steroid toxicity

toxicity includes risk of gonadal toxicity and malignancies.

Monitoring

The cumulative dose should not exceed 168 mg/kg; repeat courses are avoided. Leukocyte counts should be monitored every 2 weeks; cyclophosphamide should be discontinued if leukocyte count is below 4000/mm^3. Fluid intake should be increased and the child is encouraged to void frequently.

Concomitant steroid therapy: The dose of prednisolone is maintained at 1–1.5 mg/kg on alternate days during cyclophosphamide therapy. Subsequently prednisolone is tapered and discontinued over 2–3 months.

Chlorambucil

This is also an alkylating agent. Although effective, the medication has significant toxicity and a low margin of safety, and is therefore not recommended.

Mycophenolate Mofetil

Dose and duration: 600–1000 mg/m^2/day; 20–23 mg/kg/d in two divided doses for 12–24 months

Adverse effects: Uncommon; gastrointestinal discomfort, diarrhea and leukopenia.

Monitoring: Leukocyte counts should be monitored every 1–2 months; treatment is withheld if count falls below 4000/mm^3. Side effects of abdominal pain, vomiting and diarrhea may be difficult to distinguish from features of infectious gastroenteritis.

Concomitant steroid therapy: Tapering doses of prednisolone are administered for 6–12 months. The agent has a moderate steroid sparing potential, with steroid discontinuation in a proportion of patients.

Cyclosporine (CsA) and Tacrolimus

Therapy with either of these agents is indicated in patients with frequent relapses or steroid dependence that fail to benefit with levamisole, cyclophosphamide and mycophenolate mofetil. Therapy with these medications may be associated with significant adverse effects and cautious use under supervision of an expert is necessary.

Dose and duration: CsA 4–5 mg/kg/day; tacrolimus 0.1–0.2 mg/kg/day in two divided doses, for 12–24 months.

Adverse effects: Acute and chronic nephrotoxicity (equivalent with both agents); hirsutism, gum hyperplasia (common with CsA); hypertension; hypercholesterolemia (common with CsA); hyperglycemia (with tacrolimus); elevated transaminases; neurotoxicity with headache and seizures (common with tacrolimus); hypomagnesemia, diarrhea (common with tacrolimus).

Monitoring: Renal function is monitored every 3 months; an increase of serum creatinine >25% is of concern.

Trough levels (CsA 80–120 ng/mL; tacrolimus 4–7 ng/mL), are estimated, particularly if response is unsatisfactory, noncompliance is suspected, and there is increase in serum creatinine.

Monitoring of lipid profile is done annually and blood sugar every 3–4 months.

Renal biopsy is repeated after 2–3 yr of therapy, particularly if prolonged therapy with either of the agents is planned.

Concomitant therapy: These agents have strong steroid sparing potential, with steroids discontinued in a majority of patients over 6–9 months.

Rituximab

This is a monoclonal anti-CD20 antibody, used with moderate success in patients with steroid dependent nephrotic syndrome, with remission lasting 6–18 months. This agent is recommended in patients with marked steroid dependence that has failed other therapies, or in patients with medication related toxicity.

SUPPORT READING

Bagga A, Mantan M. Nephrotic syndrome in children. Indian J Med Res 2005; 122: 13–28

Indian Society of Pediatric Nephrology. Management of steroid sensitive nephrotic syndrome: Revised guidelines. Indian Pediatr 2008; 45: 203–14

Hodson EM, Willis NS, Craig JC. Corticosteroid therapy for nephrotic syndrome in children. Cochrane Database Syst Rev 2007; 4:CD001533

Gipson DS, Massengill SF, Yao L, et al. Management of childhood onset nephrotic syndrome. Pediatrics 2009; 124: 747–57

Hodson EM, Alexander SI. Evaluation and management of steroid-sensitive nephrotic syndrome. Curr Opin Pediatr 2008; 20: 145–50

Moudgil A, Bagga A, Jordan SC. Mycophenolate mofetil therapy in frequently relapsing steroid-dependent and steroid- resistant nephrotic syndrome of childhood: current status and future directions. Pediatr Nephrol 2005; 20: 1376–81

Gulati A, Sinha A, Hari P, Bagga A. Daily corticosteroids reduce infection associated relapses in frequently relapsing nephrotic syndrome: a randomized controlled trial. Clin J Am Soc Nephrol 2011; 6: 63–69

Gulati A, Sinha A, Jordan S, Bagga A. Efficacy and safety of treatment with rituximab for difficult steroid resistant and dependent nephrotic syndrome. Clin J Am Soc Nephrol 2010; 5: 2207–12

17 Steroid Resistant Nephrotic Syndrome

The management of patients with steroid resistant nephrotic syndrome (SRNS) is difficult, with variable response to immuno-suppression, adverse effects of prolonged therapy and high risk of progressive renal damage. In view of the complexity of treatment, patients with SRNS should be managed at centers with pediatric nephrology services.

Definition

A patient is diagnosed to have SRNS if there is lack of remission despite treatment with prednisolone, at a dose of 2 mg/kg/day (60 mg/m^2/day) for 4 weeks. This definition is based on knowledge that 95% patients with steroid sensitive nephrotic syndrome achieve remission within 4 weeks of steroid therapy,

and that longer therapies are associated with high incidence of medication related adverse effects.

Care should be taken to exclude systemic infections (e.g. peritonitis, cellulitis, respiratory tract infections), which might result in persistent proteinuria and an inappropriate diagnosis.

Initial resistance is defined by the lack of remission at the first episode of nephrotic syndrome, and late resistance is considered in patients who are steroid sensitive initially, but show steroid resistance during a subsequent relapse.

Evaluation

Investigations in a patient with SRNS are listed in Table 17.1. Baseline assessment of

Table 17.1: Investigations in steroid resistant nephrotic syndrome
Essential
Urinalysis: red and white cells; 24-hr urine protein
Blood: urea, creatinine, albumin, cholesterol, electrolytes, transaminases
Hepatitis B surface antigen, anti-HCV IgG
Renal biopsy
If required (indication)
C3, antinuclear antibodies (microscopic or gross hematuria)
Anti-HIV antibodies; anti-parvovirus IgM (collapsing variant of FSGS)
Free T3, T4, TSH
Where available
Renal histology by electron microscopy
Genetic testing: sequencing of *NPHS2, NPHS1, WT1* and other genes

renal function, blood levels of albumin and cholesterol, and quantification of urinary protein loss (spot urine protein to creatinine ratio in young children; 24-hr protein excretion in older children) guides future evaluation of response to therapy. Patients with deranged liver function should be evaluated for hepatitis B and C virus infection, or if renal histology shows membranous nephropathy or membranoproliferative glomerulonephritis.

Renal Biopsy

Children diagnosed with SRNS (initial or late) should undergo renal biopsy before instituting specific treatment. Histology in patients with SRNS shows minimal change disease (MCD, Fig. 17.1) and focal segmental glomerulosclerosis (FSGS, Fig. 17.2) in 30–40% patients each, and mesangioproliferative glomerulonephritis in a small group. While patients with MCD show a satisfactory response to therapy, the presence of FSGS with chronic tubulointerstitial changes is associated with less satisfactory outcomes. Multiple histological subtypes of FSGS are recognized, which show variable response to therapy and outcome.

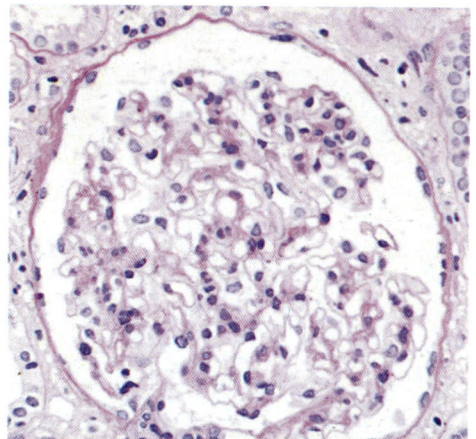

Fig. 17.1: Light microscopy (hematoxylin and eosin staining) in a 4-yr-old girl with initial steroid resistance shows no abnormality, typical of minimal change disease

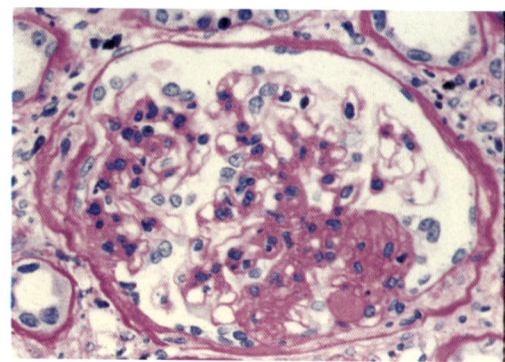

Fig. 17.2: Light microscopy (hematoxylin and eosin staining) in a 12-yr-old boy with initial steroid resistant nephrotic syndrome shows segmental sclerosis. Findings suggest focal segmental glomerulosclerosis

Approximately 15% patients with SRNS show membranoproliferative glomerulonephritis, membranous nephropathy, IgA nephropathy or amyloidosis. The diagnosis of these conditions is important, since their management differs from idiopathic MCD and FSGS.

Renal biopsy is also required before initiating treatment with potentially nephrotoxic agents, especially calcineurin inhibitors (cyclosporine or tacrolimus). Administration of calcineurin inhibitors in patients with chronic tubulointerstitial changes carries a risk of renal impairment, necessitating close monitoring of renal function.

The specimen should be examined by light and immunofluorescence microscopy. Electron microscopy helps confirm the diagnosis of MCD and enables diagnosis of early membranous nephropathy, membranoproliferative glomerulonephritis and Alport syndrome.

Genetic Studies

Patients with familial and sporadic SRNS might carry homozygous or compound heterozygous mutations in genes encoding podocyte proteins, including podocin (*NPHS2*), nephrin (*NPHS1*) and Wilms tumor

(*WT1*) genes. The disease is unresponsive to immunosuppressive medications, progresses rapidly to end stage renal disease, and unlike non-genetic FSGS (which recurs after transplantation in 30%), does not recur. Mutations in the *WT1* gene may cause Frasier syndrome, characterized by steroid resistant FSGS, male pseudohermaphroditism (female phenotype; 46, XY) and high risk for gonadoblastoma.

A significant proportion of patients with early onset nephrotic syndrome or with positive family history have mutations in these or other genes. The yield of genetic studies varies in different ethnic groups. While almost 25% Caucasian children with sporadic SRNS show mutations, their frequency in children in east and south Asia is lower.

Where facilities exist, mutational analysis should be offered to patients with: (*i*) congenital nephrotic syndrome (onset below 3 months of age), (*ii*) family history of SRNS, (*iii*) sporadic initial steroid resistance that does not respond to therapy with cyclophosphamide or calcineurin inhibitors, and (*iv*) girls with steroid resistant FSGS.

MANAGEMENT

Patients with idiopathic SRNS secondary to MCD, FSGS or mesangioproliferative glomerulonephritis are treated similarly. While patients with MCD demonstrate higher rates of remission and better prognosis, the histologies may be difficult to distinguish, and different entities may be demonstrable on sequential biopsies. *The chief factor predicting renal outcome is the response of proteinuria to therapy rather than the renal histology.*

The management of patients with membranous glomerulopathy, IgA nephropathy and membranoproliferative glomerulonephritis is discussed in Section V.

The aim of therapy in patients is to induce and maintain remission of proteinuria, while avoiding medication related adverse effects. Most regimens use a combination of an immunosuppressive agent with predni-

solone (given on alternate days) and enalapril (Table 17. 2).

Specific Therapy

Calcineurin Inhibitors (Cyclosporine or Tacrolimus)

Treatment with calcineurin inhibitors results in complete or partial remission of SRNS in a high proportion of patients with SRNS. Adverse effects are common with cyclosporine, requiring close monitoring, including for nephrotoxicity (acute and chronic), hypertension, hypertrichosis, gingival hyperplasia and dyslipidemia. Less common adverse effects include neurotoxicity, diarrhea and hyperglycemia.

The mechanism of action of tacrolimus is similar to that for cyclosporine. The rates of complete and partial remission (70–85%) are similar. Close monitoring for side effects is required; the incidence of neurotoxicity, diarrhea and impaired glucose tolerance are higher. A lower frequency of cosmetic side effects (gum hyperplasia, hirsutism) is an advantage, particularly in adolescent girls.

Cyclophosphamide

Cyclophosphamide has also been used, with modest success, either in the IV form or in combination with IV steroids (*see* Chapter 44). Intravenous cyclophosphamide, when administered monthly for six doses along with tapering doses of alternate day prednisolone, induces remission in 40–50% patients with SRNS. Oral cyclophosphamide, administered alone or with oral steroids, has limited efficacy in inducing remission.

Pulse Corticosteroids with Oral Cyclophosphamide

Pulses of IV methylprednisolone or dexamethasone have been used in combination with oral cyclophosphamide with moderate efficacy. The risk of steroid toxicity is high, with a significant proportion of patients developing systemic infections, hypertension and electro-

Nephrotic Syndrome

IV

Table 17.2: Agents used in the management of steroid resistant nephrotic syndrome

Agent	Dose	Duration	Efficacy	Adverse effects
Calcineurin inhibitors				
Cyclosporine (CsA)	4–5 mg/kg/day	12–36 months	50–80%	Acute and chronic nephrotoxicity; hirsutism and gum hyperplasia (CsA>Tac); hypertension; high
Tacrolimus (Tac)	0.1–0.2 mg/kg/day	12–36 months	70–85%	cholesterol (CsA>Tac); hyperglycemia (Tac); elevated transaminases; neurotoxicity with headache & seizures (Tac>CsA)
Cyclophosphamide				
Intravenous	500–750 mg/m^2	6 pulses	40–50%	Leukopenia; alopecia; nausea and vomiting (IV>oral); gonadal toxicity; hemorrhagic cystitis (IV>oral)
Oral	2–2.5 mg/kg/day	12 weeks	20–25%	
High dose corticosteroids with cyclophosphamide				
Methylprednisolone or Dexamethasone	20–30 mg/kg IV per dose 4–5 mg/kg/day IV per dose Administer pulses on alternate days × 6; once weekly × 8, fortnightly × 4, monthly × 8, bimonthly × 4		30–50%	Hypertension, hypokalemia, hyperglycemia, steroid psychosis, systemic infections Side effects of cyclophosphamide therapy & prolonged steroid therapy
Prednisolone	Tapering doses	18 months*		
Cyclophosphamide	2–2.5 mg/kg/day	12 weeks**		

*Prednisolone 1.5 mg/kg on alternate days for 4 weeks; 1.25 mg/kg/kg for 4 weeks; 1 mg/kg for 4 months; 0.5–0.75 mg/kg for 12–18 months
**Cyclophosphamide is administered during weeks 3–15

lyte abnormalities. Alternative protocols have been proposed with use of fewer IV doses of corticosteroids (Table 17.2).

Other Agents

Rituximab, an anti-CD20 monoclonal antibody, has been reported to be successful in inducing disease remission in 25–30% patients. Its safety and efficacy needs to be established in larger series. Other therapies that have shown promise, in anecdotal reports, include the combination of cyclosporine and mycophenolate mofetil, and plasmapheresis.

Choice of Specific Therapy

Significantly higher rates of remission are demonstrated with calcineurin inhibitors as compared to pulse IV cyclophosphamide and prednisolone. *Therefore, cyclosporine or tacrolimus are considered as the first line therapy for patients with steroid resistance.*

Adjunctive Therapy

Prednisolone

Prednisolone is a component of all regimens used in therapy of SRNS. The agent is administered on alternate days at 1 mg/kg day for 1–3 months, following which the dose may be tapered. Prednisolone may be discontinued if the child is in sustained complete remission for 6–12 months.

Angiotensin Converting Enzyme Inhibitors, Angiotensin Receptor Blockers

Therapy with angiotensin converting enzyme (ACE) inhibitors (e.g. enalapril 0.3–0.6 mg/kg/day; ramipril 6 mg/m^2 q24 h) is recommended for all patients with SRNS. This therapy is associated with 30–40% decrease in proteinuria and control of hypertension

Adverse effects of ACE inhibitors include dry cough, hyperkalemia and decline in renal function. The dose of the ACE inhibitor is decreased or therapy discontinued if hyperkalemia develops or the estimated GFR falls below <30 ml/minute/1.73 m^2.

Angiotensin receptor blockers (*e.g.*, losartan, valsartan) may be used in patients with persistent dry cough attributed to ACE inhibitors, or as an add-on therapy for better antiproteinuric effect. There are limited studies on the efficacy of the combination in children.

Statins

Annual monitoring for dyslipidemia is recommended. Persistent dyslipidemia is a risk factor for cardiovascular disease. Therapy with HMG CoA reductase inhibitors (e.g. atorvastatin 10–20 mg daily in children >5 years) is recommended in presence of biochemical abnormalities that persist for 3–6 months: total cholesterol >200 mg/dL, LDL cholesterol >130 mg/dL or triglycerides >200 mg/dL. Adverse effects of therapy include headache, muscle pain, rash, and raised levels of creatine kinase and transaminases.

Antihypertensive Drugs

The dose of ACE inhibitors is increased to permissible limits in patients with persistent hypertension, while monitoring renal function and blood levels of potassium. Other agents (calcium channel blocker, adrenergic blocker) are added if hypertension persists. Adjunctive measures include edema control, restriction of salt intake and decrease in the dose of steroids.

Calcium and Vitamin D Supplementation

Supplements of calcium carbonate (250-500 mg) with vitamin D (125-250 IU) are recommended for patients receiving prolonged treatment with steroids.

Monitoring Response to Therapy

Patients should be monitored every month until response to therapy is demonstrated, and then every 2–3 months (Table 17.3). *Complete remission* is defined as presence of trace or negative proteinuria (by dipstick) or spot urine protein to creatinine ratio (Up/Uc) <0.2

mg/mg. Patients are considered to be in *partial remission* if they show 1–2+ proteinuria (or Up/Uc between 0.2–2), blood albumin >2.5 g/dL and no edema. *Non-response* is defined as 3–4+ proteinuria (Up/Uc >2), blood albumin <2.5 g/dL or edema.

The aim of treatment in SRNS is achievement of complete remission, but occurrence of partial remission is satisfactory. Most patients who respond to treatment do so within 2–3 months. Therapy should be considered not effective and discontinued if nephrotic range proteinuria persists beyond 6 months. Patients that fail therapy with one regimen may show response to different agents.

Monitoring for Side Effects

Most agents used in the therapy of SRNS require monitoring for adverse effects (Table 17.3).

Monitoring for drug levels is recommended when using either cyclosporine or tacrolimus, because individual variations in bioavailability may result in occurrence of either subtherapeutic or toxic levels. Trough level (blood sample drawn 15–30 minutes prior to due dose) should be estimated about 2-weeks after introduction of CNI therapy, after any dose change, and if suspecting drug toxicity or poor compliance. Trough levels in the range of 80–120 ng/mL for cyclosporine and 4–7 ng/mL for tacrolimus are acceptable.

Examination of renal histology is required in patients with persistent decline in renal function (serum creatinine >50% above baseline) despite reduction in dose or discontinuation of CNI treatment. Prolonged therapy with CNI might cause histological features of nephrotoxicity, even in the absence of elevation of serum creatinine. Renal biopsy is therefore recommended in patients receiving prolonged therapy with cyclosporine or tacrolimus for 2–3 years.

Histological features of acute CNI nephrotoxicity include isometric vacuolation of tubular cells, necrosis and hyaline deposition in myocytes, endothelial vacuolation, afferent arteriolopathy and, rarely, thrombotic microangiopathy. Chronic changes include peripheral nodular hyalinosis, segmental or global glomerulosclerosis, striped interstitial fibrosis

Table 17.3: Monitoring in patients with steroid resistant nephrotic syndrome

Investigation	Frequency
Urine protein record at home	Daily or less frequent
Creatinine, albumin, electrolytes	Every 2–4 months
Urine protein & creatinine (spot, 24-hr)	Every 4–6 months
Hemogram, liver functions, glucose	Every 6 months
Lipid profile*	Annually
Creatine kinase	Annually if receiving atorvastatin; muscle pain
CNI trough level	2–4 weeks after initiation or dose change; suspected non-compliance; toxicity
Screening for infections	
Clinical	Every visit
Specific: X ray, cultures, viral serology, PCR	As required
Renal histology	
	After 2–3 years of CNI therapy; suspected nephrotoxicity

*Total cholesterol, low-density lipoproteins, very low-density lipoproteins, triglycerides
CNI calcineurin inhibitor; PCR polymerase chain reaction

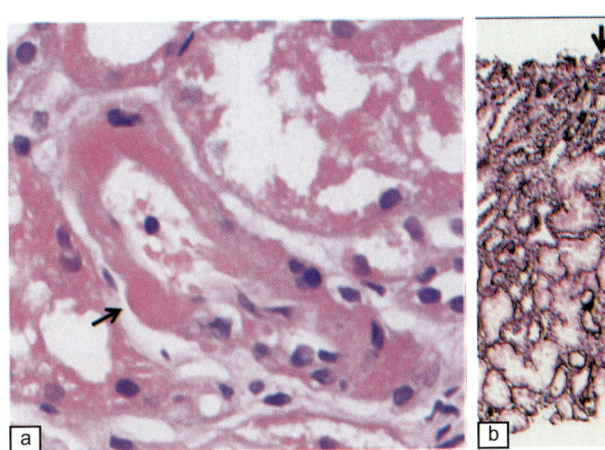 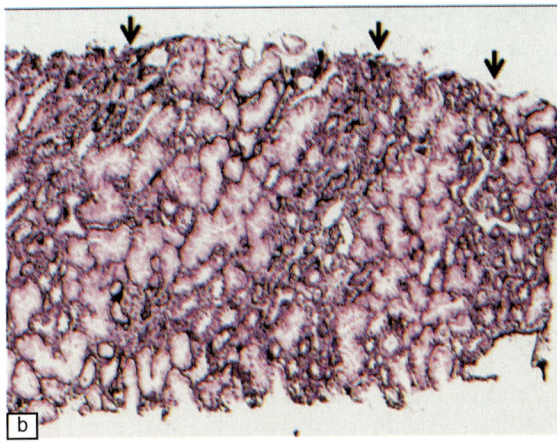

Fig. 17.3: Renal histology in a 13-yr-old girl administered cyclosporine for steroid resistant nephrotic syndrome for 3.5 years. (a) Peripheral nodular hyalinosis (arrow). (b) Silver methenamine staining shows stripes (arrows) of tubulointerstitial fibrosis

and tubular atrophy (Fig. 17.3). Prolonged duration of cyclosporine therapy (3 mg/kg/day for >24 months) and persistent heavy proteinuria beyond 30 days are risk factors for nephrotoxicity. The decision to continue CNI therapy should be reviewed in presence of these changes or the finding of increasing fibrosis.

Duration of Therapy

Consensus is lacking on the optimal duration of treatment with calcineurin inhibitors. Therapy for 2–3 years in patients that show complete or partial remission, is therefore followed by one of the following: (i) taper the dose of the CNI to the lowest effective dose, and discontinue; (ii) exclude medication-related nephrotoxicity on renal histology and continue calcineurin inhibitors; (iii) switch treatment to a less toxic agent, e.g. mycophenolate mofetil or rituximab.

Management of Disease Relapses

Patients that respond to therapy with CNI may show disease relapses, which at times are steroid sensitive. It is therefore appropriate to attempt to induce remission with oral prednisolone at 2 mg/kg/day, and increase the dose of the CNI as tolerated (based on trough levels, renal function). Patients that relapse after discontinuation of CNI may or may not respond to therapy with prednisolone and/or reintroduction of treatment.

Recurrence of FSGS after Renal Transplantation

FSGS recurs in 30–50% of children following renal transplantation, leading to graft loss in half of these patients. Risk factors for recurrence include: (i) non-genetic forms of FSGS, (ii) progression to ESRD within 2-yr of onset of disease, (iii) mesangial proliferation on the original biopsies and (iv) nephrectomy of native kidneys prior to transplant.

Pre-transplant plasmapheresis (6 treatment sessions for live related; one for deceased donor transplant) is an important preventive strategy.

There is no consensus on the optimal therapy for patients with recurrent FSGS. Options for treatment include: (i) intensive plasmapheresis; (ii) intravenous immunoglobulin (500 mg/kg/dose once a week after pheresis); (iii) rituximab (375 mg/m^2/week for 4 weeks); and (iv) oral cyclophosphamide (2–2.5 mg/kg/day for 3 months) instead of MMF.

17

Nephrotic Syndrome

IV

SUPPORT READING

Gulati A, Bagga A, Gulati S, on behalf of the Indian Society of Pediatric Nephrology. Guidelines for management of children with steroid resistant nephrotic syndrome. Indian Pediatr 2009; 46: 35–47

Benoit G, Machuca E, Antignac C. Hereditary nephrotic syndrome: a systematic approach for genetic testing and a review of associated podocyte gene mutations. Pediatr Nephrol 2010; 25: 1621–32

Choudhry S, Bagga A, Hari P, et al. Efficacy and safety of tacrolimus versus cyclosporine in children with steroid-resistant nephrotic syndrome: a randomized controlled trial. Am J Kidney Dis 2009; 53: 760–69

Hodson EM, Willis NS, Craig JC. Interventions for idiopathic steroid-resistant nephrotic syndrome in children. Cochrane Database Syst Rev 2010; (11): CD003594

Ulinski T, Aoun B. Pediatric idiopathic nephrotic syndrome: treatment strategies in steroid dependent and steroid resistant forms. Curr Med Chem 2010; 17: 847–53

Del Rio M, Kaskel F. Evaluation and management of steroid unresponsive nephrotic syndrome. Curr Opin Pediatr 2008; 20: 151–56

Colquitt JL, Kirby J, Green C, et al. The clinical and cost effectiveness of treatments for children with idiopathic steroid-resistant nephrotic syndrome: a systematic review. Health Technol Assess 2007; 11: 1–93

18 Supportive Care in Nephrotic Syndrome

Patients with relapses of steroid sensitive nephrotic syndrome as well as those with steroid resistant disease require attention for complications resulting from disease or its therapy.

Edema

Daily administration of corticosteroids results in diuresis within 2–4 days. Specific therapy for edema is not required in most patients with steroid sensitive nephrotic syndrome. Patients with significant edema and weight gain require treatment with diuretics. The occurrence of anasarca is associated with discomfort and an increased risk of infections, and should be avoided through timely treatment of relapses.

Management

Figure 18.1 shows the stepwise treatment of edema in children with nephrotic syndrome. Edema that does not respond to maximal doses of oral frusemide (loop diuretic) requires coadministration of a thiazide diuretic (e.g. hydrochlorthiazide, metolazone) given 30–60 minutes before frusemide. If frusemide is used for prolonged duration (>5–7 days) or in high doses (3–6 mg/kg/day), additional treatment with spironolactone (2–4 mg/kg/day) prevents the occurrence of hypokalemia.

Patients with refractory edema should be hospitalized and administered IV frusemide either as bolus injections (1–3 mg/kg/dose, infused over 15–20 minutes) or as continuous infusions (0.1–1 mg/kg/hr), under careful monitoring.

Infusions of albumin (20% albumin, 0.5–1 g/kg, over 2–4 hr), with an IV bolus of frusemide, administered at the end of the infusion, are useful in patients with severe hypoalbuminemia (serum albumin <1.5 g/dL). However, the effect of infusion of albumin is transient, necessitating repeat administration in patients with severe edema. Infusion of IV albumin in presence of oliguria can worsen hypertension and precipitate congestive cardiac failure. *Adequacy of urine output must be ensured prior to albumin infusion, and its administration should be avoided in individuals with respiratory distress of any cause.*

Abdominal paracentesis might be necessary in patients with refractory severe ascites and respiratory distress, but should be done carefully under aseptic precautions.

Monitoring

Patients treated on outpatient basis should be reviewed at 48–72 hr intervals. *Parents should be instructed to discontinue diuretics and review immediately if symptoms of hypovolemia (abdominal pain, dizziness) appear, or if the child has diarrhea, vomiting or poor oral intake.*

Patients receiving IV diuretics should be monitored closely for adverse effects. A daily record of weight and urine output, frequent (q4–12 hr) monitoring of vital signs (blood pressure, heart rate) and daily estimation of electrolytes (for hypokalemia, hyponatremia and metabolic alkalosis) are essential. Frequent estimation of renal function is essential, since aggressive diuresis may lead to pre-renal azotemia and acute tubular necrosis.

Hypovolemia

Hypovolemia may occur during a severe disease relapse or following administration of diuretics, particularly in children with poor oral intake, diarrhea and vomiting. Patients complain of abdominal pain, lethargy, dizziness and leg cramps. Signs include the presence of tachycardia, hypotension, delayed capillary refill, low volume pulses and cool clammy peripheries.

An elevated ratio of blood urea to creatinine and rising hematocrit suggest the presence of hypovolemia. The level of urine sodium and its fractional excretion are reduced to <20 mEq/L and 0.2–0.4% respectively. A high urinary potassium index (urine K^+/urine K^+ + urine Na^+) exceeding 0.6 also suggests aldosterone response to hypovolemia.

Therapy with diuretics should be discontinued. When signs of hypovolemia are absent, an increase in oral fluid intake alone may suffice. With features of hypovolemia, patients require admission and rapid infusion of normal saline (10–20 mL/kg) over 20–30 minutes. The bolus is repeated if features of hypovolemia persist. Patients who do not respond to two boluses of saline should receive an infusion of 5% albumin (10–15 mL/kg) or 20% albumin (0.5–1 g/kg).

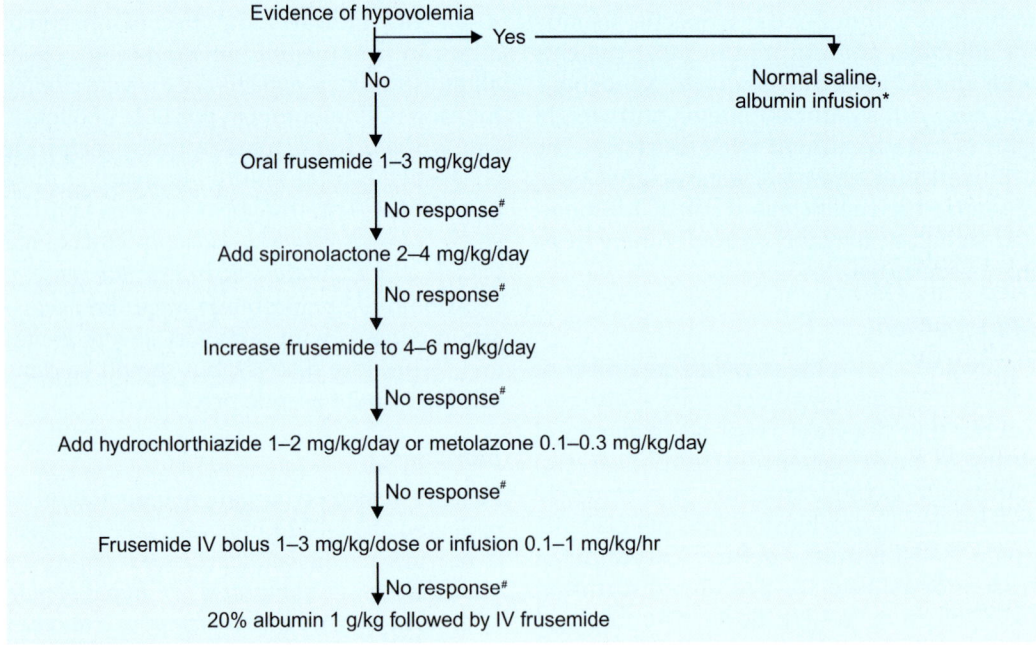

No weight loss or diuresis in 48 hr; or weight gain
*Infusion of 5% or 20% albumin is useful in subjects who do not respond to two boluses of saline

Fig. 18.1: Management of edema in patients with nephrotic syndrome. Hypovolemia is suggested by the presence of tachycardia, feeble pulses, cold extremities or hypotension. Additional features include an elevated hematocrit, high blood urea, low fractional excretion of sodium and high urinary potassium excretion.

Table 18.1: Management of systemic bacterial infections

Infection	Evaluation	Drug	Duration
Peritonitis	Abdominal pain, tenderness; diarrhea, vomiting. Ascitic fluid >100 leukocytes/mm³; >50% neutrophils	IV Cefotaxime (100–150 mg/kg/day); or Ceftriaxone (75–100 mg/kg/day)	7 days
Cellulitis	Cutaneous erythema, induration, tenderness	IV Cloxacillin (100–200 mg/kg/day) and IV Ceftriaxone (50–100 mg/kg/day) Shift to oral cloxacillin (100 mg/kg/day) or coamoxiclav (30–40 mg/kg/day) and cefixime (8 mg/kg/day) once erythema and induration resolve	10 days
Pneumonia	Fever, cough, tachypnea, intercostal recessions, crepitations	*Typical, non-severe:* Coamoxiclav (30–40 mg/kg/day); or Cephadroxil (30–40 mg/kg/day)	7–10 days
		Atypical, non-severe: Azithromycin (10 mg/kg/day)	3–5 days
		Severe: IV Cefotaxime (100–150 mg/kg/day); or Ceftriaxone (75–100 mg/kg/day)	7–10 days
		Severe infection with S. aureus: Teicoplanin (10 mg/kg/day, 3 doses q12 hr apart, then every 24 hr) or Vancomycin (40–60 mg/kg/day); and Amikacin (15 mg/kg/day)	10–14 days

Infections

Common infections include peritonitis and cellulitis. Table 18.1 provides a summary of management of these infections. During serious infections, steroids should be administered daily at stress doses, which amount to oral prednisolone 0.3–0.6 mg/kg once a day or IV hydrocortisone 50-100 mg/m² in four divided doses.

Fungal infections may develop during the course of therapy. Fungal skin rash or oral thrush responds to therapy with oral fluconazole for 10 days. Fungal sepsis is suggested by presence of pulmonary infiltrates or persistent fever unresponsive to antibiotics; supportive evidence includes sputum or urine showing septate hyphae or budding yeast cells, or positive fungal blood culture. Therapy with IV amphotericin for 14–21 days is usually effective.

Varicella may be life-threatening in patients with nephrotic syndrome receiving corticosteroids or other immunosuppressive drugs. Patients with varicella should be monitored for complications, during the illness and for 7–10 days afterwards, through periodic outpatient visits. All patients must receive oral acyclovir (80 mg/kg/day in 4 doses) for 7 days; severe illness requires admission in isolation and administration of IV acyclovir (1500 mg/m²/day in 3 doses). Administration of varicella zoster immunoglobulin (in a single dose within 96-hr of exposure) or intravenous immunoglobulin (400 mg/kg, in a single dose) prevents or lessens the severity of the disease in susceptible individuals exposed to varicella.

Children with nephrotic syndrome with positive tuberculin test should receive prophylaxis with isoniazid for six months. Patients with features of active tuberculosis should receive standard anti-tubercular therapy.

Hypertension

Hypertension may be noted at the onset of disease or develop secondarily as a result of

high dose steroid therapy. Persistent elevation in blood pressure, refractory to control
of edema and decline of corticosteroid dose,
merits treatment. An angiotensin converting
enzyme (ACE) inhibitor such as enalapril
(0.3–0.6 mg/kg/day in 2 divided doses) or
ramipril is the medication of choice. Persistent hypertension requires addition of
calcium channel blockers (e.g. amlodipine
0.1–0.6 mg/kg/day) or a vasodilator. The
target blood pressure is between the 75–90th
percentile for age, gender and height.

Thrombosis

Children with nephrotic syndrome are predis-
posed to venous thromboembolism during
relapses, due to loss of antithrombin III, low
intravascular volume (particularly with
aggressive diuretic use, or diarrheal dehydration), immobilization, indwelling vascular
catheters and puncture of deep vessels.
Thrombosis should be suspected in patients
with oligoanuria, hematuria or flank pain
(renal vein thrombosis); venous congestion,
pain, reduced mobility of limbs (deep vein
thrombosis); or seizures, vomiting, altered
sensorium and neurological deficits (saggital
sinus or cortical venous thrombosis). Deep
vein thrombosis can lead to pulmonary
embolism.

Diagnosis requires confirmation with
ultrasonography, Doppler studies and cranial
MRI if required. Therapy of thrombotic
complications includes the use of heparin (IV)
or low-molecular-weight heparin (subcutaneously) initially, followed by oral anticoagulants on the long term. Supportive care includes
correction of dehydration. There is no role for
prophylactic treatment with anticoagulants in
patients with hypoalbuminemia and edema.

Hyperlipidemia

Hyperlipidemia associated with disease
relapses does not merit treatment. However,
patients with steroid resistant nephrotic
syndrome with persistent proteinuria have

continued dyslipidemia that is undesirable,
and requires treatment with statins.

Vaccination

Primary immunization is essential since
infections form an important cause of morbidity. Vaccination may rarely precipitate
disease relapses.

The administration of live vaccines (oral
polio, varicella) should be deferred until the
child is off immunosuppressive medications
for at least 4 weeks. If essential, these vaccines
may be given to patients receiving alternate
day prednisolone at a dose <0.5 mg/kg.

The administration of pneumococcal vaccine is desirable. Children below 2 years of age
should receive the pneumococcal conjugated
vaccine, 0.5 ml intramuscularly (*age <6 months:*
3 doses 4–8 weeks apart and booster at 15–18
months; *age 6–12 months:* 2 doses 4–8 weeks
apart and booster at 15–18 months; *age between
12–23 months:* 2 doses 8 weeks apart). Above
2 years of age, one dose of the conjugate
vaccine is given followed 8 weeks later by the
polysaccharide vaccine (PPV23). Children
who continue to have relapses of nephrotic
syndrome may receive one repeat dose of
PPV23, 5 years after the primary vaccination.

Two doses of the varicella vaccine should
be administered 4 weeks apart while the child
is in remission and off immunosuppressive
medications.

Injectable polio vaccine should be administered to children with nephrotic syndrome and
their siblings. If the child has received primary
immunization with oral polio vaccine (at 6, 10
and 14 weeks), two doses of the parenteral
vaccine are given at 2 month interval followed
by a third dose 6 months after the first dose, and
a booster at 5 years (*see* Appendix 13).

Nutrition

During remission, children should eat a
balanced, nutritious diet without restrictions.
If disease relapses are associated with edema,
salt restriction is advised, by curbing the

intake of snacks and foods with high salt content. Undue restriction that makes food unpalatable is not required.

Patients with persistent or recurrent proteinuria should increase their daily intake of proteins to 2–2.5 g/kg. Increase in physical activity can help achieve desirable body weight in those with cushingoid features or obesity.

Patients receiving prolonged therapy with prednisolone (>3 months) should receive supplements of calcium carbonate (250–500 mg) and vitamin D (125–250 IU).

Stress Dose of Steroids

Patients who have received steroids at high doses for more than 2 weeks in the past year are at risk of suppression of the hypothalamo-pituitary- adrenal axis. These children require steroid supplements during surgery, anesthesia or serious infections. Corticosteroids are supplemented as parenteral hydrocortisone at a dose of 2–4 mg/kg/day, followed by oral prednisolone at 0.3–0.6 mg/kg/day. This is given for the duration of stress and then tapered rapidly.

Parent Education and Counseling

The parents are explained the natural history of the disease and its outcome, and the expected adverse effects of repeated courses of high dose steroid therapy and other medications.

The patient should return for follow up at 4 weeks of therapy of the initial episode, and during relapse. The need to examine urine protein at home (dipstick, boiling method) is emphasized. Parents should maintain a diary, recording the protein excretion, intake of medications and intercurrent illnesses. The record provides an assessment of disease status and course, including steroid threshold for relapses.

SUPPORT READING

Vasudevan A, Mantan M, Bagga A. Management of edema in nephrotic syndrome. Indian Pediatr 2004; 41: 787–95

Indian Society of Pediatric Nephrology. Management of steroid sensitive nephrotic syndrome: Revised guidelines. Indian Pediatr 2008; 45: 203–14

19 Congenital Nephrotic Syndrome

Congenital nephrotic syndrome is defined as the presence of nephrotic syndrome within the first 3 months of life. This condition can have diverse etiologies (Table 19.1). While the 'Finnish' type and other inherited defects are considered the most common forms, rare causes include intrauterine infections and maternal drugs.

Clinical Features

Patients with congenital nephrotic syndrome present with edema at or soon after birth. Infants with the classical Finnish type of nephrotic syndrome are born premature, with large placentae, and wide cranial sutures and fontanelles. Failure to thrive, delayed development, hypothyroidism and repeated infections are noted. Both hypotension (due to hypovolemia) and hypertension (with deranged renal function) are common; some may develop spontaneous vascular thrombosis. Presentation may include psychomotor retardation, hypotonia or seizures (Galloway Mowat syndrome), microcoria (Pierson syndrome) and ambiguous genitalia (Denys Drash syndrome).

Evaluation

Nephrotic range proteinuria and low serum albumin (usually <1 g/dL) are noted. Renal function is normal; deranged renal functions are found beyond infancy. Elevated thyroid

---

Table 19.1: Causes of congenital nephrotic syndrome

Known mutations

Nephrin (*NPHS1*) gene: Classic 'Finnish' type
Podocin (*NPHS2*) gene
Phospholipase C epsilon 1 (*PLCE1*) or *NPHS3* gene
Wilms tumor suppressor 1 *(WT1)* gene: Denys Drash syndrome; isolated nephrotic syndrome
Laminin β_2 *(LAMB2)* mutation: Pierson syndrome; isolated nephrotic syndrome
Laminin β_3 *(LAMB3)* mutation: Herlitz junctional epidermolysis bullosa
Lim transcription factor 1β *(LMXB1)* mutation: Nail patella syndrome

Rare causes

Galloway-Mowat syndrome: Brain malformations (microcephaly, developmental delay), hiatal hernia, diffuse mesangial sclerosis
Mitochondrial disorders
Primary focal segmental glomerulosclerosis
Congenital infections: Syphilis, toxoplasma, malaria, cytomegalovirus, rubella, hepatitis B, human immunodeficiency virus
Maternal systemic lupus erythematosus

stimulating hormone (TSH) and dyslipidemia (hypertriglyceridemia, elevated LDL and low HDL cholesterol) are common. Appropriate serology helps detect rare cases associated with congenital infections.

Genetic Testing

Genomic sequencing of *NPHS1* enables diagnosis of the classic Finnish nephrotic syndrome. Over 100 mutations in this gene have been described in non-Finnish patients, compared to two common mutations noted in individuals of Finnish ancestry. Mutations in other genes (*NPHS2*, *WT1* and *LAMB2*) might be important in patients of Asian ethnicity.

Histology

Renal biopsy shows microcysts in the cortex, representing dilatation of proximal convoluted tubules. Some glomeruli show mesangial proliferation, thickened Bowman capsule and increase in mesangial matrix. Electron microscopy reveals effacement of foot processes, thin glomerular basement membrane, mild endothelial swelling and disappearance of the slit diaphragms. *These histological changes may not be prominent if the renal biopsy is obtained early in the disease.*

Renal histology should be evaluated in context of results of genetic testing. While no single histological finding is pathognomonic for mutations in *NPHS1*, FSGS is seen in patients with *NPHS2* mutations. Patients with mutations in *WT1*, *LAMB2* and *PLCE1* genes show diffuse mesangial sclerosis.

Prenatal Diagnosis

Detection of mutation in the index case permits prenatal genetic testing by amniocentesis or chorionic villus biopsy in subsequent pregnancies. Maternal serum alpha-fetoprotein levels are elevated.

Management

A correct diagnosis is important for prognosis, therapy and genetic counseling. Management

is difficult in absence of specific treatment. The rare patient with congenital syphilis or toxoplasmosis responds to appropriate antimicrobials. Immunosuppression has no role in managing infants with congenital nephrotic syndrome.

Aggressive control of edema: This requires the use of loop and thiazide diuretics, and albumin infusions (20%, 1–4 g/kg/day, as required)

Nutritional support: A diet high in carbohydrates and polyunsaturated fats is prescribed to provide 120–130 Cal/kg/day and 3–4 g/kg/day proteins. Supplements of vitamins A, D, E and water soluble vitamins; calcium (250–500 mg) and magnesium (40–60 mg) are given. Nasogastric feeds may be necessary to ensure adequate protein and calorie intake.

Thyroxin supplements: A small dose of thyroxine (6.25–12.5 µg/day), adjusted to TSH levels corrects clinical or sub-clinical hypothyroidism.

Reduction of proteinuria: Interventions include:
1. ACE inhibitors: captopril 3–4 mg/kg/day; enalapril 0.2–0.5 mg/kg/day in divided doses
2. Indomethacin 1–2 mg/kg/day
3. Unilateral nephrectomy effectively decreases the proteinuria
4. Bilateral nephrectomy with institution of continuous peritoneal dialysis is recommended for patients planned for renal transplantation. Transplantation is offered once the body weight exceeds 9 kg.

Prognosis

Most affected children succumb to their illness during infancy, either to infections or complications of the persistent nephrotic proteinuria. Children surviving past infancy show progressive kidney disease and require renal replacement therapy. Recurrence of disease in the allograft has been rarely reported in patients with mutations in the *NPHS1* gene.

SUPPORT READING

Jalanko H. Congenital nephrotic syndrome. Pediatr Nephrol 2009; 24: 2121–28.

Glomerulonephritis

20 Acute Glomerulonephritis

Acute glomerulonephritis (AGN) or acute nephritic syndrome is an acute onset of hematuria, edema, hypertension and oliguria, with diminished glomerular filtration rate (GFR), salt and water retention and circulatory congestion. The condition usually follows a microbial infection and is often called *post-infectious* GN. AGN may also occur as part of a systemic disease (Table 20.1).

POSTSTREPTOCOCCAL ACUTE GLOMERULONEPHRITIS

AGN occurring after β-hemolytic strepto-coccal infection is the most common type in children, accounting for almost 80 percent cases. Poststreptococcal GN (PSGN) occurs following pharyngitis, impetigo or rarely, a middle ear infection caused by nephritogenic strains of group A β-hemolytic streptococci.

Table 20.1: Etiology of acute nephritic syndrome

Postinfectious

Streptococci, staphylococci, pneumococci, meningococci, *Treponema pallidum, Salmonella,* leptospira *Plasmodium malariae, P. falciparum,* toxoplasma, filaria

Hepatitis B and C, cytomegalovirus, parvovirus, Ebstein Barr virus, coxsackievirus, echovirus, varicella

Associated with severe infections; infection of shunts, prostheses, bacterial endocarditis

Systemic vasculitis

Henoch-Schönlein purpura

Microscopic polyarteritis, Wegener's granulomatosis

Others

Membranoproliferative glomerulonephritis

IgA nephropathy

Hereditary nephropathy

Systemic lupus erythematosus

The risk of developing AGN after infection with β-hemolytic streptococcus type 4 is 25 percent, and the overall risk with nephritogenic strains is 15 percent. Subclinical episodes occur 4–10 times more frequently than overt disease.

Pathology

The glomeruli are enlarged and show severe proliferative and exudative changes; obliteration of capillary lumina results in glomeruli that look bloodless (Fig. 20.1). Epithelial cell proliferation and crescents are uncommon. Immunofluorescence examination shows fine granular deposits of C3 and IgG along the capillary walls and in the mesangium (Fig. 20.2). Electron microscopy shows electron-dense subepithelial deposits or 'humps' that disappear after 6 weeks (Fig. 20.3).

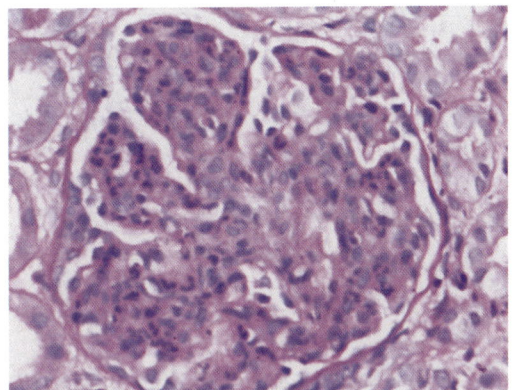

Fig. 20.1: Poststreptococcal GN. Moderately severe proliferation and exudative changes with infiltration of neutrophils. Few open capillary lumina are seen

Clinical Features

A history of sore throat or pyoderma is followed by a latent period (7–14 days in the former, 2–4 weeks in the latter), and then by the onset of the acute nephritic syndrome. During epidemics of streptococcal throat infection, subclinical cases show only microscopic hematuria and occasional gross hematuria.

PSGN usually affects children between the ages of 5 to 12 years and is rare below the age of 3 years. The presenting features are:

1. Gross hematuria and mild facial edema: Gross hematuria may last for a few hours and does not persist beyond 1–2 weeks. The symptoms may relapse following exercise or viral illness. Some degree of *oliguria* is

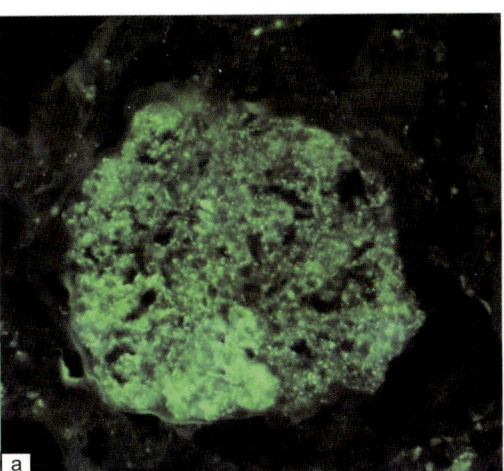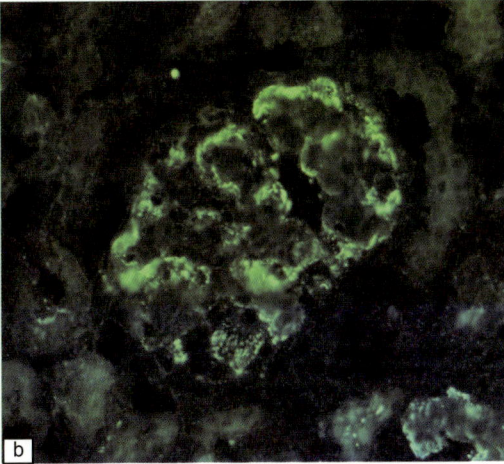

Fig. 20.2: Acute glomerulonephritis. Immunofluorescence examination showing (a) extensive fine granular deposition of IgG along the capillary wall and in mesangium with a *starry sky* appearance; and (b) dense confluent deposition along the capillary loops sparing the subendothelial and mesangial locations, in a *garland* pattern; this pattern often correlates with heavy proteinuria

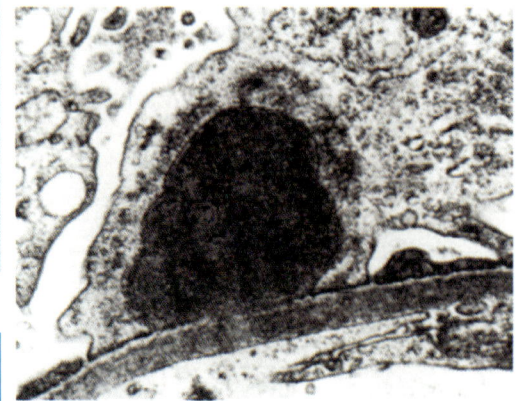

Fig. 20.3: Poststreptococcal GN. Electron micro-scopy showing electron-dense subepithelial deposits or 'humps'

associated, but anuria is infrequent and a serious sign. Edema, extending to involve hands and legs, is noted in 90% children. Hypertension, noted in 60–80% of hospi-talized patients, resolves following diuresis and loss of edema. Persistence of elevated blood pressure beyond 2–3 weeks of illness suggests chronic glomerulonephritis or rapidly progressive GN.

2. Mild cases may just have microscopic hematuria with slight proteinuria.

3. Atypical presentations: A history of sore throat and gross hematuria may be absent and the edema mild. The child may present with one or more of the complications of AGN, e.g. acute pulmonary edema, hypertensive ence-phalopathy, acute renal failure, rapidly pro-gressive GN, nephrotic syndrome or with systemic manifestations such as fever, arthri-tis, abdominal pain, purpura, rash, hepatos-plenomegaly

Investigations

Gross hematuria is present in a majority. Proteinuria is usually mild; occasionally it is in the nephrotic range. Microscopic exami-nation shows dysmorphic red cells and red cell casts. In initial stages the urine may contain a large number of neutrophils, often mistakenly regarded as urinary tract infection. The levels of blood urea and creatinine are elevated. Patients may show features of acute renal failure, with hyponatremia, hyper-kalemia and acidosis. Chest X-ray shows cardiomegaly and pulmonary congestion. Mild dilutional anemia may be noted.

Evidence of preceding streptococcal infection is indicated by rise in the anti-streptolysin O (ASO) titer in 60–80%. Early antibiotic treatment may attenuate this response. The rise in ASO titer begins 1–3 weeks after the streptococcal infection, peaks in 3–5 weeks and then reduces. In pyoderma, ASO titer is less commonly elevated whereas antihyaluronidase and anti-DNase B are raised. Streptococci can occasionally be cultured from the throat.

Approximately 90% patients have low serum C3 levels that return to normal in 6–8 weeks; C4 levels are normal. Persistent hypocomplementemia (>12 weeks) is rare in PSGN and suggests conditions such as memb-ranoproliferative GN, lupus nephritis or GN related to endocarditis or occult abscesses. The degree of C3 depression is not related to the severity of the disease.

Renal biopsy is not required in typical cases of PSGN, except when the serum complement remains depressed or if renal function is severely impaired (Table 20.2).

Management

The treatment is symptomatic. Those with moderate or severe hypertension and oliguria require hospital care. Daily weight, urine output and blood levels of urea and electro-lytes are monitored. With careful manage-ment the child should lose weight depending upon the degree of edema. Strict bed rest is not necessary.

Circulatory congestion and edema are treated with restriction of salt and water and use of diuretics. Hypertension responds to treatment with sublingual or oral nifedipine and frusemide. Hypertensive emergencies

Table 20.2: Indications for renal biopsy in acute glomerulonephritis

Systemic features: Fever, rash, joint pain, heart disease
Absence of serologic evidence of streptococcal infection; normal levels of C3 in acute illness
Mixed picture of glomerulonephritis and nephrotic syndrome
High blood levels of urea or presence of anuria requiring dialysis (rapidly progressive GN)

Delayed resolution
   Oliguria, hypertension and/or azotemia persisting past 7–10 days
   Gross hematuria persisting past 3–4 weeks; persistent microscopic hematuria beyond 12–18 months
   Nephrotic range proteinuria beyond 2 weeks; persistent proteinuria beyond 6 months
   Low C3 levels beyond 12 weeks

are managed using standard medications (IV labetalol, sodium nitroprusside, nicardipine). Beta-adrenergic blockers (atenolol) and angiotensin converting enzyme inhibitors (enalapril) are effective in lowering blood pressure, but can precipitate hyperkalemia in children with impaired function. Patients with acute renal failure require correction of fluid and electrolyte abnormalities, with dialytic support as required. Patients presenting with RPGN should be managed with IV methylprednisolone (see Table 20.2).

If oliguria is present and the level of blood urea is elevated, dietary protein should be restricted. Penicillin may be administered for 7 days if active pyoderma or residual pharyngitis is present. Antibiotic therapy has no influence on the course of the disease but may prevent spread of streptococcal infection from patients with positive cultures.

Follow up

The long-term outcome of PSGN is excellent. Risk factors for an unfavorable outcome include older age, high serum creatinine at presentation, features of nephrotic syndrome, and extensive crescents on renal biopsy.

Patients with AGN without evidence of a preceding streptococcal infection should be closely followed for several years with periodic urine examinations and measurements of blood pressure.

ACUTE NEPHRITIC SYNDROME

The features of acute GN can be caused by several conditions (Table 20.1). Infections with methicillin-resistant *Staphylococcus aureus,* and other bacterial, viral and parasitic agents have been implicated. In patients with AGN associated with infections other than group A streptococcus, the onset is often insidious and the course protracted. It is important to distinguish these patients from PSGN because appropriate antimicrobial therapy might lead to resolution of the disease.

Other conditions that may cause the acute nephritic syndrome include Henoch-Schönlein purpura, membranoproliferative GN, systemic lupus erythematosus, bacterial endocarditis, infected hydrocephalus shunt, polyarteritis, idiopathic crescentic GN, Alport syndrome, IgA nephropathy, acute interstitial nephritis and acute exacerbation of chronic GN. The possibility of these disorders should be considered if their characteristic features are associated with those of AGN.

Since patients with PSGN usually recover between 1–2 weeks, persistence of abnormalities, or a rapid deterioration should prompt consideration of other conditions (Table 20.2).

Nephritis associated with Subacute Bacterial Endocarditis or Infected Shunts

The illness in patients with bacterial endocarditis, and infected prosthetic valves,

20

ventriculoatrial shunt (occasionally ventri-culoperitoneal shunt) or long-term indwelling catheters may be complicated by the occur-rence of the acute nephritic syndrome. Fever, joint pain, pallor and purpuric rash is asso-ciated.

Complement C3 and C4 levels are depressed and blood urea may be elevated. Blood culture may grow causative organisms, usually coagulase negative staphylococci; culture from the shunt or the catheter is usually positive. Renal histology shows features of postinf-ectious AGN; in some, the abnormalities resemble membranoproliferative GN.

Treatment consists of removal of shunt or indwelling catheter, and eradication of infec-tion with use of appropriate antibiotics. Some patients have residual renal impairment.

Glomerulonephritis associated with Hepatitis B or C

Renal involvement in hepatitis B is common in many countries. While the usual lesion is membranous nephropathy, membranopro-liferative GN, mesangioproliferative GN and vasculitis may occur. Hepatitis C virus infec-tion is more commonly associated with membranoproliferative GN. The patients generally develop nephrotic syndrome but may present with acute GN. These entities are discussed in chapter 27.

ACUTE INTERSTITIAL NEPHRITIS

Acute interstitial nephritis may show fea-tures similar to acute glomerulonephritis. Gross hematuria and leukocyturia may be caused by medications (ampicillin, fluo-roquinolones, rifampicin, phenytoin, fruse-mide, NSAIDs). Fever, rash, arthralgia and flank pain may be present. While some patients show renal dysfunction, this is non-oliguric. Eosinophilia and eosinophiluria may be observed. The offending agent should be promptly removed. A short course of prednisolone, 1–2 mg/kg/d and tapered over 3–4 weeks, may hasten recovery. In patients with renal failure, 4–6 pulses of IV methylprednisolone (30 mg/kg/d) may lead to improvement of renal function.

SUPPORT READING

Kanjanabuch T, Kittikowit W, Eiam-Ong S. An update on acute postinfectious glomerulo-nephritis worldwide. Nat Rev Nephrol 2009; 5 : 259–69

Eison TM, Ault BH, Jones DP, et al. Post-strepto-coccal acute glomerulonephritis in children: clinical features and pathogenesis. Pediatr Nephrol 2011; 26 : 165–80

Ahn SY, Ingulli E. Acute poststreptococcal glomerulonephritis: an update. Curr Opin Pediatr 2008; 20: 157–62

Barratt J, Feehally J. Treatment of IgA nephro-pathy. Kidney Int 2006; 69: 1934–38

21 Rapidly Progressive Glomerulonephritis

Rapidly progressive glomerulonephritis (RPGN) is characterized by clinical features of glomerulonephritis and rapid loss of renal function, and histologically by crescent proliferation in glomeruli. RPGN is a medical emergency, which if untreated progresses to irreversible loss of renal function. Prompt evaluation and therapy are necessary for satisfactory outcome.

Definition

RPGN is a clinical syndrome characterized by an acute nephritic illness accompanied by a rapid loss of renal function over days to weeks. The pathological correlate is the presence of crescents (crescentic GN) involving 50% or more glomeruli.

The presence of crescents is a marker of severe glomerular injury, which may occur in a number of conditions including post-infectious GN, IgA nephropathy, SLE, renal vasculitis and membranoproliferative GN. The severity of clinical features correlates with the proportion of glomeruli that show crescents. While patients with circumferential crescents involving more than 80% glomeruli present with advanced renal failure, those with crescents in less than 50% glomeruli, particularly if the crescents are noncircumferential, have an indolent course.

Even though the terms RPGN and crescentic GN are used interchangeably, similar clinical presentation might occur in conditions without crescents, including hemolytic uremic syndrome (HUS), diffuse proliferative GN and acute interstitial nephritis.

Classification

Based on renal histology and patterns on immunofluorescence staining, crescentic GN is classified into three types, reflecting different mechanisms of glomerular injury:

1. Immune-complex GN with deposits of immune complexes along capillary wall and mesangium
2. Pauci-immune GN with minimal or no immune deposits, with or without systemic vasculitis
3. Anti-GBM GN with linear deposits of anti-GBM antibodies

Table 21.1 lists the common conditions that present with various forms of crescentic GN. Immune complex GN is the most common pattern of crescentic GN in children. Pauci-immune crescentic GN, while common in adults, is less frequent in children, accounting for 15–20% cases.

Clinical Features

The chief complaints are similar to severe postinfectious GN with the course extending over several days. Clinical features include macroscopic hematuria (60–90% patients), oliguria (60–100%), hypertension (60–80%) and edema (60–90%). The illness may be complicated by the occurrence of hypertensive emergencies, pulmonary edema and cardiac failure. Occasionally, RPGN has an

Table 21.1: Common causes of rapidly progressive glomerulonephritis

Immune complex GN

Postinfectious GN: Poststreptococcal GN, infective endocarditis, visceral abscesses, *S. aureus* sepsis, human immunodeficiency virus, hepatitis B and C

Systemic disease: Systemic lupus erythematosus, Henoch-Schönlein purpura, rheumatoid arthritis

Primary GN: IgA nephropathy, membranoproliferative GN, C1q nephropathy

Pauci-immune crescentic GN

Microscopic polyangiitis, Wegener's granulomatosis, renal limited vasculitis

Idiopathic crescentic GN

Medications: penicillamine, hydralazine, hydrocarbons, propylthiouracil

Anti-glomerular basement membrane (GBM) GN

Anti-GBM nephritis, Goodpasture syndrome, post-renal transplantation in Alport syndrome

insidious onset with the initial symptoms being fatigue or edema.

Systemic complaints, involving the upper respiratory tract (cough, sinusitis), skin (vasculitic rash), musculoskeletal (joint pain, swelling) and/or the nervous system (seizures, altered sensorium) are common in patients with pauci-immune crescentic GN, with or without ANCA positivity. Sixty to seventy five percent patients with Wegener's granulomatosis patients have crescentic GN, and 80% show pulmonary features.

Microscopic polyangiitis is characterized by glomerulonephritis in 90% patients, pulmonary capillaritis and gastrointestinal involvement in 40–50% each; and skin and musculoskeletal features in 60% each.

Patients with anti-GBM antibody disease present with hemoptysis and, less often, pulmonary hemorrhage. Similar complications may be found in Wegener's granulomatosis, SLE, Henoch Schonlein purpura and severe GN with pulmonary edema.

Investigations

Gross or microscopic hematuria with red cell casts is characteristic. Most patients show variable degree of non-selective proteinuria (2+ to 4+), with leukocyte, granular and epi-

thelial casts. Renal failure is present at diagnosis in almost all cases.

Serology

Serological investigations assist in evaluation of the cause and in monitoring disease activity (Table 21.2). Low levels of complement 3 (C3) are seen in postinfectious GN, SLE and membranoproliferative GN, and inversely correlate with disease activity. Positive antistreptolysin O titers and anti-deoxyribonuclease B suggests streptococcal infection in the past 3 months. Patients with SLE show antinuclear (ANA) and anti-double stranded DNA autoantibodies.

Elevated levels of ANCA suggest underlying vasculitis, and are present in patients with pauci-immune crescentic GN. Most ANCA have specificity for myeloperoxidase (MPO) or proteinase-3 (PR3). ANCA should be screened by indirect immunofluorescence and PR3-ELISA and MPO-ELISA. Wegener's granulomatosis is associated with PR3 ANCA, which produces a cytoplasmic staining pattern on immunofluorescence (c-ANCA) in 85% cases. Renal limited vasculitis and drug induced pauci-immune GN are associated with MPO ANCA that shows perinuclear staining on immunofluorescence (p-ANCA). Patients with microscopic polyangiitis have

Table 21.2: Diagnostic evaluation of patients with rapidly progressive GN

Complete blood counts; peripheral smear for type of anemia; reticulocyte count
Blood levels of urea, creatinine, electrolytes, calcium, phosphate
Urinalysis: proteinuria; microscopy for erythrocytes and leukocytes, casts
Complement C3, C4, CH50
Antistreptolysin O, antinuclear antibody (ANA), anti-double stranded DNA antibodies
Antinuclear cytoplasmic antibodies (ANCA): immunofluorescence, ELISA
Renal biopsy: light microscopy, immunofluorescence, electron microscopy

Required in specific instances

Anti-GBM IgG antibodies
Blood levels of cryoglobulin, hepatitis serology
Radiograph, CT of chest (suspected Goodpasture syndrome and vasculitides)
Radiograph, CT of sinuses (suspected Wegener's granulomatosis)

almost equal distribution of MPO ANCA and PR3 ANCA. Approximately 10% patients with Wegener's granulomatosis or microscopic polyangiitis have negative assays for ANCA.

Apart from diagnosis, ANCA titers are used for monitoring activity of systemic vasculitis. The risk of relapse in patients who show persistently negative ANCA titers is low. On the other hand, persistent or reappearing ANCA positivity in patients in remission may be associated with disease relapse.

High titers of anti-GBM IgG antibodies are seen in anti-GBM nephritis or Goodpasture syndrome and correlate with disease activity. About 5% of ANCA positive samples are also anti-GBM positive and approximately 20–30% of anti-GBM positive samples are ANCA positive.

Renal Histology

A glomerular crescent is an accumulation of two or more layers of cells that partially or completely fill the Bowman's space. Crescents in anti-GBM nephritis or ANCA associated disease are usually circumferential, while they are often segmental in immune complex GN. Once the glomerular capillary loop is compressed by the crescent, tubules that derive their blood flow from that efferent arteriole show ischemic changes.

Crescents may be completely cellular or show variable scarring and fibrosis (Fig. 21.1). Biopsies from patients with vasculitis show crescents in various stages of progression indicating episodic inflammation. Early lesions have segmental fibrinoid necrosis, while severe acute lesions show focal or diffuse necrosis in association with circumferential crescents. Features of small vessel vasculitis, affecting interlobular arteries might be seen.

Immunofluorescence examination assists in determining the cause of crescentic GN, based on location and nature of immune deposits. Crescents stain strongly for fibrin. Mesangial deposits of IgA are seen in IgA nephropathy and Henoch Schonlein purpura; granular, subepithelial deposits of IgG and C3 in post-infectious GN; mesangial, subendothelial and intramembranous deposits of IgG and C3 in MPGN; and *full house* capillary wall and mesangial deposits of granular IgG, IgA, IgM, C3, C4 and C1q in SLE. Glomeruli of patients with vasculitis, with and without ANCA positivity, have few or no immune deposits. Anti-GBM disease shows linear staining of the GBM with IgG (rarely IgM and IgA) and C3.

Diagnosis

It is necessary to make an accurate and rapid diagnosis in RPGN as treatment strategies

Glomerulonephritis

V

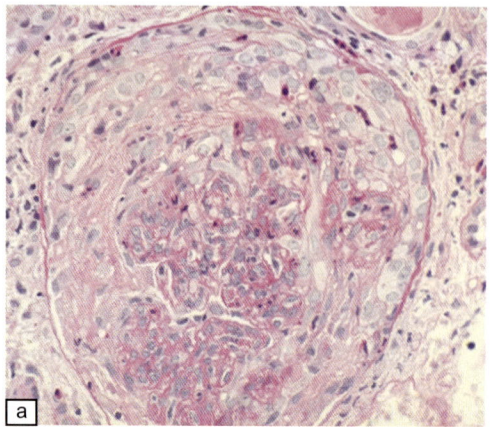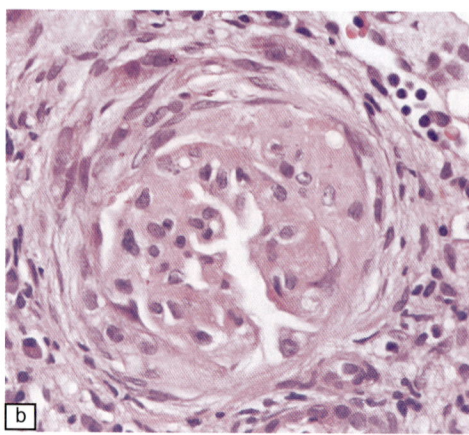

a b

Fig. 21.1: (a) Large cellular crescent with compression of glomerular tuft (Masson Trichome × 200); (b) Fibrocellular circumferential crescent with admixture of collagen fibers and membrane proteins amongst the cells (hematoxylin and eosin X 200)

vary and delay in instituting treatment results in irreversible disease. *All patients with RPGN should undergo a kidney biopsy promptly.*

The diagnosis of the etiology of crescentic GN depends on integration of clinical data and findings on serology and renal histology (Fig. 21.2). Timely and appropriate therapy is indicated in view of the widely recognized unsatisfactory outcome in untreated patients.

Treatment

Supportive management includes maintenance of fluid and electrolyte balance, providing adequate nutrition, and control of infections and hypertension. The specific treatment of RPGN comprises two phases: *induction* of remission and its *maintenance* (Table 21.3). The first phase aims at control of inflammation and the associated immune response. The maintenance phase attempts to prevent further renal damage and relapses.

Induction

Therapy with high dose corticosteroids and cyclophosphamide is used initially. Treatment includes IV pulses of methylprednisolone (15–20 mg/kg, maximum 1 g/day) for 3–6 days, followed by high-dose oral prednisone (1.5–2 mg/kg daily) for 4 weeks, with tapering to 0.5 mg/kg daily by 3 months and alternate day prednisone for 12–24 months.

Cyclophosphamide is administered IV, beginning at a dose of 500 mg/m^2 and increased every 3–4 weeks to a maximum dose of 750 mg/m^2. The dose is adjusted to maintain a nadir leukocyte count, two weeks' post treatment of 3000–4000/mm^3. An alternative is oral cyclophosphamide (2 mg/kg/day) for 3–6 months. The former is preferred in view of similar efficacy, but fewer side effects.

Since intensive immunosuppression is associated with risk of infections, prophylactic antimicrobials especially against *Pneumocystis carinii* and *Candida* may be required during induction.

The patients are transferred to *maintenance therapy* at 3 months when receiving oral cyclophosphamide and at 3–6 months when receiving IV medication, once disease remission is achieved.

Plasmapheresis: During induction, double volume plasmapheresis is recommended for patients with the following:

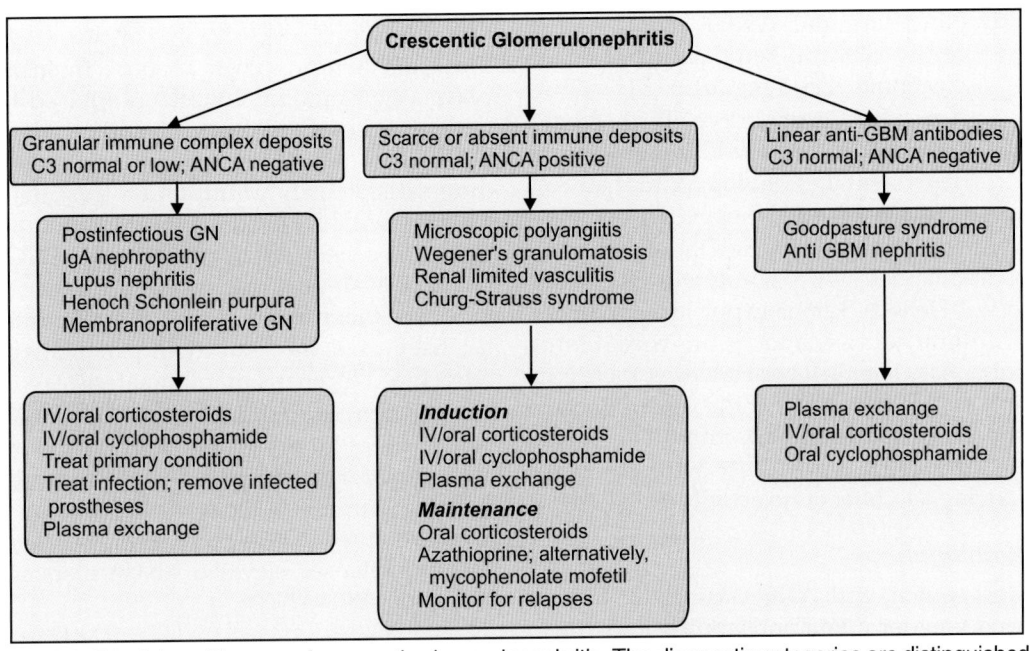

Fig. 21.2: Principles of therapy of crescentic glomerulonephritis. The diagnostic categories are distinguished based on immunofluorescence findings and serology. Therapy is tailored to the specific diagnosis. The role of long-term immunosuppression and/or plasma exchange is limited in immune complex GN

Table 21.3: Treatment of crescentic glomerulonephritis

Induction phase (3–6 months)

Methylprednisolone 15–20 mg/kg (maximum 1 g) IV daily for 3–6 doses
Prednisolone 1.5–2 mg/kg/day PO for 4 weeks; taper to 0.5 mg/kg daily by 3 months; 0.5–1 mg/kg on alternate day for 3 months
Cyclophosphamide 500–750 mg/m^2 IV every 3–4 weeks for 6 pulses*
Plasmapheresis (double volume) on alternate days for 2 weeks#

Agents for refractory disease

Intravenous immunoglobulin, TNF-α antibody (infliximab), anti CD20 (rituximab)

Maintenance phase (2–5 yr)

Azathioprine 1.5–2 mg/kg/day, *or*
Mycophenolate mofetil (1000–1200 mg/m^2/day) *and*
Prednisolone 0.5–1 mg/kg on alternate days; later taper

*The dose of cyclophosphamide is increased to 750 mg/m^2 if no leukopenia. Dose reduction is necessary in patients showing impaired renal function.
#Plasmapheresis should begin early, especially if patient is dialysis dependent at presentation or if biopsy shows severe histological changes (>50% crescents). Plasma exchange is useful in anti-GBM nephritis and ANCA-associated vasculitis

1. Pauci-immune, ANCA positive crescentic GN and renal failure (serum creatinine >2.5–3 mg/dL)
2. Anti-GBM disease, especially those who are anuric with severe azotemia, dialysis dependent and having more than 85% crescents on renal biopsy

Anecdotal reports confirm the effectiveness of plasmapheresis in patients with RPGN due to SLE, Henoch-Schönlein purpura and severe proliferative GN, and in life-threatening pulmonary hemorrhage. However, there is no firm evidence to support the role of plasmapheresis in patients with immune complex crescentic GN, or in those with extensive scarring and little or no activity on biopsy.

Maintenance

Most patients with ANCA-associated disease need long-term immunosuppression, due to the risk of relapses. Once disease is in remission (usually after 4–6 months of induction), therapy with cyclophosphamide is discontinued and switched to azathioprine or mycophenolate mofetil during the maintenance phase.

The duration of maintenance treatment is debatable, with most patients of pauci-immune crescentic GN treated for two or more years. The length of maintenance therapy is extended in those with Wegner's granulomatosis or persistent PR3-ANCA positivity.

Immune Complex Crescentic GN

Poststreptococcal GN presenting with extensive crescents is rare and the benefits of intensive immunosuppressive therapy are unclear, since most patients recover spontaneously. Despite the lack of evidence-based data, we propose that patients with immune complex RPGN and crescents involving 50% or more glomeruli be treated with 3–6 IV pulses of methylprednisolone, followed by tapering doses of oral steroids for 6 months. Therapy should be combined with cyclophosphamide.

Pauci-immune Crescentic GN

Induction therapy is given as above. Intensive plasma exchange for 2 weeks is advised for patients who are dialysis dependent, those with pulmonary hemorrhage or not responding satisfactorily to induction treatment. Therapy with intravenous immunoglobulin should be considered in patients with ANCA positive systemic vasculitis, refractory to induction therapy. Treatment with rituximab has been used successfully in patients with refractory Wegener's granulomatosis.

Treatment during the maintenance phase comprises of tapering doses of oral prednisolone and azathioprine for at least 24 months. A longer duration of therapy, extended up to 5 yr, is required in Wegener's granulomatosis showing relapses, elevated ANCA titers and those with PR3-ANCA.

Anti-GBM Crescentic GN

Double volume plasma exchange is done daily, and subsequently on alternate days until anti-GBM antibodies are no longer detectable (usually 2–3 weeks). Patients are also treated with IV steroids followed by oral prednisolone, with tapering over 6–9 months. Co-administration of cyclophosphamide (2 mg/kg daily for 3 months) suppresses further antibody production. Maintenance therapy is not required.

Outcome

Patients with poststreptococcal crescentic GN have a better prognosis, with most showing spontaneous improvement. The outcome in patients with pauci-immune crescentic GN, membranoproliferative glomerulonephritis and idiopathic RPGN is less favorable than Henoch Schonlein purpura or systemic lupus erythematosus.

The potential for recovery corresponds with the relative proportion of cellular or fibrous crescents, and extent of tubular atrophy, interstitial fibrosis and glomerulosclerosis. The presence of normal glomeruli is a positive predictor of dialysis independence and recovery of renal function, suggesting that the unaffected part of the kidney is vital in determining renal outcome.

SUPPORT READING

Chen M, Yu F, Wang SX, Zou WZ, Zhao MH, Wang HY. Antineutrophil cytoplasmic antibody-negative pauci-immune crescentic glomerulonephritis. J Am Soc Nephrol 2007; 18: 599–605

de Groot K, Jayne D, Tesar V, Savage C; EUVAS investigators. Randomised controlled trial of daily oral versus pulse cyclophosphamide for induction of remission in ANCA-associated systemic vasculitis. Kidney Blood Press Res 2005; 28: 103

Jayne DRW, Gaskin G, Rasmussen N, et al; on behalf of the European Vasculitis Study Group. Randomized trial of plasma exchange or high-dosage methylprednisolone as adjunctive therapy for severe renal vasculitis. J Am Soc Nephrol 2007; 18: 2180–88

Lapraik C, Watts R, Bacon P, et al, on behalf of the BSR and BHPR Standards, Guidelines and Audit Working Group. BSR and BHPR guidelines for the management of adults with ANCA associated vasculitis. Rheumatology 2007; 46: 1615–16

Tam FWK. Current pharmacotherapy for the treatment of crescentic glomerulonephritis. Exper Opin Investig Drugs 2006; 15: 1353–69

Brogan P, Eleftheriou D, Dillon MJ. Small vessel vasculitis. Pediatr Nephrol 2010: 25; 1025–35

22 Lupus Nephritis

Systemic lupus erythematosus is an uncommon, multisystem disorder that requires prompt evaluation, appropriate therapy and long-term follow up. It is characterized by widespread inflammation of connective tissues affecting the skin, joints, kidneys, heart, lungs and nervous system, with a higher rate and more severe involvement than in adults. Biopsy proven lupus nephritis, seen in 80% cases of childhood-onset SLE, is an important determinant of prognosis.

Clinical Features

The presence of 4 of 11 criteria proposed by the American College of Rheumatology suggests definite SLE; three criteria suggests probable SLE; and two criteria possible SLE (Table 22.1).

Nephritis is seen in a significant proportion of children with SLE. In the majority, renal disease manifests within 2-yr of onset of the disease. Clinical features of lupus nephritis range from minor abnormalities on urinalysis to severe renal insufficiency, proteinuria (including nephrotic syndrome, 55%), microscopic or macroscopic hematuria (80%), hypertension (40%) and decreased GFR (50%). Lupus nephritis may rarely present with acute renal failure or rapidly progressive glomerulonephritis.

The *antiphospholipid syndrome,* characterized by anticardiolipin antibodies and/or lupus anticoagulant, is relatively common in children. Patients are prone to develop both arterial and venous thrombosis. Children with

---

Table 22.1: American College of Rheumatology criteria for classification of systemic lupus erythematosus

Malar rash
Discoid rash
Photosensitivity
Oral ulcers
Arthritis
Serositis: pleuritis, pericarditis
Renal disorder: proteinuria, red blood cell casts
Neurological disorder: seizures, psychosis (after excluding other causes)
Hematological disorder: hemolytic anemia, leukopenia ($<4 \times 10^9$/L on two occasions), lymphopenia ($<1.5 \times 10^9$/L on two occasions), thrombocytopenia ($<100 \times 10^9$/L)
Immunological disorder: elevated anti-double stranded DNA, elevated anti-Smith antibodies, positive antiphospholipid antibodies
Elevated antinuclear antibodies (after excluding drug-induced lupus)

the antiphospholipid syndrome might show renal thrombotic microangiopathy and severe renal disease.

Disease activity scoring systems, such as the SLE Disease Activity Index (SLEDAI) and Systemic Lupus Activity Measure (SLAM), are helpful in monitoring disease activity and organ damage.

Investigations

Table 22.2 provides a list of investigations that help determine the severity and extent of the disease in a new patient with SLE.

Antinuclear antibody (ANA) is positive in 95% by ELISA. On immunofluorescence, a homogenous diffuse pattern is usual, while peripheral pattern is associated with active disease. The titer usually exceeds 1:80 and persists despite treatment.

Anti-double stranded DNA is specific for SLE (Table 22.3); presence of high titers is related with active lupus nephritis. Anti-Smith (Sm) antibody is specific to SLE and proposed to be a marker of central nervous system disease. Anticardiolipin antibody (IgM, IgG) should be examined in patients with recurrent thrombosis, livedo reticularis, chorea, cerebrovascular accidents and hypertension; lupus anticoagulant is also estimated. Estimation of complement C3, C4 is useful for monitoring activity.

In addition to standard care, the assessment of patients includes regular evaluation for disease activity, organ damage, general quality of life, drug toxicity and risk factors for cardiovascular events.

Renal Biopsy

The indications for kidney biopsy include the presence of: *(i)* active urinary sediment, *(ii)* proteinuria, and *(iii)* elevated serum creatinine. The current classification of lupus nephritis, proposed by the International Society of Nephrology (ISN) and Renal Pathology

Table 22.2: Investigations at onset of systemic lupus erythematosus
Blood investigations
Hemoglobin, total and differential leukocyte count, platelets
Erythrocyte sedimentation rate (ESR) and C-reactive protein (CRP)
Urea, creatinine, electrolytes; calcium, phosphate, alkaline phosphatase
Transaminases, protein, albumin
Serology
Antinuclear antibody (ANA), anti-double stranded DNA
Complement C3, C4
Anti-Ro, anti-La, anti-ribonucleoprotein, anti-Smith, anti-phospholipid antibodies
Urinalysis
Microscopy
Urine protein to creatinine ratio (Up/Uc); 24-hr protein and creatinine excretion
Others
Lipid profile; thyroid functions (T3, T4, TSH)
Chest X-ray, tuberculin test
Renal ultrasound
Bleeding time, clotting time, prothrombin time
Pulmonary function tests, electrocardiography, echocardiography in selected cases
Screening for hepatitis B, hepatitis C, human immunodeficiency virus

Society (RPS) in 2002, attempts to standardize definitions, emphasize clinically relevant lesions and encourage uniform and reproducible reporting (Table 22.4).

Up to half (50–80%) of all children with lupus nephritis have the most severe class (class IV or diffuse lupus nephritis) (Fig. 22.1). The subgroup of diffuse global sclerosing lupus nephritis is associated with unsatisfactory outcome.

Active and chronic histological lesions should be defined. Features of activity, which are potentially reversible, include the presence of cellular crescents, endocapillary proliferation, fibrinoid necrosis, karyorrhexis, thrombi and wire loops. The presence of glomerulosclerosis, fibrous crescents, and

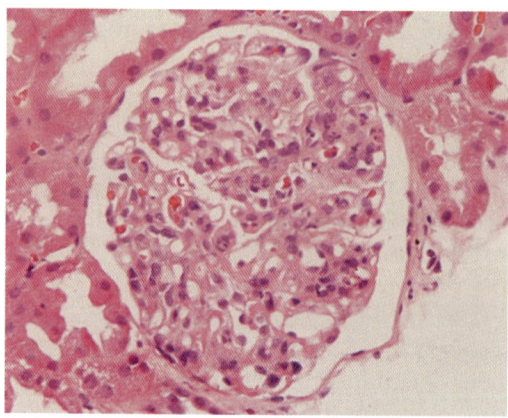

Fig. 22.1: Light microscopy (hematoxylin and eosin) showing endocapillary and mesangial proliferation, with luminal occlusion, suggestive of diffuse proliferative lupus nephritis (Class IV)

Table 22.3: Autoantibodies in patients with lupus nephritis

	Frequency	Specificity	Association with disease activity
Anti-ds DNA	40–90%	High	Yes
Anti-SSA/Ro	35%	Low	No
Anti-SSB/La	15%	Low	No
Anti-Sm	5–30%	High	No
Anti-C1q	80–100%	High	Yes

C1q complement factor 1q; ds-DNA double stranded DNA; SSA Sjögren syndrome A; SSB Sjögren syndrome B; Sm Smith

Table 22.4: Classification of International Society of Nephrology/ Renal Pathology Society (ISN/RPS)

WHO Class	ISN/RPS Histological class
Class I	*Minimal mesangial lupus nephritis:* Normal glomeruli by LM; mesangial immune deposits by IF or EM
Class II	*Mesangial proliferative lupus nephritis:* Pure mesangial hypercellularity of any degree or mesangial matrix expansion by LM with mesangial immune deposits, with none or few isolated subepithelial or subendothelial deposits by IF or EM
Class III	*Focal lupus nephritis* involving <50% glomeruli: III (A); III (A/C); III (C)
Class IV	*Diffuse lupus nephritis segmental (IV-S) or global (IV-G)* involving >50% glomeruli: IV-S (A); IV-S (A/C); IV-S (C); IV-G (A); IV-G (A/C); IV-G (C)
Class V	*Membranous lupus nephritis:* pure membranous; V+III; V+IV depending on degree of proliferation
Class VI	*Advanced sclerosing lupus nephritis:* >90% glomeruli show global sclerosis with no evidence of ongoing active glomerular disease

A active; C chronic; S segmental; G global
LM light microscopy; IF immunofluorescence; EM electron microscopy

tubular and interstitial fibrosis are features of chronicity.

Severity of SLE

For purpose of management, non-renal involvement in SLE is classified as mild, moderate and severe:

Mild: Arthritis, mild cutaneous lesions, non-active pleuritis or pericarditis

Moderate: Active pleuritis and pericarditis, thrombocytopenia, severe cutaneous lesions

Severe: Pulmonary hemorrhage, central nervous system disease.

TREATMENT OF LUPUS NEPHRITIS

Histological grading of the renal biopsy is helpful in deciding therapy.

Class II Lupus Nephritis

Prednisolone (1 mg/kg/d) is tapered to maintenance dose, administered along with azathioprine (2–2.5 mg/kg/day) for 12–24 months.

Class III/IV/III+V/IV+V Lupus Nephritis

Prolonged therapy is necessary for patients with proliferative lupus nephritis. Therefore, an initial *induction treatment* (5–6 months) is followed by prolonged *maintenance therapy* (for 3–5 years, even longer). The goals of continued immunosuppressive therapy are to avoid relapse and flares of disease activity, avoid smoldering activity resulting in chronic damage and prevent long-term side effects of therapy.

Induction Therapy

The choice between administration of IV methylprednisolone (500 mg/m^2, maximum dose 1 g; for 3–5 consecutive days) or high dose prednisolone is dictated by the severity of the illness. Therapy is then switched to prednisolone (1–2 mg/kg/d, maximum dose 60 mg) for 6–8 weeks.

Therapy should simultaneously include the use of IV cyclophosphamide (500–750 mg/m^2 monthly for 6 months) beginning soon after initiation of corticosteroid treatment. It is necessary to keep the child well hydrated and to administer MESNA to reduce the risk of hemorrhagic cystitis. Details on administration of these medications are provided in Chapter 43.

After 8 weeks, the dose of prednisolone is reduced by 2.5 mg every week for doses above 20 mg, by 2.5 mg every 2–4 weeks for doses between 10–20 mg and 2.5 mg every 4–8 weeks for doses below 10 mg. Alternate day doses are used once prednisolone dose is below 10 mg.

Patients who do not show remission despite 6-doses of IV cyclophosphamide might benefit from treatment with mycophenolate mofetil (MMF, 1000 mg/m^2 daily in two divided doses).

There is increasing evidence from studies in adults that oral MMF may be equally good for induction treatment as IV cyclophosphamide. Patients treated with the former show similar efficacy but significantly lower side effects compared to those receiving cyclophosphamide.

Patients with severe and refractory SLE, e.g. crescentic glomerulonephritis and/or cerebral lupus may be treated with 5-10 sessions of plasma exchange, often combined with IV rituximab (two IV doses of 500–750 mg/m^2 given 1–2 weeks apart). Treatment with intravenous immunoglobulin (2 g/kg; maximum 70 g) should be considered for patients with severe hematological disease, ascending polyneuritis and severe cardiac failure.

Maintenance therapy

Patients with class III and IV lupus nephritis require maintenance therapy for prolonged periods. It is recommended to use the lowest and best tolerated immunosuppressive agent. Any of the following regimens might be used for maintenance therapy:

1. *Prednisolone and MMF:* MMF is used at a dose of 500–1000 mg/m²/day, in 2 divided doses. Patients with gastrointestinal side effects benefit either by substituting to mycophenolate sodium or giving MMF 3 times a day. The dose of prednisolone is tapered to 5–10 mg daily or on alternate days

2. *Prednisolone and azathioprine:* The dose of prednisolone is tapered as above. Azathioprine (2–2.5 mg/kg/day) is safe and well tolerated. Both azathioprine and MMF show efficacy in maintaining remission and preventing relapses. The equivalence of MMF and azathioprine for maintenance therapy is demonstrated in recent studies that show similar rates of remission and disease flares.

Class V Lupus Nephritis

For patients with pure membranous lupus nephritis (Fig. 22.2), therapy is provided with a combination of prednisolone and either of the following: *(i)* MMF; *(ii)* cyclosporine or tacrolimus; *(iii)* azathioprine; or *(iv)* IV cyclophosphamide. Treatment with prednisolone and MMF might be preferred at the first instance.

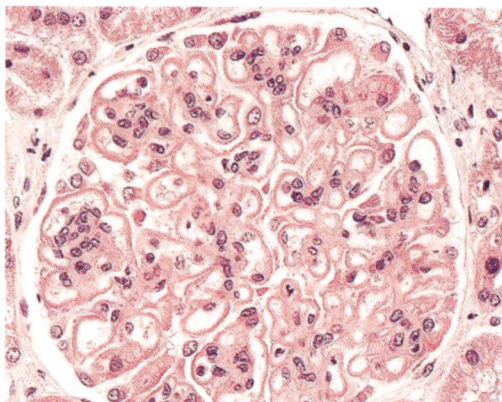

Fig. 22.2: Light microscopy (hematoxylin and eosin) showing glomerulus with stiff and diffusely thickened capillary walls, patent capillary lumina and lack of proliferation, suggesting membranous lupus nephritis (Class V)

The combination of MMF and a calcineurin inhibitor may be useful for patients with refractory class IV or V lupus nephritis or a combination of these lesions.

Duration of Treatment

Maintenance doses of corticosteroids are administered for 5 years after remission, following which they may be tapered and stopped. Surveillance for disease reactivation should continue indefinitely.

General Management

All patients are advised the following:

1. Sunscreen with sun protection factor (SPF) >15

2. Hydroxychloroquine sulfate (HCQ) is beneficial in children with skin disease and arthritis, and has a steroid sparing effect. HCQ reduces steroid induced hyperlipidemia and the risk for atherosclerosis. Color vision should be checked annually.

3. Treatment with naproxen (15–20 mg/kg/d) or ibuprofen (40 mg/kg/d) is recommended for patients with systemic and musculoskeletal features. Prolonged therapy is not necessary.

4. Angiotensin converting enzyme inhibitors (ACEI) are preferred agents for the management of hypertension and/or proteinuria.

5. HMG CoA reductase inhibitors are recommended for patients with dyslipidemia.

6. Patients receiving long term steroids should receive supplements of calcium and vitamin D.

7. Immunization: Live vaccines are contraindicated in patients taking prednisolone at a dose of 2 mg/kg per day or, for patients weighing >10 kg, a maximum of 20 mg/day. Patients receiving other immunosuppressive medications should also not be given live vaccines. The following killed vaccines are not associated with disease flares and the

majority of patients develop protective antibodies: *(i)* flu, *(ii)* pneumococcal, *(iii)* hepatitis B, and *(iv)* tetanus toxoid. Pneumococcal vaccination is recommended for patients on long term corticosteroids (Appendix 13).

8. Management of infections: Children on immunosuppressive treatment are susceptible to severe infections, including septicemia, disseminated varicella and tuberculosis. Prompt medical advice should be sought in these cases; most patients with serious infections require stress doses of corticosteroids.

Antiphospholipid Syndrome

A high proportion of patients with SLE have IgG antiphospholipid antibodies, without evidence of thrombosis. Patients with the antiphospholipid syndrome (APS) show radiological or histological features of arterial, venous or small vessel thrombosis. The detection of any of the following antibodies is necessary: (i) lupus anticoagulant; (ii) anticardiolipin antibodies; and (iii) anti-β_2 glycoprotein-1 antibody.

Patients with SLE and persistent high titer of antiphospholipid antibodies are at risk of a thrombotic event, and should receive low dose aspirin (3–5 mg/kg/d). Concomitantly, HCQ should be administered since it has a modest anticoagulant role. Prophylaxis with low molecular weight heparin is considered during high risk situations such as surgery and prolonged immobilization.

The management of acute thrombosis is similar to that from other causes. In the acute phase, patients are treated with either unfractionated IV heparin or low molecular weight heparin subcutaneously. The latter is preferred in view of ease of administration, predictable dose response and need for less rigorous monitoring. The activated partial thromboplastin time is inaccurate for monitoring, since it may be altered by the lupus anticoagulant.

Patients subsequently receive long term therapy with warfarin, aiming for a target international normalized ratio (INR) of 2–3 for patients with venous or non-cerebral arterial thrombosis, and 1.4–2.8 in ischemic stroke. Patients with recurrent thrombosis may benefit from the use of rituximab. Thrombotic features and complications may recur during pregnancy.

Monitoring

Patients with no evidence of activity, and in the absence of organ damage and comorbidities should be assessed every 6 months. During these evaluations, emphasis is given to discussion of preventive measures such as sun avoidance, adequate vitamin D and calcium intake, weight control and measures to reduce cardiovascular risk. Patients in whom immunosuppressive therapy is being reduced need to be monitored for reactivation of disease, especially those with renal disease, which may recur without symptoms.

Follow up visits need to be more frequent in patients with lupus nephritis. The following investigations are recommended every 6–12 months:

1. Complete blood count, erythrocyte sedimentation rate, C-reactive protein
2. Blood creatinine, albumin
3. Urinalysis, estimation of urine protein to creatinine ratio
4. Anti-ds DNA, C3, C4.

An elevated CRP that exceeds 20 mg/dL suggests complicating infection, serositis or arthritis. Values exceeding 50 mg/dL indicate a superimposed infection. While increase in anti-ds DNA antibody titers correlate with disease activity, therapy need not be modified in the absence of clinical activity. Anti-Ro/Sjögren syndrome antigen A (SSA) and anti-La (SSB) antibodies are associated with occurrence of neonatal lupus.

Glomerulonephritis

Table 22.5: Diagnosis and management of renal flares

Flare	Manifestation	Therapy
Mild	Increase in hematuria; stable serum creatinine; no proteinuria	Pre-flare prednisolone dose <15 mg/d: Increase dose to 0.5 mg/kg/d (maximum 25 mg) Pre-flare prednisolone dose >15 mg/d: Treat as moderate flare
Moderate	Serum creatinine <1.5 mg/dl; increased proteinuria to 2+	Increase prednisolone dose to 1 mg/kg/d (maximum 40 mg)
Severe	Serum creatinine >1.5 mg/dl; increased proteinuria to 3+/4+	Increase prednisolone dose to 2 mg/kg/d (maximum 60 mg) for 4–6 weeks; taper

Renal Flares

Reactivation of lupus nephritis should be classified and treated as shown in Table 22.5. Abnormalities on urinalysis should be confirmed on 2 occasions, 1–2 weeks apart.

A repeat renal biopsy is not required for renal flares that are successfully managed. A biopsy, indicated if there is failure to respond to 4–6 weeks of appropriate therapy, aims to examine for histological activity and its severity. A renal biopsy also enables exclusion of conditions requiring major modification of treatment, *e.g.*, advanced glomerular or interstitial fibrosis, or the appearance of thrombotic glomerulopathy.

Support Reading

Weening JJ, D'Agati VD, Schwartz MM, et al, on behalf of the ISN/RPS Working Group on the Classification of Lupus Nephritis. The classification of glomerulonephritis in systemic lupus erythematosus revisited. Kidney Int 2004; 65: 521–30

Mosca M, Tani C, Aringer M, et al. European League Against Rheumatism recommendations for monitoring patients with systemic lupus erythematosus in clinical practice and in observational studies. Ann Rheum Dis 2010; 69: 1269–74

Bomback AS, Appel GB. Updates on the treatment of lupus nephritis. J Am Soc Nephrol 2010; 21: 2028–35

23

Henoch-Schönlein Purpura

Henoch-Schönlein purpura (HSP) is an immunoglobulin-A mediated systemic vasculitis. The disease usually has a self-limited course affecting the skin, joints, gastrointestinal tract and the kidneys.

Etiology

The etiology is unclear. Since HSP often follows an upper respiratory tract infection and occurs commonly in winters, numerous pathogens, particularly β-hemolytic streptococci, are reported to trigger HSP. Other associated conditions include infections such as measles, parvovirus B19, rubella, mumps, Coxsackie virus, mycoplasma, adenovirus, staphylococci and *Campylobacter jejuni*; insect bites and food allergens. The pathogenesis of nephritis is mediated by increased IgA1 concentration in the serum and deposition of polymeric IgA1 in the glomerular mesangium.

Clinical Features

HSP commonly affects children between 3 and 10 years, with a male predominance. The onset is acute with major features occurring over a period of weeks. Typically, purpuric rash, joint involvement and abdominal pain appear within 1–2 days of each other.

Cutaneous: Palpable, purpuric rash appears in crops over dependent or pressure-bearing areas, particularly malleoli of ankles, dorsum of legs (Fig. 23.1) and glutei. Young children (<3 year old) may present with subcutaneous

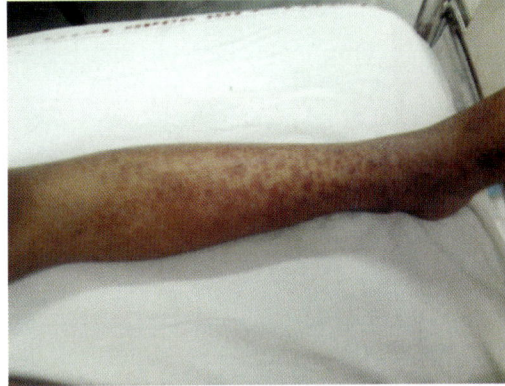

Fig. 23.1: Henoch-Schönlein purpura in a 6-yr-old girl admitted with severe abdominal pain. Note purpuric rash over the lower limbs

edema over scalp, periorbital region, dorsa of hands and feet and scrotum.

Gastrointestinal: Abdominal pain and gastrointestinal hemorrhage are common features, preceding the rash or occurring within 1–4 weeks of its onset. Colicky and periumbilical abdominal pain occurs in over two-thirds of patients.

Gastrointestinal hemorrhage may be occult, or cause hematemesis, melena or frank bleeding per rectum. Intussusception (2–3%), bowel ischemia and infarction, fistula, stricture and hemorrhagic pancreatitis are uncommon.

Joints: Joint involvement, seen in two-thirds of the patients, is the first symptom in 25%. Knees and ankles are commonly affected; the involvement of wrists, elbows and small joints of fingers is less common. There is periarticular swelling, joint pain, tenderness and limitation of movement. The symptoms resolve in a few days without sequelae.

Renal: Renal involvement (*Henoch-Schönlein nephritis*) occurs in 20–40% patients. Renal manifestations usually present within 3 months of onset; in less than 10% they may occur after other systemic features have resolved. Usual renal manifestations include microscopic hematuria (4–100%), macroscopic hematuria (8–80%) and proteinuria (45–100%). Rarely, rapidly progressive renal failure may be seen. Risk factors for the occurrence of nephritis are:

1. Age at onset greater than 7 years
2. Severe abdominal pain with gastrointestinal bleeding
3. Persistent purpura for over 1 month
4. Coagulation factor XIII activity less than 80%.

Genitourinary complications: These include orchitis (2–35% patients) and epididymitis. Periureteral vasculitis, ureteral ischemia and priapism are uncommon.

Other complications: Rare systemic manifestations include neurological involvement (behavioral changes, seizures, altered sensorium, Guillain Barre syndrome) and pulmonary hemorrhage.

Infantile HSP

HSP during infancy (Seidelmayer syndrome) is less common and has distinctive clinical features. An acute onset of purpura is noted with ecchymoses and inflammatory edema of limbs and face. Skin manifestations occur in a medallion-like pattern on the face, auricles and extremities. Renal disease and other visceral manifestations are uncommon.

Course and Recurrences

The average duration of the disease is 4 weeks. The disease may have a protracted course over many years with remissions and recurrences. Almost half of the patients have one or more recurrences in the initial 6 weeks. These episodes are similar to but milder as compared to the initial episode. Cutaneous, renal and gastrointestinal involvement is common during recurrences.

Diagnosis

The diagnosis of HSP is predominantly based on clinical features. A set of criteria for the diagnosis of Henoch-Schönlein purpura are listed in Table 23.1.

Table 23.1: Classification criteria for Henoch-Schönlein purpura

Mandatory criterion	
Purpura	Purpura (palpable, in crops) or petechiae with lower limb predominance*, not related to thrombocytopenia
And at least 1 out of the following	
Abdominal pain	Diffuse, acute, colicky pain; may include intussusception and gastrointestinal bleeding
Histopathology	Leukocytoclastic vasculitis with predominant IgA deposits; proliferative glomerulonephritis with predominant IgA deposits
Arthritis or arthralgia	Acute joint pain with or without swelling or limitation on motion
Renal involvement	Proteinuria >0.3 g/24 hr; or ≥ 2+ on dipstick Hematuria, red cell casts

*If purpura has atypical distribution, demonstration of IgA deposit on biopsy is required

Investigations

1. *Complete blood count:* Normocytic normochromic anemia, leukocytosis with shift to the left, mild elevation of platelet count; increased erythrocyte sedimentation rate
2. *Blood urea and creatinine:* Increased levels suggest acute nephritic syndrome or rapidly progressive glomerulonephritis
3. *Urinalysis:* Microscopic or gross hematuria; variable proteinuria (trace to nephrotic range)
4. *Antinuclear antibody* and *rheumatoid factor* are negative and *complement levels* (C3 and C4) are normal
5. *Elevated serum IgA* is seen in more than 50% patients, but is not required for the diagnosis. Patients may show IgA antinuclear cytoplasmic antibodies and/or antiendothelial cell antibodies
6. *Biopsy of the involved skin* shows leukocytoclastic vasculitis involving capillaries and venules of the upper and mid-dermis. Immunofluorescence shows perivascular IgA, and occasionally C3 and fibrinogen deposits (Fig. 23. 2).

Indications for Kidney Biopsy

A renal biopsy is required in patients with HSP with:

1. Nephrotic range proteinuria and/or nephrotic syndrome
2. Nephritic syndrome (hematuria, proteinuria) and impaired renal function

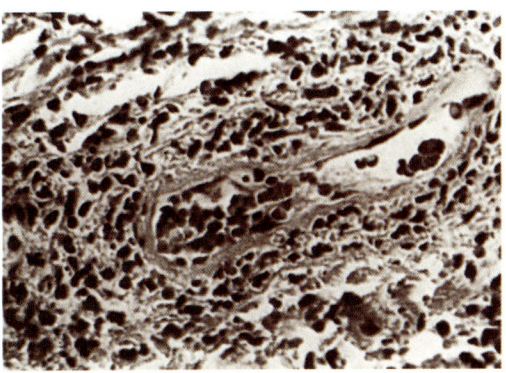

Fig. 23.2: Leukocytoclastic vasculitis. The characteristic nuclear dust is seen as granular, darkstained material in the vessel wall (hematoxylin and eosin)

3. Rapidly progressive renal failure.

Table 23.2 shows a histological classification of Henoch-Schönlein nephritis.

Management

HSP is usually a self-limiting condition with more than 50% patients undergoing spontaneous remissions. Most patients require only supportive treatment (Table 23.3).

Joint involvement (arthritis, arthralgia or inflammatory soft tissue edema) is managed with analgesics like acetaminophen or nonsteroidal anti-inflammatory drugs.

Severe *gastrointestinal manifestations*, including acute abdomen or gastrointestinal bleeding resolve rapidly with a short course of prednisolone at a dose of 1 to 2 mg/kg per day for one

Table 23.2: Histological classification of Henoch-Schönlein nephritis

Grade I	Minor glomerular abnormalities
Grade II	Pure mesangial proliferation (a, focal; b, diffuse)
Grade III	Minor glomerular abnormalities or mesangial proliferation with crescents/segmental lesions in less than 50% glomeruli (a, focal; b, diffuse mesangial proliferation)
Grade IV	Similar to grade III but with crescents/segmental lesions in 50–75% of glomeruli (a, focal; b, diffuse mesangial proliferation)
Grade V	Similar to grade III but with crescents/segmental lesion in more than 75% of glomeruli (a, focal; b, diffuse mesangial proliferation)
Grade VI	Lesion resembling membranoproliferative glomerulonephritis

Table 23.3: Therapy of patients with Henoch-Schönlein purpura

Clinical features	Supportive care	Corticosteroids		Plasmapheresis
		Per oral	Intravenous	
Rash, edema, arthritis	X , NSAIDs			
Rash, severe edema	X	X		
Severe colic	X	X		
Orchitis	X	X		
Nephrotic syndrome	X	X*	?X	
RPGN	X	X*	X	X
Pulmonary bleed	X	X*	X	X

NSAIDs: nonsteroidal anti-inflammatory drugs; RPGN: rapidly progressive glomerulonephritis
*Along with immunosuppressive drugs

week followed by tapering over the next 2 to 3 weeks (Table 23.3). Orchitis may benefit from a 2–3 weeks course of corticosteroids.

Long-term morbidity and mortality in patients with HSP is exclusively attributed to renal manifestations. *There is no evidence that a short course of corticosteroid therapy is effective in preventing nephritis in subjects with HSP.* In the absence of evidence based guidelines on therapy of Henoch Schönlein nephritis, therapy is guided by clinical presentation.

Minor urinary abnormalities (microscopic hematuria, non-nephrotic range proteinuria with normal renal function): These patients need close follow up for 12 months to monitor progression of renal involvement.

Nephrotic or acute nephritic syndrome: Therapy is started with a combination of prednisolone (2 mg/kg daily for 4 weeks, 1.5 mg/kg alternate days for 4 weeks, subsequent tapering to 0.5 mg/kg on alternate days) and azathioprine (1–2 mg/kg daily) for 6–12 months.

Rapidly progressive (crescentic) glomerulonephritis: Three to six intravenous pulses of high dose methylprednisolone (20–30 mg/kg) are administered, followed by oral prednisolone (2 mg/kg/d for 4 weeks, subsequently 1–1.5 mg/kg on alternate days for the next 8 weeks, and tapered to 0.5 mg/kg for 12–18 months). Co-administration of cyclophosphamide (2 mg/kg/d for 12 weeks) followed by azathioprine for 12–18 months is beneficial. Patients who do not show improvement in renal function despite high dose IV or oral corticosteroids may benefit from 10–12 sessions of intensive plasmapheresis.

Other medications that have been used for nephritis include cyclosporine and mycophenolate mofetil. A combination of IV urokinase, warfarin, dipyridamole, prednisolone and cyclophosphamide was found useful in subjects with rapidly progressive glomerulonephritis. Fish oil (1g twice a day) has been used to decrease proteinuria, with equivocal results.

ACE inhibitors (enalapril, lisinopril, ramipril) are effective in treating hypertension and reducing proteinuria, and delaying the progression of renal disease.

Prognosis

Most patients with HSP have a satisfactory outcome. While the majority of patients with hematuria and non-nephrotic proteinuria maintain normal renal function, about 5% progress to end stage renal disease over 10–25 years. Patients with a nephritic or nephrotic syndrome at the onset, and/or more than 50% crescents on renal histology, have a poorer prognosis. Over 50% of these patients have hypertension and impaired renal function and 20% progress to chronic renal failure and end stage renal disease.

Henoch-Schönlein nephritis accounts for almost 2% of pediatric renal transplants. Following transplant, histological recurrence may occur in nearly 50% cases. Clinical recurrence is uncommon (20%) and graft failure or loss is rare.

SUPPORT READING

Brogan P, Bagga A. Leukocytoclastic vasculitis. In: Cassidy JT, Petty RE, Laxer RM, Lindsay CB, eds. Textbook of Pediatric Rheumatology, 6th edn. Philadelphia, Saunders Elsevier, 2011; pp 483–97

Gedalia A. Henoch-Schönlein purpura. Current Rheumatol Reports 2004; 6: 195–202

Ballinger S. Henoch-Schönlein purpura. Curr Opin Rheumatol 2003; 15: 591–94

Ozen S, Ruperto N, Dillon MJ, et al. The EULAR/ PRES endorsed consensus criteria for the classification of childhood vasculitides. Ann Rheumatol Dis 2006; 65: 936–41

24 IgA Nephropathy

Definition

IgA nephropathy is characterized by the presence of predominant IgA deposits in the glomeruli. The diagnosis of primary IgA nephropathy is made in the absence of systemic disease (Henoch-Schönlein purpura, systemic lupus erythematosus), cutaneous or liver disease, and malabsorption syndromes, which are associated with similar immunofluorescence findings.

Clinical Features

The onset of primary IgA nephropathy is usually in the teens. The disease may have a variety of presentations ranging from microscopic or gross hematuria (isolated, or accompanied by non-nephrotic proteinuria), to nephrotic syndrome, acute nephritic syndrome and rapidly progressive glomerulonephritis with extensive crescent formation on biopsy (Table 24.1). Although microscopic hematuria is the most common presentation, gross hematuria occurs in 30–40% children. Recurrent episodes of gross hematuria occur concomitant with upper respiratory tract infections, vaccination or heavy physical exercise.

Evaluation

The diagnosis is suspected in patients showing persistent microscopic hematuria, recurrent episodes of gross hematuria, and

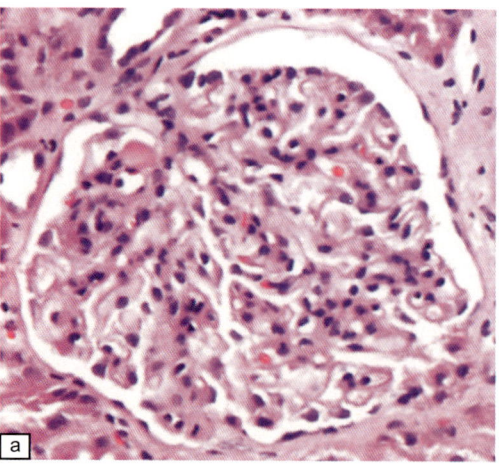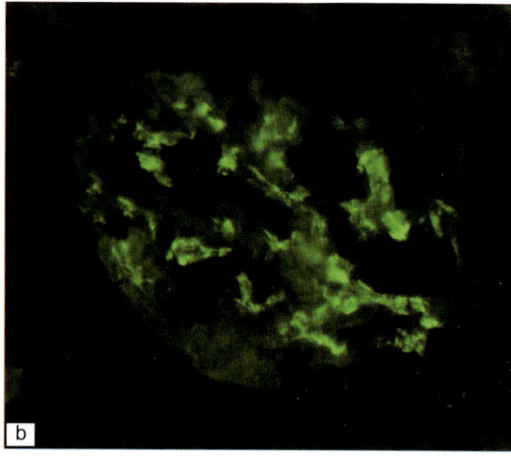

Fig. 24.1: IgA nephropathy. (a) Light microscopy showing moderate mesangial proliferation (H&E); (b) Immunofluorescence showing positive staining for IgA in mesangial areas.

nephrotic syndrome with hematuria. Uncommon presentations include an acute nephritic syndrome or rapidly progressive glomerulonephritis.

High levels of IgA are present in almost one-third patients. Complement levels (C3, C4) are normal. Blood levels of urea and creatinine correlate with the degree of renal dysfunction.

Urinalysis shows proteinuria and presence of red blood cells with or without red cell or granular casts. Estimation of 24-hr urine protein excretion or urinary protein/creati-nine ratio should be done at initial evaluation and follow up.

Renal Histology

In order of increasing severity of renal damage, the renal histology in IgA nephropathy has been classified as follows:

1. Minimal or no mesangial hypercellularity without glomerular sclerosis
2. Focal and segmental glomerulosclerosis without active cellular proliferation
3. Focal proliferative glomerulonephritis

Table 24.1: Treatment of IgA nephropathy based on clinical presentation

Clinical presentation	Therapy
Isolated microscopic* or gross hematuria; normal renal function, no proteinuria	No specific treatment; regular surveillance (monitor urine protein 3–6 monthly)
Microscopic or gross hematuria with non-nephrotic proteinuria	
Proteinuria <0.5 g/1.73 m²/day	No specific treatment
Proteinuria 0.5–1 g/1.73 m²/day	ACEI or ARB**
Nephrotic range proteinuria or onset with nephrotic syndrome	Prednisolone 2 mg/kg/d for 4 wk, with taper (1.5 mg/kg alternate day for 4 wk; 1 mg/kg alternate day for 6 months; 0.5 mg/kg alternate day for 1 yr), with Cyclophosphamide 2 mg/kg/day for 3 months, followed by Azathioprine 1.5–2 mg/kg/day for 2 yr, and ACEI or ARB
Acute nephritic syndrome; no crescents on biopsy	Prednisolone (1 mg/kg alternate day for 6 months; 0.5 mg/kg alternate day for at least 1 year) and Azathioprine 1.5–2 mg/kg/day for 2 years
Rapidly progressive glomerulonephritis; with crescents involving >30% glomeruli	Induction[#] Methylprednisolone (3–5 alternate day pulses; 10 mg/kg), followed by Prednisolone (1 mg/kg alternate day for 6 months; 0.5 mg/kg alternate day for 1 year) and Cyclophosphamide (500 mg/m² IV q month for 6 month Maintenance Prednisone tapering as above and Azathioprine 1.5–2 mg/kg/day for 2 years
Advanced disease; GFR <30 mL/min/1.73 m², high chronicity index	Immunosuppression not useful; supportive therapy

* Isolated microscopic hematuria is often detected at routine medical examination
** Angiotensin converting enzyme inhibitors (ACEI) or angiotensin receptor blockers (ARB) benefit patients with hypertension and proteinuria
# Plasmapheresis might be considered in patients with dialysis dependency

24

4. Diffuse proliferative glomerulonephritis
5. Biopsy showing ≥40% globally sclerotic glomeruli, and/or ≥40% cortical tubular atrophy

Recently, the International IgA Nephropathy Network and Renal Pathology Society have proposed the Oxford Classification that defines and scores four parameters based on changes in the mesangium (M), endocapillary proliferation (E), glomerulosclerosis (S) and tubular atrophy and interstitial fibrosis (T). Severity of these histological changes is associated with unsatisfactory outcome.

Therapy

While usually benign, children with IgA nephropathy and nephrotic range proteinuria are at risk for progressive disease. The treatment of IgA nephropathy depends on the clinical features (Table 24.1).

Prognosis

Important factors determining progression of disease are presence of heavy proteinuria, reduced renal function at onset, persistent hypertension and significant changes on biopsy (sclerosis in >20% of glomeruli, crescents, tubulointerstitial disease).

SUPPORT READING

Hogg RJ. Idiopathic immunoglobulin A nephropathy in children and adolescents. Pediatr Nephrol 2010; 25: 823–29

Roberts IS, Cook HT, Troyanov S. The Oxford classification of IgA nephropathy: pathology definitions, correlations and reproducibility. Working Group of the International IgA Nephropathy Network and the Renal Pathology Society. Kidney Int 2009; 76: 546–56

Haas M. Histologic subclassification of IgA nephropathy: a clinicopathologic study of 244 cases. Am J Kidney Dis 1997; 29: 829–42

25 Membranous Nephropathy

Membranous nephropathy (MGN) is uncommon in childhood, responsible for <2% cases of nephrotic syndrome. Most patients present in later childhood or adolescence. The majority (40–75%) presents with nephrotic syndrome, occasionally with asymptomatic proteinuria with or without microscopic hematuria.

Etiology

Although idiopathic in many cases, the condition may be secondary to systemic lupus erythematosus, viral infections (hepatitis B or C; Ebstein Barr virus), sickle cell hemoglobinopathy and medications (penicillamine, gold salts).

Diagnosis

The diagnosis of MGN is based on the characteristic histology. The glomerular capillary wall is thickened and shows spikes on silver methenamine and periodic acid-Schiff stains. On immunofluorescence, granular staining for IgG and complement C3 is found along the capillary wall. Electron microscopy shows multiple, finely granular, electron dense deposits along the subepithelial surface.

Evaluation

Findings of mesangial or endocapillary proliferation, a "full-house" pattern of immunoglobulin and C1q staining on immunofluorescence suggest the diagnosis of lupus erythematosus. Deposits in drug induced MGN may be subendothelial, rather than subepithelial and intramembranous.

The diagnosis of idiopathic MGN follows exclusion of specific etiologies. The evaluation includes:

1. Complete blood counts; levels of urea, creatinine, albumin and cholesterol
2. Urinalysis for microscopic hematuria and proteinuria
3. Complement C3 levels
4. Hepatitis B surface antigen, hepatitis C antibody, anti HIV antibody, antinuclear antibodies.

Treatment

Asymptomatic, Non-nephrotic Proteinuria

For patients with no edema, normal serum albumin and urine protein to creatinine ratio (Up/Uc) 0.2–2, immunosuppression is not required. Therapy with angiotensin converting enzyme inhibitors (ACEI) or angiotensin receptor blockers (ARB) achieves reduction in proteinuria. Enalapril or ramipril are effective agents.

Nephrotic Syndrome

Therapy is instituted with oral prednisolone at 1.5 mg/kg on alternate days for 4 weeks, then 1 mg/kg for 12-24 months and tapered.

Additionally, these patients should receive treatment with oral cyclophosphamide (2 mg/kg/day for 12 weeks), with close monitoring for side effects. Alternatively patients may receive therapy with cyclosporine (3–5 mg/kg/day) or tacrolimus (0.1–0.2 mg/kg/day) with oral steroids for 12–24 months. Cyclosporine is known to induce partial or complete remission in 50-60% of patients, but relapses are common when discontinued. Prolonged therapy with low dose cyclosporine or tacrolimus should be considered for patients with partial remission.

In patients with deteriorating renal function and/or persistent heavy proteinuria, calcineurin inhibitors may be preferred as first line therapy.

Mycophenolate mofetil (600–1000 mg/m^2 per day) and rituximab (375 mg/m^2 once weekly for 4 weeks) have also been used with beneficial effects in uncontrolled trials in adults with idiopathic MGN.

Monitoring

Blood levels of albumin, cholesterol and creatinine, and urinary protein excretion (24–hr, spot specimens) are monitored every 3 months. Spontaneous remission and relapses are noted.

Outcome

Features associated with a better prognosis include onset in childhood, non-nephrotic proteinuria, normal renal function at onset, and favorable response to treatment. Poor prognostic factors on histology include: *(i)* segmental glomerular sclerosis, *(ii)* tubulo-interstitial damage and *(iii)* ultrastructural findings of intramembranous deposits with thickening and dissolution of the basement membrane.

SUPPORT READING

Menon S, Valentini RP. Membranous nephropathy in children: clinical presentation and therapeutic approach. Pediatr Nephrol 2010; 25: 1419–28

Ponticelli C, Passerini P. Management of idiopathic membranous nephropathy. Expert Opin Pharmacother 2010; 11: 2163–75

Membranoproliferative Glomerulonephritis

Membranoproliferative or mesangiocapillary glomerulonephritis (MPGN) refers to a pattern of glomerular injury seen in a variety of diseases characterized by complement activation.

Classification

Light microscopy shows diffuse mesangial cell proliferation and thickening of capillary walls due to subendothelial extension of the mesangium. Based on findings on immunofluorescence and electron microscopy, 3 types are recognized.

Type I (classical MPGN): This is the most common type, characterized by subendothelial immune complexes deposits, secondary to activation of the classic complement pathway.

Type II (dense deposit disease): This type shows dense deposits within the glomerular basement membrane and absence of immune complexes. An immunoglobulin, the *C3 nephritic factor (C3NeF)*, stabilizes C3 convertase (C3bBb) resulting in activated alternative complement pathway. Some patients show C3, but no dense deposits in the basement membrane (C3 glomerulonephritis).

Type III MPGN: Considered a variant of type I, this subtype has subendothelial and subepithelial deposits.

Clinical Features

MPGN accounts for 5–7% of primary nephrotic syndrome in children. Features include nephrotic syndrome (40–70%), asymptomatic proteinuria and hematuria (20–30%), hypertension (30–50%), acute nephritic syndrome (16–30%), recurrent gross hematuria (10–20%) and azotemia (rare). The presence of partial lipodystrophy or retinal deposits of *drusen* (macular degeneration) suggests MPGN type II.

Histology

Findings include enlarged hypercellular glomeruli with lobular accentuation, increase in mesangial matrix and cellularity, and neutrophilic and monocytic infiltration (Fig. 26.1). A tram track or double contoured appearance of the capillary wall, resulting from subendothelial extension of mesangium (mesangial interposition) is best seen on methenamine silver (Fig. 26.1) or periodic acid-Schiff staining.

Immunofluorescence examination in type I MPGN shows C3 and IgG deposits in a granular pattern, predominantly on capillary walls and variably in mesangium. In type II disease, C3 is deposited in an irregular granular pattern on either side of the basement membrane.

Electron microscopy in type II MPGN reveals deposits in the sites described above, in addition to discontinuous, amorphous electron dense deposits within the glomerular basement membrane (Fig. 26.2).

Evaluation

The diagnosis of idiopathic MPGN follows exclusion of specific etiologies, including

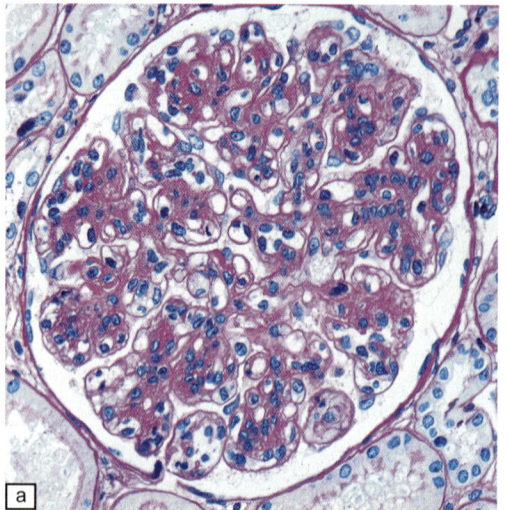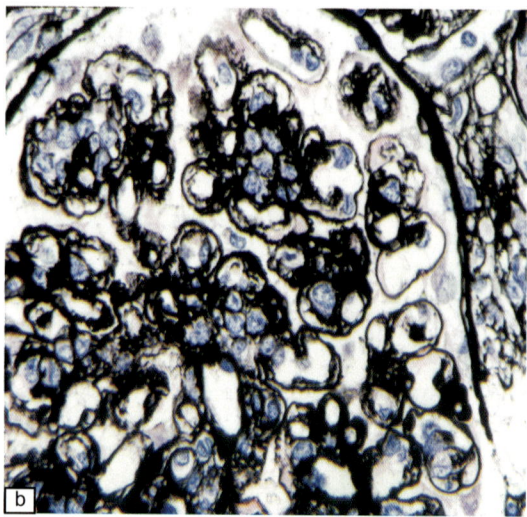

Fig. 26.1: Membranoproliferative glomerulonephritis. (a) Light microscopy shows prominent lobular accentuation, mesangial expansion and neutrophilic infiltration. (b) Silver methenamine stain showing tram track or double contoured appearance of the capillary wall

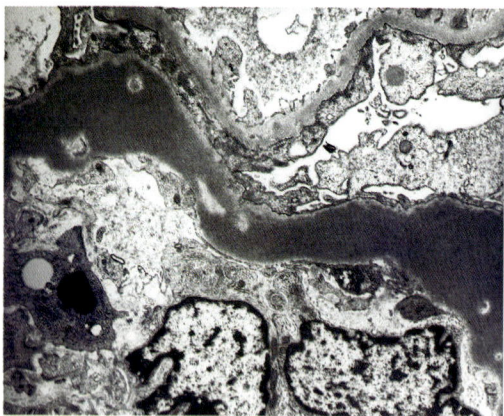

Fig. 26.2: Membranoproliferative glomerulo-nephritis type II (dense deposit disease). Electron micrograph shows elongated dense in amembranous densities and subepithelial hump shaped deposits

infections (hepatitis B and C, human immuno-deficiency virus, shunt nephritis, visceral abscesses, infective endocarditis, malaria, schistosomiasis, leprosy, mycobacteria) and autoimmune diseases (systemic lupus, sclero-derma).

The initial evaluation includes the follo-wing:

1. Blood levels of urea, creatinine; lipid profile; transaminases
2. Urinalysis: proteinuria, dysmorphic red blood cells, RBC casts
3. 24-hr or spot urinary protein, creatinine ratio
4. Low complement C3 is noted in 50-70% cases; C3 is persistently low in type II MPGN
5. Low C4 indicates activation of classical complement pathway (MPGN type I). Low levels of factor H with normal C4 and presence of C3NeF suggests MPGN type II
6. Hepatitis B surface antigen; hepatitis C; HIV antibodies; antinuclear antibodies
7. If required: chest X ray, cultures, ultra-sound abdomen, echocardiography

Treatment

There is lack of consensus on the management of MPGN. Figure 26.3 provides an approach to management. Therapy with ACE inhibitors

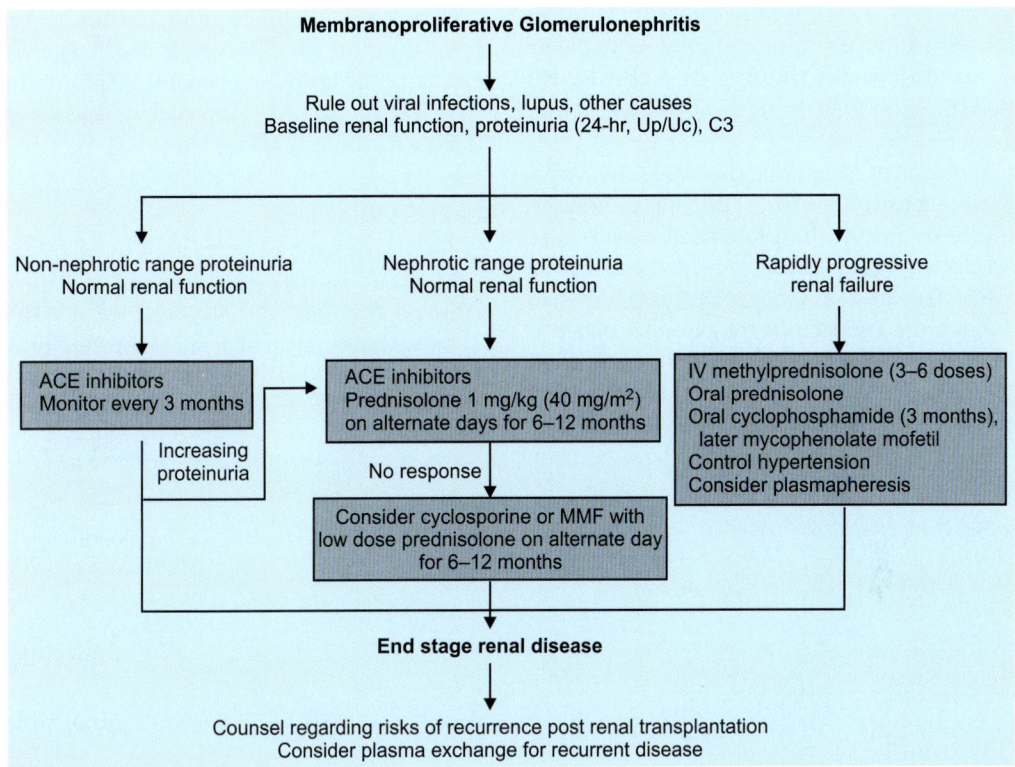

Fig. 26.3: Therapy for membranoproliferative glomerulonephritis. ACE angiotensin converting enzyme, MMF mycophenolate mofetil

is effective in reducing proteinuria and managing hypertension.

Following exclusion of secondary causes, patients with nephrotic range proteinuria should receive a trial of therapy with oral prednisolone at a dose of 30–40 mg/m² on alternate days. The same dose is continued for at least 18–24 months and tapered depending upon the response. Anecdotal reports suggest that therapy with mycophenolate mofetil (600–1000 mg/m²/day) or cyclosporine (4–5 mg/kg/day) in combination with alternate day prednisolone might reduce proteinuria and preserve renal function.

Patients with rapidly progressive glomerulonephritis are treated initially with IV methylprednisolone (20–30 mg/kg/day IV for 3–6 pulses) followed by oral prednisolone. Supportive care including dialytic support might be necessary. Therapy with cyclophosphamide might be rarely used.

Patients with factor H deficiency, MPGN type II with circulating C3 nephritic factor (C3NeF) and post transplantation recurrence might benefit from plasmapheresis.

Monitoring

Nephrotic range proteinuria disappears in the responders by 6–12 months. Microscopic hematuria can persist for 12 months. Serum C3 levels improve in 3 months and normalize by 6 months in the majority. Blood levels of creatinine, lipids and urinary protein to creatinine ratio are estimated every 6–12 months.

Outcome

MPGN secondary to an inciting condition, e.g. infection, usually responds to management of

Glomerulonephritis

the infection. Treatment of hepatitis C infection with interferon, or removal of catheter and antimicrobial therapy in a child with infected shunt results in resolution of glomerulonephritis.

All forms of idiopathic disease show a progressive clinical course, with fluctuations in disease severity. Complete remission is rare and about 40% patients progress to ESRD within 10 years of diagnosis. Features linked to adverse outcome include the presence of nephrotic syndrome, renal dysfunction or persistent hypertension, type II MPGN, and presence of chronic interstitial damage on biopsy.

Treatment outcomes are better for MPGN type I than for MPGN type II or III. The risk of recurrence following renal transplantation varies from 20–30% for type I disease to 80–90% for type II MPGN.

SUPPORT READING

Andrésdóttir MB. Recommendations for the diagnosis and treatment of dense deposit disease. Nat Clin Pract Nephrol 2008; 4: 68–69

Levin A. Management of membranoproliferative glomerulonephritis: evidence-based recommendations. Kidney Int Suppl 1999; 70: S41–46

27 Hepatitis B and C Associated Nephropathies

Infections due to hepatitis B (HBV) and C (HCV) viruses are an important cause of morbidity and mortality in developing countries. Chronic HBV infection is an important infection in South and South East Asia, where HBV carriers constitute up to 1–5% of the population. Children are often affected through perinatal transmission. Chronic infection with either of these viruses can result in significant glomerular disease.

HEPATITIS B RELATED NEPHROPATHY

Extrahepatic manifestations of HBV infection include glomerulonephritis, polyarteritis nodosa and reactive arthritis. Glomerular involvement is more common in children than adults. Common pathologies include membranous nephropathy and membranoproliferative glomerulonephritis. Evaluation for HBV infection is also a consideration when (i) evaluating candidates for renal replacement therapy and (ii) managing patients with diseases that require immunosuppression (e.g. nephrotic syndrome, lupus nephritis).

Evaluation

Investigations following the detection of hepatitis B surface antigen (HBsAg) are as follows:

1. *Anti-hepatitis B core (HBc) IgM:* This assesses acute infection. If anti-HBc IgM is detected, repeat testing usually shows the HBsAg to be negative and anti-hepatitis B surface antibody (anti-HBs) is positive. This suggests clearance of HBV infection.

2. *Tests for viral replication:* If anti-HBc IgM is negative, hepatitis B extracellular antigen (HBeAg) and quantitative PCR for HBV are required to determine the level of viral replication.

3. *Tests for liver function:* These include blood counts, transaminases, albumin and prothrombin time. Ultrasonography of the liver and portal system is necessary. Decision regarding liver biopsy is taken in consultation with a hepatologist.

4. Serological tests should be done for co-infection with human immunodeficiency virus and hepatitis C virus. Siblings and parents should be screened for HBsAg.

Therapy

The therapy for hepatitis B disease is based on levels of transaminases and HBV DNA, HBeAg status and liver histology.

Immunocompromised individuals: In these patients, e.g. transplant recipients, treatment with nucleos(t)ide analog is initiated when the HBV DNA level is at or above 10^5 copies/mL irrespective of transaminase levels, or at 10^2 to 10^5 copies/mL if transaminases are elevated.

Non immunosuppressed subjects: While guidelines for treatment are evolving, HBV

DNA levels of 10^4 to 10^5 copies/mL are regarded as the threshold in most cases.

Hepatitis B induced nephropathy should not be treated with corticosteroids, since it is ineffective, delays viral clearance and might worsen liver disease. Agents recommended for management of hepatitis B related nephropathies include interferon, lamivudine and newer oral nucleos(t)ide analogues. Most regulatory authorities have approved interferon alpha (IFN-α) and lamivudine for use in children.

Interferon: IFN-α is administered at a dose of 6 MU/m² three times a week subcutaneously for 6 months. Studies in children have shown clearance of HBeAg in 20–40% and HBV DNA in 25–60% patients. Therapy accelerates the spontaneous resolution of HBV infection and loss of HBsAg is seen in ≥25% responders.

Adverse effects of therapy include flu like symptoms, anxiety, weight loss, bone marrow suppression, thyroid disorders and induction of autoantibodies. Patients should be monitored for levels of hemoglobin, blood counts, transaminases and thyroid function.

Lamivudine is administered at 3 mg/kg/day (maximum 100 mg) for 1 year. Therapy is associated with clearance of HBeAg and HBV DNA in 25% patients. The development of drug-resistant mutations in the YMDD motif of the HBV polymerase gene is an important cause of resistance to therapy.

Combination of IFN and lamivudine may be associated with faster normalization of transaminases and clearance of HBV DNA, but with limited benefit on final response rate.

Other agents that have been examined include famciclovir, adefovir dipivoxil, and pegylated interferon. Agents such as entecavir or adefovir are effective in patients with lamivudine resistance; the latter should be used with caution in patients with renal impairment.

Outcome

The resolution of proteinuria in HBV mediated nephropathies is associated with clearance of HBeAg and/or HBsAg, and usually occurs within 6 months of seroconversion. A favorable response to antiviral treatment is more likely in *(i)* children compared to adults, and *(ii)* patients with hepatitis flare. Poor outcomes are predicted by the persistence of active viral replication.

HBsAg-positive Kidney Transplant Recipients

Since IFN treatment may lead to a high incidence of renal allograft failure, therapy is initiated with nucleos(t)ide analogs. Patients are prescribed treatment, either *(i)* prophylactically, starting at the time of kidney transplantation, or *(ii)* preemptively, when the level of HBV DNA increases, with or without abnormal transaminase levels. The latter approach requires frequent monitoring of HBV DNA. Salvage treatment given after the onset of liver dysfunction is associated with inferior outcomes. Treatment is continued for an indefinite duration.

HEPATITIS C RELATED NEPHROPATHY

Chronic hepatitis C virus (HCV) infection is usually acquired by perinatal transmission, or less commonly, through infected blood products. Extrahepatic manifestations of infection include membranoproliferative glomerulonephritis (MPGN) with or without cryoglobulinemia; rarely, severe vasculitis, fibrillary GN, focal segmental glomerulosclerosis and thrombotic microangiopathy in association with anticardiolipin antibodies have been reported. As for HBV, the HCV status impacts the management of candidates for renal replacement therapy (before and after transplantation).

Evaluation

Investigations for suspected HCV infection include:

1. Screening with third-generation, enzyme-linked immunosorbent assay for anti-HCV antibody
2. Quantitative polymerase chain reaction for HCV RNA; genotyping
3. Evaluation for liver disease, screening of family members and screening for co-infections.

Therapy

Children older than 2 years are considered for treatment with antiviral agents in presence of viremia and demonstration of inflammation on liver biopsy. Options for treatment include:

1. *Interferon alpha (IFN-α)* is administered at 3–5 million units (MU) 3 times a week for 12–18 months. The medication should not be given following transplantation due to high risk of allograft rejection.
2. *Pegylated IFN-α* is given at 1 µg/kg weekly for 48 weeks.
3. *Ribavirin* is administered at 8–15 mg/kg/d orally. It should be used cautiously in patients with estimated GFR <50 mL/min/1.73 m^2 due to the risk of hemolysis.

The combination of pegylated IFN-α and ribavirin (given for 18 months) is proposed as initial therapy for patients with infection due to HCV genotype 1.

Outcome

Higher rates of sustained viral response are observed in children compared to adults, and for non-genotype 1 disease than infection with genotype 1.

SUPPORT READING

Schwarz KB. Pediatric issues in new therapies for hepatitis B and C. Curr Gastroenterol Rep 2003, 5: 233–39

Chan TM. Hepatitis B and renal disease. Curr Hepatitis Rep 2010; 9: 99–105

28 Urinary Tract Infections

Urinary tract infections (UTI) cause significant morbidity in childhood, affecting 3–10% girls and 1–3% boys, and are an important "occult" bacterial infection in febrile infants. A significant proportion of children with UTI have an underlying urinary tract anomaly, most often vesicoureteric reflux (VUR). Early recognition and appropriate management of UTI and severe VUR is necessary to prevent renal scarring (reflux nephropathy).

Definition

The diagnosis of UTI is based on the growth of significant number of organisms of a single species in the urine, *in the presence of symptoms*. The number of organisms required to be present to define UTI depends on the site from which urine has been collected. *Significant bacteriuria* is defined as a colony count of $>10^5$/mL of a single species of bacteria in a midstream clean catch sample. In samples taken by urethral catheterization, a colony count of $>5 \times 10^4$ colony forming units/mL is considered significant bacteriuria. The culture of any pathogens from a superpubic aspirate is considered significant.

The occurrence of significant bacteriuria in the absence of symptoms is termed *asymptomatic bacteriuria*.

The distinction between simple and complicated UTI has importance for the modality of therapy. *Complicated UTI* is diagnosed in the presence of high fever (>39 °C), systemic toxicity, persistent vomiting, dehydration, renal angle tenderness or raised creatinine. Patients with low grade fever, dysuria, frequency and urgency, and absence of symptoms of complicated UTI are considered to have *simple UTI*.

Clinical Features

The symptoms of UTI in young children are nonspecific. Neonates may present with features of sepsis including lethargy, temperature instability, hyperbilirubinemia and shock. Unexplained fever may be the only symptom in young children. Older children present with fever, dysuria, urgency, frequency and abdominal or flank pain. Adolescents may have symptoms restricted to the lower urinary tract.

It is often difficult to distinguish between infection localized to the bladder (cystitis) and upper tracts (pyelonephritis). However, this distinction is not necessary since radionuclide imaging shows that almost 70–75% of UTI in children below 5 yr of age involve the kidney and upper tracts. *UTI in children is thus always*

Urinary Tract Infections

considered to involve the upper tract and should be treated promptly to avoid renal parenchymal injury.

Diagnosis

While urinalysis enables a presumptive diagnosis of UTI and facilitates initiation of empirical treatment, the diagnosis of UTI must be confirmed by urine culture.

Urinalysis

Urine examination is a useful screening test for UTI. The presence of >10 leukocytes per mm^3 in a fresh uncentrifuged sample, or >5 leukocytes per high power field in a centrifuged sample, is considered significant. *The detection of leukocyturia in absence of significant bacteriuria is not sufficient to diagnose a UTI.*

Rapid dipstick based tests, which detect leukocyte esterase and nitrite, are useful in screening for UTI. A combination of these tests has moderate sensitivity and specificity for detecting UTI in children, and is diagnostically as useful as microscopy.

Urine Culture

A clean catch midstream sample is advised for urine culture in toilet-trained children. It is sufficient to clean the genitalia with soap and water prior to sample collection; antiseptic washes are not required. In neonates and infants, the specimen should be obtained by suprapubic aspiration or transurethral catheterization. Culture of a bag specimen is not recommended.

The specimen should be processed promptly and plated within an hr of collection. If delay of more than 2-hr is anticipated, the specimen should be stored in a refrigerator at 4 °C (not frozen) for up to 12–24 hr.

Etiology

Nearly 90% of the first UTI and 70% of recurrent infections are caused by *Escherichia coli*. Organisms like *Klebsiella, Staphylococci epidermidis* and *Streptococcus fecalis* are occasionally incriminated. UTI following instru-mentation and nosocomial infections may be due to *Proteus* and *Pseudomonas*. Fungal UTI should be suspected in hospitalized newborns and infants who are either immunocompromised or have received prolonged parenteral antimicrobials. Tuberculosis of the urinary tract is extremely rare in children.

Evaluation

History regarding prior episodes of UTI, and bowel and bladder habits should be elicited. Assessment of hydration, ability to retain oral intake, signs of systemic toxicity and blood pressure are necessary.

Features that suggest an underlying abnormality include: *(i)* urinary incontinence; *(ii)* surgery for meningomyelocele or anorectal malformation; *(iii)* poor urinary stream, straining at micturition; *(iv)* palpable kidney(s), distended bladder; *(v)* tight phimosis, vulval synechiae; and *(vi)* neurological deficit in lower limbs. History may suggest bowel bladder dysfunction, in form of constipation or impacted stools, infrequent (<3 times) or frequent (>8 times) daytime voiding, straining during micturition and holding maneuvers to postpone voiding.

Children with complicated UTI should be evaluated with complete blood counts, creatinine and blood culture.

Treatment

Treatment of UTI should be initiated promptly to prevent potential renal parenchymal injury. Empiric therapy is started once a sample for culture has been taken.

Except for afebrile adolescents with chiefly lower tract symptoms, all children with UTI should be treated as for pyelonephritis. The mode of therapy depends on the age of the child, and whether the UTI is complicated or uncomplicated.

Complicated UTI

Infants below 3 months of age and children with complicated UTI should be treated with

28

parenteral antibiotics. The choice of antibiotic is guided by local sensitivity patterns. A third generation cephalosporin (cefotaxime or ceftriaxone) is preferred (Table 28.1). Parenteral therapy with a single daily dose of aminoglycoside is also safe and effective for treatment of complicated UTI. A single antimicrobial should be used in community acquired infections, and combinations reserved for more sick patients. Once the result of antimicrobial sensitivity is available, the treatment may be modified.

Once oral intake improves and symptoms abate, therapy is switched to an oral antibiotic, usually after 48–72 hr. The duration of treatment for complicated UTI should be 10–14 days.

Uncomplicated UTI

Children above 3 months of age who are accepting by mouth and not toxic (simple UTI) are treated with oral antibiotics for 7–10 days. Coamoxiclav, amoxicillin or cefixime may be used for initial treatment, and treatment modified following availability of sensitivity reports. Adolescents with cystitis may receive shorter duration of antibiotics, lasting 72 hours.

Supportive Care

It is important to maintain adequate hydration during the infection. Admission for intravenous fluids may be required if the child appears sick, dehydrated or is unable to take orally. Routine alkalization of the urine is not necessary.

Assessing Response to Therapy

With adequate therapy, resolution of toxicity occurs within 24–48 hr and fever by 48–72 hr. A repeat urine culture is *not required* during or following treatment, unless: (*i*) symptoms fail to resolve despite 48–72 hr of adequate antibiotic therapy; (*ii*) symptoms recur, suggesting recurrent UTI, or (*iii*) contamination of the initial urine culture is suspected.

Antibiotic Prophylaxis

After a course of antimicrobial therapy, long-term low dose antibiotic prophylaxis is administered to patients with: (*i*) UTI below 1-yr of age, while awaiting imaging studies; (*ii*) VUR; and (*iii*) frequent febrile UTI (3 or more episodes in a year), even if the urinary tract is normal.

The medication is given as a single bedtime dose (Table 28.2). The antibiotic used should

Table 28.1: Antimicrobials for treatment of urinary tract infections

Medication	Dose, mg/kg/day
Parenteral	
Ceftriaxone	75–100, in 1–2 divided doses IV
Cefotaxime	100–150, in 2–3 divided doses IV
Amikacin	10–15, single dose IV or IM
Gentamicin	5–6, single dose IV or IM
Ampicillin	100, in 3–4 divided doses IV
Oral	
Cefixime	8–10, in 2 divided doses
Coamoxiclav	30–40 of amoxicillin, in 2 divided doses
Cotrimoxazole	6–10 of trimethoprim, in 2 divided doses
Ciprofloxacin	10–20, in 2 divided doses
Ofloxacin	15–20, in 2 divided doses
Cephalexin	50–70, in 2–3 divided doses

Table 28.2: Antimicrobials for prophylaxis of urinary tract infections*

Medication	Dose, mg/kg/day	Remarks
Cotrimoxazole	1–2 of trimethoprim	Avoid in infants <3 months-old, glucose-6-phosphate dehydrogenase (G6PD) deficiency
Nitrofurantoin	1–2	May cause vomiting and nausea; avoid in infants <3 months old, G6PD deficiency, renal insufficiency
Cephalexin	10	Drug of choice in first 3–6 months of life
Cefadroxil	5	An alternative agent in early infancy

*Usually given as single bedtime dose

be effective, non-toxic with few side effects and not alter the bacterial flora or induce bacterial resistance. Agents that can be used include cotrimoxazole and nitrofurantoin. Cephalexin or cefadroxil is preferred in young infants and those with deficiency of the enzyme, glucose-6-phosphate dehydrogenase.

Antibiotic prophylaxis is not advised for patients with urinary tract obstruction (e.g. posterior urethral valves), urolithiasis or neurogenic bladder, and patients on clean intermittent catheterization.

Breakthrough UTI on Prophylactic Antibiotics

Breakthrough UTI results either from poor compliance or associated voiding dysfunction. The UTI should be treated with appropriate antibiotics. A change of the medication being used for prophylaxis is usually not necessary. There is no role for cyclic therapy, where the antibiotic used for prophylaxis is changed every 6–8 weeks.

Asymptomatic Bacteriuria (ABU)

ABU refers to significant bacteriuria in a child who has no symptoms of UTI. The frequency of ABU is about 1–2% in girls and 0.05–0.2% in boys. The organisms isolated in most cases are usually *E. coli* of low virulence. The condition is benign, does not cause renal injury and remits spontaneously. On the other hand, eradication of these non-pathogenic organisms may be followed by symptomatic

infection with more virulent strains. Use of antibiotics to treat asymptomatic bacteriuria or antibiotic prophylaxis is not indicated. *The presence of asymptomatic bacteriuria in a patient previously treated for UTI should not be considered as recurrent UTI.*

Evaluation after the First Episode of UTI

The aim of imaging studies is to identify urologic anomalies that predispose to pyelonephritis and detect evidence of renal scarring. These investigations should be performed judiciously (Table 28.3), so that the evaluation is completed at minimum risks of radiation exposure and other iatrogenic complications. The modalities for evaluation are described below.

Renal ultrasonography provides information on kidney size, number and location, presence of hydronephrosis, urinary bladder anomalies and post-void residual urine. An ultrasound may be performed even during therapy of the urinary tract infection.

Radiocontrast micturating cystourethrogram (MCU) is the standard for diagnosing and grading the severity of VUR (Fig. 28.1) and defining urethral and bladder anatomy. When required, the MCU may be carried out within 2–3 weeks of the treatment of the UTI.

Direct radionuclide cystography (DRCG) is chiefly used for follow up studies (Fig. 28.2a).

Dimercaptosuccinic acid (DMSA) scintigraphy is a sensitive test for detecting renal scars, characterized by decreased uptake with loss of renal contours or presence of cortical

Table 28.3: Evaluation following the first episode of urinary tract infection

Age	Evaluation*
Below 1 yr	Ultrasound
	Micturating cystourethrogram (MCU)
	Dimercaptosuccinic acid (DMSA) renal scan
1-5 yr	Ultrasound
	DMSA scan
	If ultrasound or DMSA scan is abnormal: MCU
Above 5 yr	Ultrasound
	If ultrasound abnormal: MCU and DMSA scan

*Patients with recurrent UTI need detailed evaluation with ultrasonography, DMSA scan and MCU

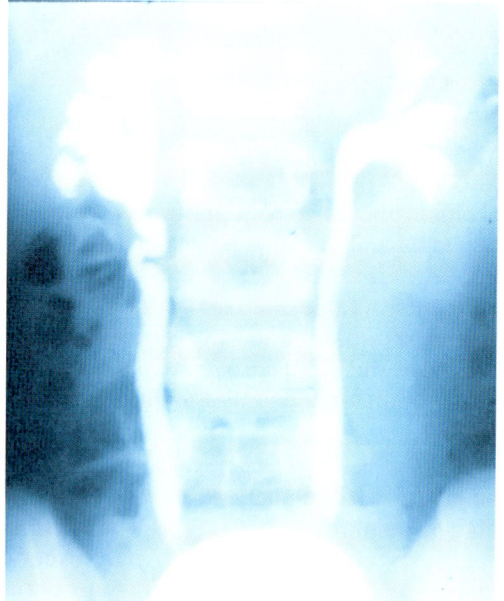

Fig. 28.1: Bilateral grade IV and V vesicoureteric reflux in a girl with recurrent UTI. Note the dilatation, tortuosity of ureters and loss of cupping of the calyces

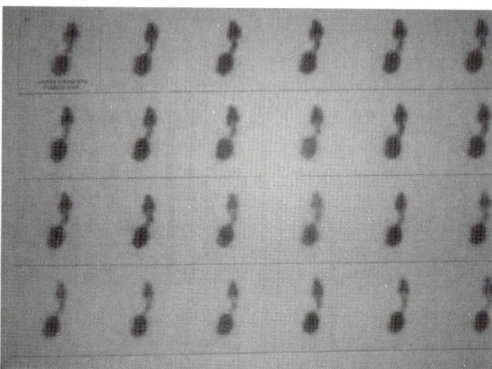

Fig 28.2a: Radionuclide scintigraphy in a 4-yr old with bilateral grade V VUR on MCU performed at 18 months. The images suggest persistence of severe reflux on the right side

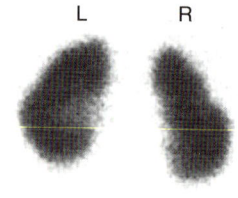

Fig. 28.2b: ^{99m}Tc-DMSA scintigraphy showing multiple scars and loss of volume in the right (R) kidney. The left kidney is normal

thinning with decreased volume (Fig. 28.2b). In order to differentiate these from changes of acute pyelonephritis, the procedure is recommended 3 months after therapy for urinary tract infection.

Magnetic resonance urography is a highly sensitive tool for evaluation of the kidneys and urinary tract, without risks of radiation exposure. The risk of nephrogenic systemic fibrosis with use of gadolinium-based contrast agents in patients with impaired kidney function should be considered (Chapter 37).

Recommendations for Evaluation

Recommendations for imaging following the first UTI are variable. All patients are screened with the aim to identify patients at high risk of renal damage, chiefly those below 1-yr of age, and those with VUR or urinary tract obstruction. A 'high-risk' approach should be followed to avoid subjecting children with no abnormality to multiple investigations. However, this approach is now tempered with the knowledge that intensive imaging and subsequent management do not significantly alter the long-term outcome of children with reflux nephropathy diagnosed following a UTI. In addition, the routine use of antenatal screening has resulted in majority of the significant anomalies to be detected and managed after birth.

The recommendations of the Indian Society of Pediatric Nephrology on evaluation following the first UTI are summarized in Table 28.3. All infants (<1-yr) need to be evaluated aggressively using ultrasonography, MCU and DMSA scan. Many at-risk children would show the sequelae of pyelonephritis that are detected by scintigraphy. The early detection of scarring, high grade VUR or obstructive uropathy is likely to enable interventions that prevent progressive kidney damage. Since infants are at the highest risk, it is necessary that this group undergo focused evaluation.

A DMSA scan and ultrasound are required between 1–5 years, and ultrasound above 5 years of age. Further imaging with MCU is necessary if scintigraphy or ultrasound examination is abnormal. A milder grade of reflux, which may be missed by this approach, is not likely to contribute to renal scarring.

The above recommendations are based on the assumption that early detection of urologic abnormalities shall result in improved out-

comes. The policy for radiological evaluation following UTI is under review. It is possible that application of antenatal ultrasonography and availability of non invasive methods for evaluating the lower urinary tract might result in modification of the existing recommendations in the future.

Recurrent UTI

Recurrent UTI are observed in 30–50% children, more commonly infants. Most recurrences occur within 3 months of the initial episode. Predisposing factors include: *(i)* female sex; *(ii)* age below 6 months; *(iii)* obstructive uropathy; *(iv)* severe (grade III-V) VUR; *(v)* repeated episodes of pyelonephritis; *(vi)* voiding dysfunction; *(vii)* constipation; and *(viii)* repeated catheterization in neurogenic bladder.

Patients with recurrent UTI at any age should undergo detailed imaging with ultrasonography, MCU and DMSA scintigraphy.

Prevention

Interventions that have been associated with a decrease in incidence of UTI include relief of constipation and voiding dysfunction. Adequate fluid intake and frequent voiding is advised.

Antibacterial prophylaxis is indicated in children with recurrences, even in the absence of VUR. Breakthrough UTI may result either from poor compliance or associated voiding dysfunction. UTI should be treated with appropriate antibiotics. A change of the medication being used for prophylaxis is usually not necessary.

Increased periurethral bacterial colonization in uncircumcised boys may be a risk factor for UTI. Circumcision reduces the risk of recurrent UTI in infant boys, and might have benefits in patients with high grade VUR.

Voiding Dysfunction and Bowel Bladder Dysfunction

Normal micturition requires complex neuromuscular coordination, autonomic innervation and control by higher centers. Loss of innervations, as in meningomylocele and spinal dysraphism, may predispose a child to recurrent UTI. On the other hand, *voiding dysfunction* refers to abnormal patterns of micturition in the presence of intact neuronal pathways without congenital or anatomical abnormalities (Chapter 29). When constipation is associated with a functional voiding disorder, the condition is referred to as *bowel bladder dysfunction (BBD)*.

Children with recurrent UTI are likely to have dysfunctional voiding. A diagnosis of voiding dysfunction can be made based on history of the voiding pattern and urodynamic studies. A record of frequency and voided volume and fluid intake for two to three days is useful. The urinary stream should be observed, including for post void dribbling in boys. Voiding dysfunction should be suspected in children with: (*i*) persistent high grade VUR; (*ii*) thickened urinary bladder wall >2 mm; (*iii*) post-void urine >20 mL, and (*iv*) spinning top configuration of bladder on MCU.

The child and parents are explained to follow a structured voiding pattern, with frequent voids and double micturition. Constipation is managed with dietary modifications and medications as required. Patients with large post-void residues benefit from timely voiding, bladder retraining and clean intermittent catheterization. In patients with an overactive bladder, therapy with anticholinergic medications (e.g. oxybutinin) effectively reduces the bladder tone and increase bladder capacity.

VESICOURETERIC REFLUX

VUR refers to the retrograde flow of urine from bladder to ureters and pelvis at rest or during micturition. Reflux allows pathogenic organisms in the bladder to initiate inflammation in the renal parenchyma. VUR may be an isolated anomaly (primary) or associated with other anomalies of the urinary tract (secondary). Its severity is graded using the International Study Classification from grade I to V, based on the appearance of the urinary tract on MCU (Fig. 28.3). Primary VUR tends to

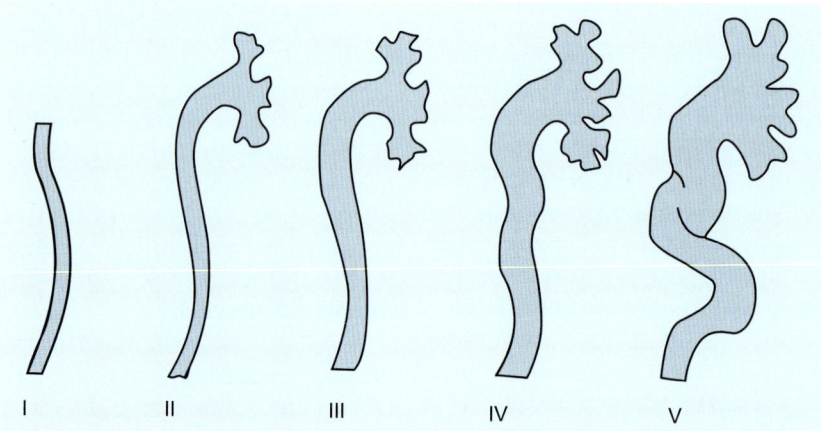

Fig. 28.3: Grading of vesicoureteric reflux (VUR) on micturating cystourethrogram. *Grade I*: VUR does not reach the renal pelvis; *Grade II*: VUR extending up to the renal pelvis without dilatation of pelvis or calyceal fornices; *Grade III*: VUR extending up to the kidney, with mild dilatation or tortuosity of the ureter and renal pelvis, with no or minor blunting of the calyceal fornices; *Grade IV*: Moderate dilatation or tortuosity of the ureter, renal pelvis and fornices, with complete obliteration of the sharp angles of the calyceal fornices, but normal appearance of the papillary impressions; *Grade V*: gross dilatation and tortuosity of the ureter, renal pelvis and calyces, with loss of papillary impressions on calyces

resolve by 6–10 yr of age. Factors favoring resolution are younger age, low grade VUR and unilateral involvement. The rate of resolution is 70–90% for grades I-III and 10–35% for higher grades. Secondary VUR is often related to bladder outflow obstruction, as with posterior urethral valves, neurogenic bladder or a functional voiding disorder.

Recognition of significant reflux is important since urinary tract infections in this setting predispose to renal parenchymal damage and renal scarring (reflux nephropathy), an important cause of hypertension and progressive renal injury in later life. However, it has been increasingly recognized that not all children with VUR benefit from diagnosis or treatment. In some patients, the reflux is innocuous and self limiting, while in others VUR is accompanied with renal damage with onset during the intrauterine period and dysplastic kidneys at birth.

Therapy for Primary VUR

Conventional therapy for VUR includes antibiotic prophylaxis and surgical inter-vention. In patients with dilating reflux, the outcomes following surgical repair *versus* prophylaxis are similar in terms of the number of breakthrough UTI and risk of renal scarring. Experts recommend that the management of patients with VUR should depend on the patient age, grade of reflux and whether there are any breakthrough infections.

The proposed guidelines for management of VUR are outlined in Fig. 28.4. *It is reco-mmended that patients should initially receive antibiotic prophylaxis while awaiting spontaneous resolution of VUR.* A close follow up is required for occurrence of breakthrough UTI. Repeat imaging is required after 18–36 months in patients with grade III-V VUR. Radionuclide cystogram, with lower radiation exposure, has higher sensitivity for detecting reflux and is therefore preferred for follow-up evaluation. Since the risk of recurrent UTI and renal scarring is low after 4–5 years of age, it is advised that prophylaxis be discontinued in children older than 5 years with normal bowel and voiding habits, even if mild to moderate reflux persists.

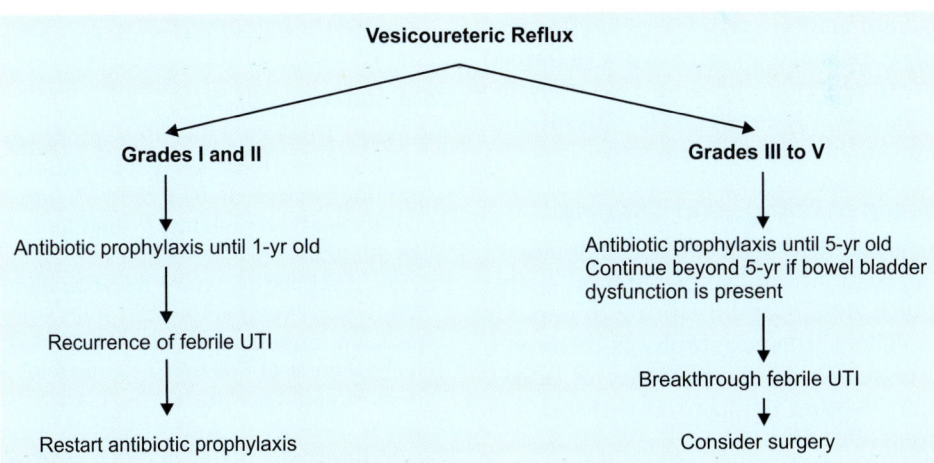

Fig. 28.4 Management of vesicoureteric reflux. Medical therapy of VUR is based on the principle that VUR resolves over time, and prophylactic antibiotics maintain urine sterility and prevent infections while awaiting spontaneous resolution. Reflux takes longer to resolve if associated with bowel bladder dysfunction or if high grade reflux is present; such patients require prolonged prophylaxis. Surgical correction of VUR is indicated if breakthrough infections occur, since significant parenchymal injury may occur with pyelonephritis

Disorders of the Urinary Tract

VI

While evidence from few studies suggests that the strategy of prompt diagnosis and treatment of UTI might be as effective as antibiotic prophylaxis, this approach requires validation in controlled trials. The clinician should discuss the benefits and risks of withholding antibiotic prophylaxis with the parents.

Patients with grade III to V reflux may be offered surgical repair if they have break-through febrile UTI, appearance of new scars, if parents prefer surgical intervention to prophylaxis, or in patients who show deterioration of renal function. An evaluation for voiding dysfunction (based on history, voiding diary) should be done before surgery. Antibiotic prophylaxis is continued for 6 months after surgical repair.

The availability of dextranomer/hyaluronic acid copolymer (Deflux) endoscopic treatment has been proposed as an alternative to surgical repair for patients with VUR. While results are satisfactory if the surgeon is experienced with the procedure, a significant proportion of patients, particularly those with bowel bladder dysfunction, may show persistence and/or recurrence of reflux and progressive renal damage. In view of limited prospective randomized controlled trials, the use of endoscopic correction is currently not recommended as first line therapy.

Screening of Siblings and Offspring

Reflux is inherited in an autosomal dominant manner with incomplete penetrance; almost one-third siblings and offspring of patients show VUR. Ultrasonography is recommended to screen for the presence of reflux. Further imaging is required if ultrasonography is abnormal.

Long Term Follow-up

Patients with a renal scar (reflux nephropathy) are counseled regarding the need for early diagnosis and therapy of UTI and regular follow up. Physical growth and blood pre-

ssure is monitored every 6–12 months, through adolescence. Investigations include urinalysis for proteinuria and estimation of blood levels of creatinine. Annual ultrasound examinations are done to monitor renal growth.

SUPPORT READING
Urinary Tract Infections

National Collaborating Centre for Women's and Children's Health. Urinary tract infection in children diagnosis, treatment and long-term management. RCOG Press, London 2007; http://www.rcpch.ac.uk/Research/ce/Clinical-Audit/Urinary-Tract-Infection accessed 17 March 2011

American Academy of Pediatrics. Urinary Tract Infections: Clinical practiceguideline for the diagnosis and management of the initial UTI in febrile infants and children 2 to 24 months. Pediatrics 2011; 128 : 595–610

Indian Society of Pediatric Nephrology Group. Indian Academy of Pediatrics. Consensus statement on management of urinary tract infections. Indian Pediatr 2011; 48: 709–17

Williams GJ, Lee A, Craig JC. Long-term antibiotics for preventing recurrent urinary tract infection in children. Cochrane Database Syst Rev 2006; 3: CD001534

Vesicoureteric Reflux

Lebowitz RL, Olbing H, Parkkulainen KV, et al; International system of radiographic grading of vesicoureteric reflux: International Reflux Study in Children. Pediatr Radiol 1985; 15: 105–09

Peters CA, Skoog SJ, Arant BS, et al; American Urological Association Education and Research, Inc. Summary of the AUA Guideline on management of primary vesicoureteral reflux in children. J Urol 2010; 184: 1134–44

Skoog SJ, Peters CA, Arant BS, et al; American Urological Association Education and Research. Pediatric vesicoureteral reflux guidelines panel summary report: clinical practice guidelines for screening siblings of children with vesicoureteral reflux and neonates/infants with prenatal hydronephrosis. J Urol 2010; 184: 1145–51

Holmdahl G, Brandström P, Läckgren G, *et al;* The Swedish reflux trial in children: II. Vesicoureteral reflux outcome. J Urol 2010; 184: 280–85

Hodson EM, Wheeler DM, Smith GH, *et. al;* Interventions for primary vesicoureteric reflux. Cochrane Database Syst Rev 2007; 3: CD 001532

Nevéus T, von Gontard A, Hoebeke P, *et al.* The standardization of terminology of lower urinary tract function in children and adolescents: report from the standardization committee of the International Children's Continence Society. J Urol 2006; 176: 314–24

29 Voiding Disorders

The lower urinary tract, consisting of urinary bladder, bladder neck and sphincter and urethra, works as a coordinated unit; voiding disorders occur when this functioning is disturbed. Voiding disorders, including enuresis, are common in childhood, occurring either in isolation or in conjunction with bowel disturbances. In addition to impairing the quality of life, they are associated with an increased risk of urinary tract infections, constipation and delayed resolution of vesicoureteral reflux.

Normal Physiology

During infancy, micturition is autonomous, mediated by a spinal vesicovesical reflex. Once the bladder fills up to an intrinsic volume threshold, spontaneous bladder contraction is triggered by relaxation of the bladder neck and external urethral sphincter. Thus complete voiding is achieved at low bladder pressures about 20 times a day. As the child grows older, the maturation of cortical pathways inhibits the vesicovesical reflex, and coordination of voiding is mediated by the pons and midbrain. Children between 1–2 years old are aware of bladder fullness, and urinate less frequently due to an increase in the functional bladder capacity. Between 2 and 3 years of age, an adult pattern of daytime urinary control emerges, such that voiding can be postponed volitionally as well as initiated at low bladder volumes. The time course for attaining continence varies, with full control achieved between 3 and 5 years.

Etiology

Abnormal voiding can be caused by an underlying disease process (organic incontinence), or can have no underlying associated abnormality (functional voiding disorder) (Table 29.1). Organic urinary incontinence is caused by an underlying structural or neurogenic abnormality. Structural causes include developmental, iatrogenic, and traumatic or anatomic abnormalities that interfere with the bladder's ability to store or evacuate urine. Neuropathic urinary incontinence includes congenital or acquired abnormalities of bladder or urinary sphincter innervation.

The term voiding disorders is reserved for functional problems in which no structural or neurologic abnormality can be identified. The majority of cases of urinary incontinence in children are included in this category. Nocturnal enuresis is particularly common.

EVALUATION

Assessment of children with lower urinary tract symptoms should include a detailed history, a voiding diary and physical examination. It is important to distinguish voiding disorders from structural and neuropathic bladder dysfunction. Figs. 29.1 and 29.2 summarize an approach for evaluating a child suspected to have a voiding disorder. Table 29.2 provides a list of important definitions that assist in evaluation.

Table 29.1: Causes of abnormal voiding

Structural abnormalities

Congenital	Bladder exstrophy, posterior urethral valves, prune belly syndrome, ectopic ureter
Acquired	Traumatic stricture, damage to the sphincter or urethra

Abnormalities of neurological innervation

Congenital	Myelomeningocele, spina bifida occulta, caudal regression syndrome, tethered cord syndrome, sacral agenesis
Acquired	Cerebral palsy, transverse myelitis, spinal cord injury

Detrusor and sphincter muscle dysfunction

Congenital	Muscular dystrophy
Acquired	Chronic bladder distension; fibrosis of the detrusor and bladder wall

Functional voiding disorders

Urge syndrome (overactive bladder)
Dysfunctional voiding
    Staccato voiding
    Fractionated voiding
    Lazy bladder: poor bladder emptying secondary to underactive detrusor
    Non-neurogenic neurogenic bladder (Hinman-Allen syndrome)
    Dysfunctional elimination syndrome

Voiding postponement
Giggle incontinence
Vesicovaginal entrapment: vaginal reflux voiding

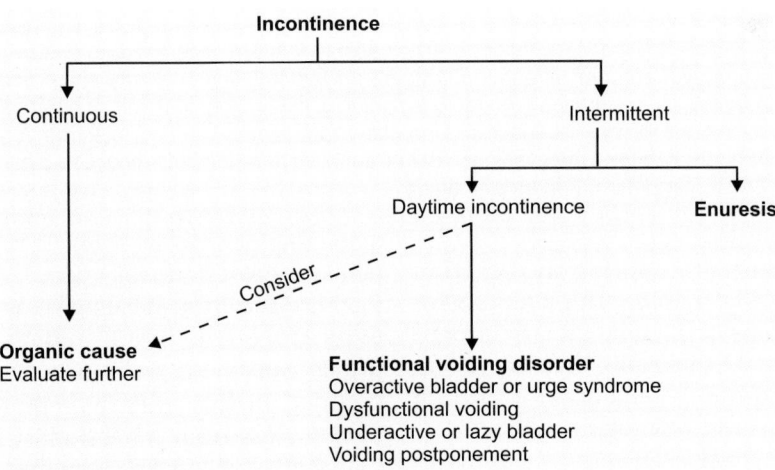

Fig. 29.1: Classification of childhood incontinence, as proposed by the International Children's Continence Society. Patients with intermittent daytime incontinence usually have a functional voiding disorder, but an organic cause should be ruled out

Disorders of the Urinary Tract

VI

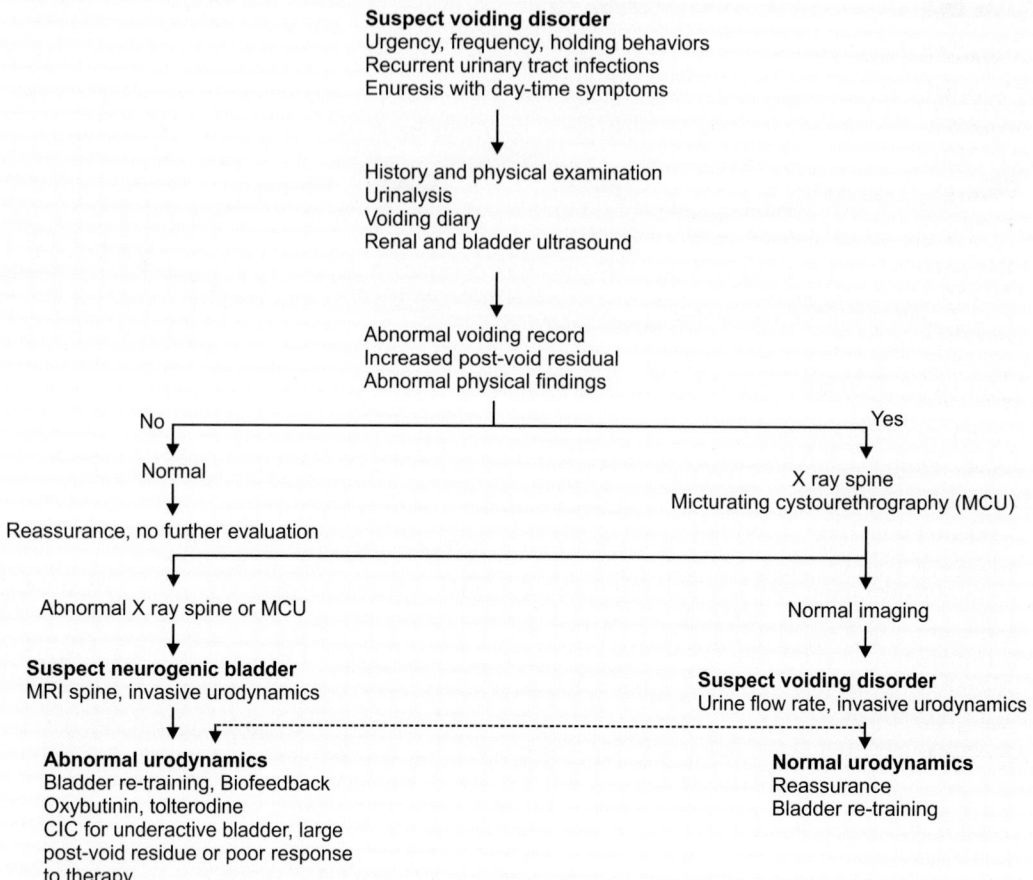

Fig. 29.2: Evaluation of childhood incontinence. If the patient's initial medical history, physical examination, urinalysis or renal and/or bladder ultrasound suggest an abnormality, an X ray spine and micturating cystourethrography (MCU) are obtained. An MCU is useful for confirming anatomic or neuropathic etiology, and when vesicoureteral reflux is suspected. Urine flow rate with pelvic floor electromyogram, with or without cystometrography, allows the evaluation of functional daytime incontinence. CIC clean intermittent catheterization, MRI magnetic resonance imaging

Clinical Features

Most children with voiding dysfunction present after toilet training with symptoms of either night time or daytime urinary incontinence or both. Occasionally they are recognized early, during evaluation for urinary tract infection or vesicoureteric reflux.

History includes relevant questions to define the pattern of voiding and wetting. Symptoms of urgency, frequency (eight or more times per day), holding behaviors (squatting or crossing legs), or urge incontinence suggest detrusor overactivity. Symptoms of difficulty in initiating voiding, the need to push or strain during voiding, or a weak urinary stream suggest functional or organic bladder outflow obstruction. Infrequent voiding (three or less times per day) suggests hypocontractile or lazy bladder. History of encopresis, constipation and fecal impaction is important, since bowel dysfunction may coexist.

Table 29.2: Important definitions (International Continence Society for Children, 2006)

Decreased daytime frequency: 3 or fewer voidings per day

Increased daytime frequency: 8 or more voidings per day

Polyuria: 24-hour urine output of more than 2 L/m^2 body surface area

Maximum voided volume: The largest voided volume, as documented in a bladder diary

Expected bladder capacity: Age related maximum voided volume, (age +2) × 30 mL

Incontinence: Uncontrollable leakage of urine

Continuous: Continuous leakage of urine, not in discrete portions; indicates malformations

Intermittent: Leakage of urine in discrete portions during the day and/or night

Enuresis: Intermittent incontinence while sleeping

Monosymptomatic: Enuresis without any (other) lower urinary tract symptoms

Non-monosymptomatic: Enuresis with (other) lower urinary tract symptoms, e.g. daytime incontinence, urgency, holding maneuvers

Primary: Enuresis without ever having been dry for less than 6 months

Secondary: Enuresis after being dry for at least 6 months

Overactive bladder: Condition afflicting patients with urgency (replaces term bladder instability)

Underactive bladder: Condition afflicting patients with low voiding frequency and the need to increase intra-abdominal pressure to void (replaces term underactive, lazy bladder)

Dysfunctional voiding: Contraction of the urethral sphincter during voiding, as observed by uroflow measurements

Detrusor-sphincter dyssynergia: Detrusor voiding contraction with involuntary contraction of the urethra

Residual urine: Urine left in the bladder after voiding residual urine in excess of 5 to 20 mL (or 10% of expected bladder capacity) indicates incomplete bladder emptying

Examination of lower spine, abdomen and external genitalia is essential. Spinal dysraphism is suggested by asymmetric gluteal folds, hairy patches, dermovascular malformations and lipomatous abnormalities in lower spine. Perianal and perineal sensation and anal tone are assessed. A palpable bladder is abnormal and suggests a neurogenic bladder or obstruction.

Voiding Diary

This home record of the voiding pattern and bladder symptoms provides useful information on lower urinary tract function (Table. 29.3). The diary provides information on the number of voids, their time and distribution, voided volumes and any episodes of urgency and leakage. It is desirable to have a 48-hr record, including assessment of night-time volumes. The expected voided volume is estimated as follows:

Infants:

Bladder capacity (mL) = 38 + 2.5 × age in months

Older children:

Bladder capacity (mL) = (Age in years + 2) × 30

Imaging Studies

Ultrasonography of kidneys and urinary bladder is the first investigation in children with voiding dysfunction. Apart from anatomic information about lower and upper urinary tract, it provides important information on the bladder volume, post void residue and wall thickness.

Other studies include a plain radiograph and MRI of the spine for the possibility of a neurogenic cause of bladder sphincter dysfunction, and micturating cystourethrogram for detecting vesicoureteric reflux and outflow obstruction.

29

Table 29.3: Voiding diary in a 7-yr-old girl showing small and frequent voids and voiding accidents

Time	Urine volume	Fluid intake	Comments
7:00 am [first void]	200 mL	200 mL	Undergarments wet
9:30 am	60 mL		Rushed to pass urine
10:00 am	50 mL	300 mL	
11:00 am	100 mL		
12:30 pm	140 mL	300 mL	Lunch
2:00 pm	80 mL		Undergarments wet
4:00 pm	80 mL		
5:00 pm	30 mL	100 mL	
7:00 pm	60 mL	200 mL	
8:00 pm		200 mL	Dinner
8:30 pm	60 mL		
9:30 pm	100 mL	100 mL	
Overnight			Passed urine twice in bed; 1 am, 5 am

The voiding diary should be maintained for atleast 48-hr (1-night, 2-day), usually over the weekend.

Urodynamic Evaluation

Uroflowmetry should precede invasive evaluation, and in many cases is the only urodynamic evaluation required in children. It gives information on normal flow rates and the pattern of the flow curve (Fig. 29.3). The shape of the flow curve is determined by detrusor contractility and presence of abdominal straining. Uroflowmetry is performed when the child experiences a normal desire to void and does so in the correct sitting or standing position.

Invasive urodynamic studies are pressure flow studies carried out during filling and voiding phases. Indications for these studies include: *(i)* suspected neurogenic bladder; *(ii)* unsatisfactory response to treatment predicted on noninvasive evaluation; *(iii)* prior to surgery for persistent vesicoureteric reflux; *(iv)* anorectal anomalies with suspected voiding disorder; *(v)* abnormal voiding with fecal incontinence; and *(vi)* bladder trabeculation or sphincter spasm noted during micturating cystourethrography.

NEUROGENIC BLADDER

Common causes of neurogenic bladder dysfunction are abnormalities of the spinal cord, including myelomeningocele, diastematomyelia and tethered conus medullaris. Other causes include spinal cord injury, transverse myelitis, cerebral palsy and demyelinating neuropathies.

Children with neurogenic bladder require prompt management in order to preserve renal function and achieve urinary and fecal continence to the extent possible. Long term outcomes are improved by regular clean intermittent catheterization (CIC) and, when required, timely surgical intervention. Urodynamic studies are recommended before and after therapy of the spinal defect. Intravesical pressures greater than 40 cm H_2O at urinary leakage (detrusor leak point pressure, DLPP) are associated with reflux, hydronephrosis and upper tract damage; sustained intravesical pressures as low as 20 cm H_2O increase the likelihood for bladder damage.

Patients with low intravesical pressures are followed closely with clinical examination and biannual ultrasonography to detect any dilatation of upper tract or symptoms suggesting detrusor sphincter dyssynergia. Children with high intravesical pressures or uninhibited bladder contractions should be treated

Voiding Disorders

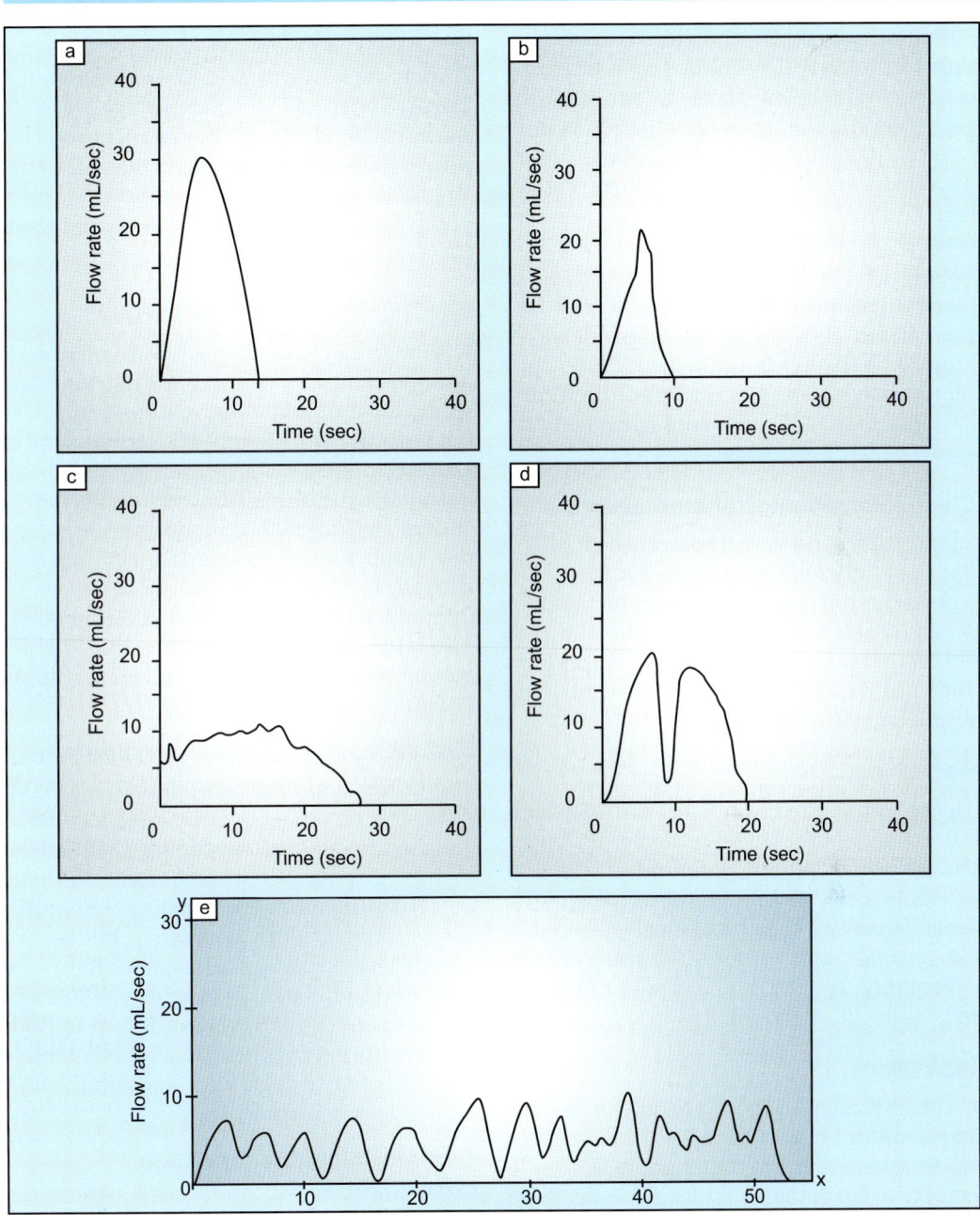

Fig. 29.3: Results of uroflowmetry. (a) *Bell-shaped curve:* The normal urinary flow curve of a healthy child is bell shaped in which a smooth increase and subsequent decrease in flow rate is observed. (b) *Tower-shaped curve* is produced by an explosive voiding contraction, seen in overactive bladder. (c) *Plateau-shaped curve* suggests outlet obstruction. (d) *Staccato pattern* of voiding is seen with sphincteric overactivity during voiding, with peaks and troughs throughout voiding. (e) *Interrupted flow* is seen in underactive bladder with decreased contractility

29

with anticholinergics and clean intermittent catheterization (CIC). The dosage is increased until pressures below 40 cm H_2O and areflexia are achieved. Bladder augmentation is indicated in patients with hydronephrosis and/or reflux with end-filling pressures greater than 40 cm H_2O (low capacity, high pressure bladder) despite medical management.

Sphincter incompetence is diagnosed in incontinent children with pressures less than 40 cm H_2O and detrusor areflexia. A bladder neck revision with a 360° tight rectus fascial sling with appendicovesicostomy may make the child continent and facilitate CIC.

Clean Intermittent Catheterization

Clean intermittent catheterization (CIC) involves catheterization of the bladder, with a clean but not sterile technique, in a regular schedule several times a day. The aim is to empty the bladder, prevent its overdistension and improve bladder function by maintaining physiological volumes.

Frequency

The recommended frequency of CIC is between 4 and 6 times in 24-hr. Intervals longer than 8 hours should be avoided. Careful scheduling of CIC through the day, including lunch hours and class breaks, can ensure that CIC can be done without disruption of the school day. If available, a school nurse can help with CIC at school.

Indications

CIC is indicated in those not able to feel the sensation of bladder filling, e.g. neurogenic bladder secondary to meningomyelocele, in cases with incomplete bladder emptying (high post void residues on ultrasound; >10% of bladder capacity) and for high pressure bladders on urodynamic evaluation. By allowing timely drainage of urine, CIC helps prevent urinary tract infection, reflux and toileting accidents.

Self Catheterization

Parents are taught to do CIC until the child is at least 5 years old. Beyond that age, the child can be encouraged to participate in parts of the procedure, such as washing hands or organizing CIC equipment. At about seven or eight years of age, the child is often able to carry out CIC on his or her own.

FUNCTIONAL VOIDING DISORDERS

It is important to distinguish between normal developmental variations of the bladder-sphincter unit and abnormal lower urinary tract function in children. The terminology of voiding disorders proposed by the International Children's Continence Society is shown in Table 29.2. Incontinence means uncontrollable leakage of urine; it is *continuous* if there is constant dribbling of urine, or *intermittent,* if urine leaks in discrete amounts. The latter includes conditions like *daytime incontinence* and *enuresis* (incontinence during sleep).

Dysfunctional Elimination Syndrome

The terms dysfunctional elimination syndrome and bowel bladder dysfunction (BBD) are used to denotes functional disturbances in the urinary tract that result from functional bowel disturbances. These include: *(i) Functional disorder of filling:* overactive bladder or overdistension of the bladder associated with fecal impaction and *(ii) Functional disorder of emptying:* over-recruitment of pelvic floor activity during voiding, causing incomplete emptying; associated with defecation difficulties or pain on defecation.

Overactive Bladder and Urge Incontinence

This is characterized by frequent attacks of sudden sensations of urge even with small bladder capacities (Fig. 29.3b), represented by detrusor overactivity during the filling phase. The child may show holding maneuvers, e.g. *Vincent's curtsey,* during which the child attempts to voluntarily contract the pelvic floor muscles and externally compress the urethra to counteract the involuntary contractions either by crossing the legs or squatting. The condition is associated with an increased risk of urinary tract infections. Constipation is often present. Detrusor contractions may be triggered by stimulation of stretch receptors in the bladder wall by the extrinsic fecal mass, or colonic contractions may increase detrusor contractions *via* shared neural pathways.

Dysfunctional Voiding

Dysfunctional voiding is characterized by incomplete relaxation or involuntary intermittent contractions of pelvic floor muscles during voiding in neurologically intact children. Staccato voiding is interrupted voiding that is caused by periodic bursts of pelvic floor muscle activities during voiding. The flow time is usually prolonged and bladder emptying is incomplete (Fig. 29.3d). Fractionated voiding involves several small, discontinuous voids that result from poor and unsustained detrusor contractions characterized by infrequent and incomplete emptying.

Underactive Bladder (Lazy Bladder)

Patients with underactive bladder show infrequent voiding (every 8–10 hr or longer). This results in a large, floppy bladder with inefficient emptying. Urodynamics shows unsustained, low-pressure detrusor contractions (Fig 29.3e). Abdominal muscles are used to increase the bladder pressure during voiding (Valsalva voiding). The urine flow rate is irregular but continuous; the voiding frequency is low and bladder capacity large. Large volume of residual urine predisposes patients to recurrent UTI and overflow incontinence.

Hinman Syndrome

Non-neurogenic neurogenic bladder (Hinman-Allen syndrome), an acquired form of bladder-sphincteric dysfunction characterized by a combination of bladder decompensation with incontinence, poor emptying, and recurrent urinary infections. Urodynamic studies show decreased bladder capacity and poor compliance with marked sphincteric overactivity and abrupt contractions of the pelvic floor as the child attempts to control incontinence from uninhibited bladder contractions. A neurologic abnormality must be ruled out.

Treatment of Voiding Disorders

Anatomic or neurological causes should be excluded by history and examination, and assessment of voiding diary, uroflowmetry and ultrasonography (Fig. 29.2).

Therapy should include education of the child and family regarding bladder and bowel dysfunction. Constipation should be managed by enemas, followed by use of laxatives. Concurrent urinary tract infections are treated. Dietary advice is given to ensure adequate water and high fiber intake. The patients are encouraged to void every 3–4 hr. Correct posture during voiding is important and caregivers at home and school must allow adequate toilet time and access to clean and safe toilet.

Drug Therapy

For children with detrusor overactivity, anticholinergic agents (oxybutynin, tolterodine) can increase functional bladder capacity and suppress uninhibited contractions during filling (Table 29.4).

Biofeedback Therapy

Biofeedback programs give the child an indication of physiologic processes controlled by the central nervous system that is otherwise not perceived accurately. Through watching urine flow rates, pelvic floor EMG, or detrusor pressures in real time, children can learn to relax the pelvic floor during voiding.

Clean Intermittent Catheterization

Children with dysfunctional elimination syndrome or the Hinman syndrome with recurrent urinary tract infections or upper tract damage occasionally require CIC for effective emptying, just like patients with organic neurogenic bladders.

Enuresis

Enuresis refers to intermittent incontinence during sleep that occurs beyond 5-years of age. Enuresis without any other lower urinary tract symptoms and without history of bladder dysfunction is termed *monosymptomatic*. Enuresis in the presence of lower urinary tract symptom is defined as *non-monosymptomatic*. *Primary* enuresis refers to enuresis in a child who has never been dry whereas *secondary* enuresis is when a child has had a previous dry period of at least 6 months.

Evaluation

It is important to differentiate monosymptomatic from non-monosymptomatic enuresis, since they differ in management and outcome. History is taken for excessive daytime voiding, thirst and urinary tract infections, and for voiding frequency, urgency, holding maneuvers, interrupted micturition, weak stream and straining, and for constipation or fecal incontinence. A family history of enuresis, difficult sleep arousal and a family event or stress, which might have precipitated secondary enuresis is obtained.

A clinical examination is done. The voiding diary provides objective data on voiding frequency, volumes, urgency and incontinence and excludes non-monosymptomatic enuresis.

Urinalysis is done to screen for abnormalities. Blood tests, radiology and urodynamic studies are not necessary.

Management
Behavioral Therapy

This includes the use of voiding diary and general advice to all bed-wetting children such as adequate duration of sleep for age, restricting fluid intake for several hours before sleep, and voiding before sleep. The parents should be advised not to punish the child for wetting episodes. Incentives for a positive *star chart*, as a record of dry and wet nights, can be useful. Counseling of the child and the parents ensures motivation for treatment.

Active Treatment

This is considered beyond 6 years of age and comprise of:

Alarm therapy: It is a therapy based on a device that provides a strong sensory signal, usually acoustic, immediately upon the occurrence of incontinence. It is usually used during night-time sleep. Enuresis alarms are activated by micturition and are intended to change the meaning of the sensation of having a full bladder from a signal to urinate to a signal to inhibit urination and waken.

Types of alarms which can be used are a standard bed-pad-and –bell or a "mini-alarm' which is a discrete portable body-worn alarm with a sensor placed in the pants. Alarms condition children before they wet the bed. Alarms appear more effective than desmopressin or tricyclics as around half the children remain dry after alarm treatment stops. Over learning (giving extra fluids at bedtime after successfully becoming dry using an alarm), dry bed training and avoiding penalties may further reduce the relapse rate.

Alarm therapy should be preferred over pharmacologic therapy because of lack of side effects and better long term results.

Pharmacological therapy: Desmopressin is an analog of vasopressin with increased anti-diuretic activity but no vasopressor activity. It has higher relapse rates than alarm therapy. A short course of desmopressin is also beneficial in children while on alarm therapy (Table 29.4). It is available as a nasal spray (10 µg per puff) and 0.2 mg oral tablets and the dose used is 20–40 µg intranasal at bedtime usually as short

Table 29.4: Medications for functional bladder disorders

Drug	Dose	Duration
Desmopressin		
DDAVP nasal spray	20–40 µg/d nasally at bedtime	until 4 weeks dry
Oral tablets	0.2 to 0.4 mg	until 4 weeks dry
Oxybutinin*	5–20 mg/d	3–6 months
Tolterodine*	1 mg twice daily	3–6 months
Imipramine*	0.9–1.5 mg/kg/d (25–50 mg)	3–6 months

*For use in children> 6 yr

term treatment which is withdrawn every 3 months to reassess for a week. The use of anticholinergic agents (oxybutinin, tolterodine) is limited. Therapy with tricyclic antidepressants (imipramine) is required in cases refractory to all other therapy.

SUPPORT READING

Aubert D, Berard E, Blanc JP, *et al;* Isolated primary nocturnal enuresis: International evidence based management. Consensus recommendations by French Expert Group. Prog Urol 2010; 20: 343–49

Neveus T, Eggert P, Evans J, et al; International Children's Continence Society. Evaluation of and treatment for monosymptomatic enuresis: a standardization document from the International Children's Continence Society. J Urol 2010; 183: 441–47

Jones EA, Vemulakonda VM. Primer: Diagnosis and management of uncomplicated daytime wetting in children. Nat Clin Prac Urol 2006; 3: 551–60

Nevéus T. Nocturnal enuresis - theoretic background and practical guidelines. Pediatr Nephrol 2011; 26: 1207–14

30 Obstructive Uropathy

Obstructive uropathy is an important cause of chronic kidney disease in children. Common causes of obstruction include pelviureteric junction obstruction, vesicoureteric junction obstruction, ureterocele and posterior urethral valves. Intermittent obstruction may be caused by calculi in the bladder or urethra.

Clinical Features

Most cases are detected on antenatal ultrasonography as unilateral or bilateral hydronephrosis. Presentation in late childhood includes dribbling of urine, poor urinary stream, fever and/or urinary tract infections. Examination may reveal a palpable bladder or kidney(s).

Newborns with severe lower urinary tract obstruction present at birth. These patients show additional abnormalities secondary to oligohydramnios, such as Potter sequence, pulmonary hypoplasia and orthopedic complications.

Evaluation

Ultrasonography detects dilated urinary tract, renal and bladder anomalies and calculi. Dynamic scintigraphy is useful for estimating differential renal function in terms of uptake and excretion of radionuclides, including DTPA, LLEC or MAG-3. A post-frusemide scan may show evidence of obstruction. DMSA scintigraphy allows assessment of renal scarring while magnetic resonance urography allows delineation of anatomy in complex malformations.

Pelviureteric Junction (PUJ) Obstruction

PUJ obstruction affects 1 in 500–800 newborns, and is a common cause of hydronephrosis. The condition is more common in boys and is usually unilateral. Ipsilateral or contralateral vesicoureteric reflux, vesicoureteric obstruction or a duplex system may be associated.

Many cases are detected during evaluation for antenatally diagnosed hydronephrosis. Others present later with asymptomatic flank mass, flank pain, urinary tract infection, calculi, or hematuria following minor abdominal trauma. *Dietl crisis* refers to abdominal pain and palpable renal mass that resolve with passage of large amounts of urine.

Diagnosis

Ultrasound shows hydronephrosis with a dilated renal pelvis (>20–30 mm) and normal sized ureter (Fig. 30.1). Diagnosis is confirmed on diuretic renal scintigraphy, which evaluates differential renal function and drainage times. A reduction in split renal function to <40% with prolonged t½ of more than 20 minutes indicates high grade obstruction.

If scintigraphy is not available, intravenous pyelography shows distended renal pelvis and calyces with an abrupt cut off at the PUJ. Micturating cystourethrography (MCU) is indicated if: (*i*) hydronephrosis is bilateral, (*ii*) ureter is dilated, or (*iii*) history suggests urinary tract infections.

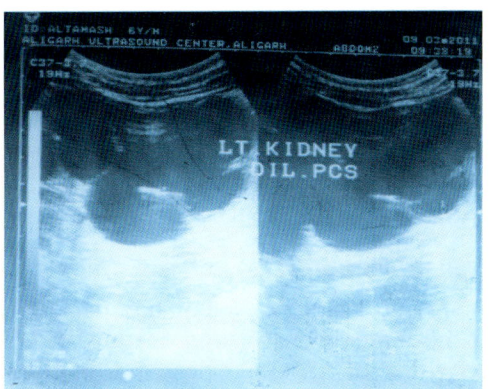

Fig. 30.1: Pelviureteric junction obstruction. Axial ultrasound image of a 4-yr-old child with palpable abdominal lump reveals gross hydronephrosis of left kidney and disproportionately dilated renal pelvis; the ureter was not visualized

Management

Anderson Hynes pyeloplasty, performed using an extraperitoneal approach, is successful in over 95% cases. A double-J stent is placed if the ureter is hypoplastic. Laparoscopic pyeloplasty is less popular. Percutaneous nephrostomy is beneficial in patients with extremely poor renal function (<10%). Unilateral nephrectomy may be required if renal function does not recover with drainage and the patient has refractory hypertension.

Patients without reduction in renal function (differential function >40%) are managed conservatively. Close follow-up is essential. Surgical intervention is planned if differential function declines by >10% on follow up scintigraphy, or there is increasing dilatation or cortical thinning on ultrasonography.

Megaureter

Causes of dilatation of ureter(s) include: *(i)* vesicoureteric junction (VUJ) obstruction; *(ii)* ureterocele, isolated or with a duplex system; *(iii)* vesicoureteric reflux (VUR); *(iv)* non-refluxing unobstructed primary megaureter; and *(v)* prune belly syndrome. Bilateral hydroureteronephrosis with dilated and/or thickened bladder are noted with a neurogenic bladder and urethral obstruction (posterior urethral valves, urethral stricture).

Primary VUJ obstruction is secondary to an aperistaltic segment of the ureter near VU junction that cannot propel urine into the bladder. Constituting 5% cases of neonatal hydronephrosis, the condition is common in males and on the left side. It is often associated with an ureterocele or VUR.

Ureterocele is a congenital condition in which the terminal part of the ureter distends within the bladder to form a sac, due to an abnormality in the submucosal part of the ureter and stenosis of the ureteric orifice (Fig. 30.2). Ureteroceles are more common in girls, occurring usually in association with a duplex system and affecting the upper moiety. Vesicoureteric reflux is common in the lower moiety. Single system ureteroceles are usually seen in boys.

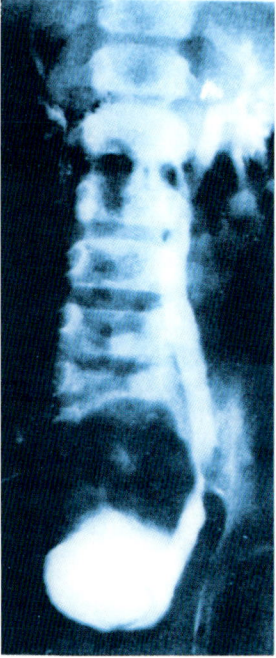

Fig. 30.2: Ureterocele. Intravenous pyelography (IVP) showing single moiety in the left kidney with 'cobra head' appearance of the ureterovesical junction

Primary non-refluxing megaureter is a non-obstructive condition, secondary to functional obstruction at the lower end of the ureter. The ureteric orifice is normal and a ureteric catheter passes easily. Patients with *prune belly syndrome* have degeneration of the abdominal wall musculature and cryptorchidism, bilateral VUR and bladder distension.

Evaluation

VUJ obstruction is suggested by ultrasound finding of a dilated ureter (>7 mm) and absence of reflux on MCU. Obstruction is confirmed on DTPA diuretic renography. In cases where obstruction cannot be excluded, cystoscopy and retrograde pyelogram are performed. On ultrasound, ureterocele is seen as a cystic dilation of the intravesical portion of the ureter. A duplex system must be excluded by DTPA scan or intravenous pyelography.

Management

Surgical treatment of VUJ obstruction consists of excision of the obstructing lower segment of ureter and its reimplantation. Nephro-ureterectomy may be required in patients with very poor renal function and recurrent urinary tract infections.

A ureterocele is managed by endoscopic deroofing. In a duplex system, the upper moiety draining into the ureterocele is excised. Postoperative reflux and obstruction should be excluded by MCU and ultrasound. Rare cases require total excision of the upper moiety (dysplastic kidney, ureter and ureterocele) with reimplantation of the lower moiety ureter.

Definitive surgical treatment for megaureter involves refashioning the lower end of the affected ureter so that a tunnelled reimplantation into the bladder can be done to prevent VUR.

Posterior Urethral Valves

The most common cause of lower urinary tract obstruction in boys is posterior urethral valves (PUV), located at the junction of the anterior and posterior urethra. Obstruction to the urinary stream causes dilatation of posterior urethra, hypertrophy of the bladder neck and trabeculations of the bladder wall. Secondary VUR results in pyelonephritis and reflux nephropathy.

Clinical Features

Infants have variable presentation, depending on the degree of obstruction. Features include dribbling of urine, weak urinary stream, urinary retention, recurrent urinary infections, straining during micturition and a palpable bladder. Infants may show dehydration, urosepsis and dyselectrolytemia. Patients may present later with advanced stages of chronic kidney disease.

Diagnosis

PUV are suspected on antenatal ultrasound, which shows bilateral hydroureteronephrosis and thick walled bladder, with or without oligohydramnios. Postnatally, MCU shows dilated and elongated posterior urethra, enlarged bladder with or without trabeculations and VUR (Fig. 30.3).

Management

Occasional cases with severe PUV, severe hydronephrosis and oligohydramnios benefit from antenatal intra-amniotic shunting. This decision is taken if major extrarenal abnormalities have been excluded and fetal karyotype is normal. Shunt placement might reverse oligohydramnios and ensure prolongation of pregnancy, but is associated with risk of preterm labor, and may not influence the long term outcome.

Infants with PUV require resuscitation at birth, particularly if oligohydramnios is associated with pulmonary hypoplasia. Immediate drainage of the urinary bladder is provided with a 6F feeding tube. Catheterization might be difficult due to coiling of the catheter in the dilated

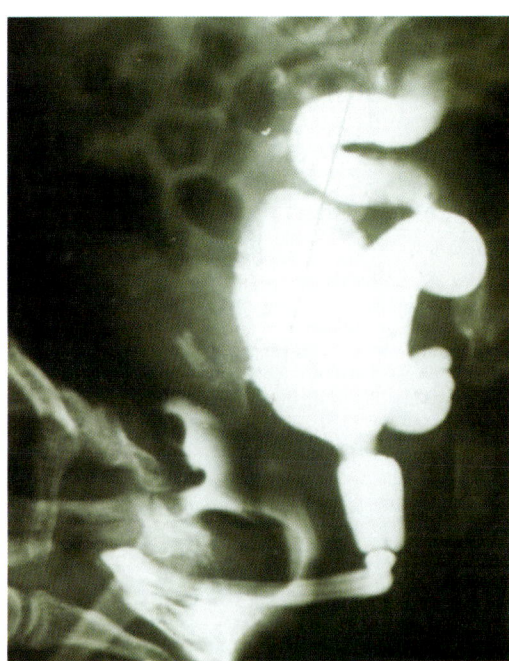

Fig. 30.3: Posterior urethral valves. Micturating cysturethrogram shows dilated posterior urethra, bladder neck hypertrophy and bladder diverticuli. High grades of VUR are often associated

posterior urethra; a suprapubic catheter may be required. A postnatal ultrasound and MCU are performed within 24–48 hr of birth.

Management of acidosis, dehydration and sepsis takes precedence. Endoscopic incision or resection of the valves or tubeless drainage (vesicostomy, ureterostomy) is performed once the neonate is stable, in absence of electrolyte abnormalities and with declining serum creatinine. Valve ablation is carried out in neonates by cystoscopy using small resectoscopes.

If an appropriate sized cystoscope or resectoscope is not available, expertise is lacking or gross pyuria is present, vesicostomy should be carried out. High urinary diversion, such as a high loop ureterostomy, may be considered if the child is sick, has gross pyuria and a trial of bladder drainage has failed. The valves are ablated and the vesicostomy closed when the boy is 1-yr-old.

Complications

VUR is observed in up to 80% cases, with bilateral reflux in 30%. Frequent and double voiding helps decrease reflux associated damage.

Renal dysplasia often begins *in utero*. Progression to end stage renal disease is noted in 30–50%. The success of renal transplantation is determined by the degree of bladder dysfunction.

Bladder dysfunction is common, with manifestations including delay in achieving continence, poor bladder sensation and detrusor instability. The term *valve-bladder syndrome* describes the combination of persistent dilation of the upper urinary tracts, a thick-walled, noncompliant bladder and urinary incontinence seen in patients with PUV. Therapy is directed towards ensuring a low pressure good volume bladder without outflow obstruction. Bladder augmentation, clean intermittent catheterization and reimplantation for VUJ obstruction might be required.

Follow up

Evaluation at each visit includes measurement of blood pressure and assessment of growth, hydration and nutrition. Renal function tests, electrolytes, pH, bicarbonate and urinalysis (proteinuria) are carried out every 6–12 months, and more frequently with advanced renal dysfunction. Urodynamic studies are often necessary.

Complications of Obstruction

Tubular Dysfunction: Obstructive uropathy results in tubulointerstitial injury that presents with polyuria, salt wasting and renal tubular acidosis. Bony abnormalities result from progressive renal insufficiency and metabolic acidosis. Tubular insufficiency also causes severe growth retardation which is disproportionate to the degree of renal impairment.

Increase in fluid intake, supplements of sodium chloride and alkali, and a calorie dense diet is advised.

Hypertension and proteinuria: Hypertension is common with reflux associated scarring. ACE inhibitors are preferred, since most patients also have glomerular hyperfiltration with proteinuria.

Urinary tract infections: Prompt diagnosis and treatment are essential to prevent pyelonephritis. Long-term antibiotic prophylaxis may help patients with recurrent UTI. Asymptomatic bacteriuria should not be treated.

Stones: Magnesium ammonium phosphate (struvite) stones and calcium phosphate stones form in the presence of infected urine. Underlying infection with *Proteus* sp is common.

SUPPORT READING

Riccabona M. Obstructive diseases of the urinary tract in children: lessons from the last 15 years. Pediatr Radiol 2010; 40: 947–55

Sarhan O, El-Ghoneimi A, Hafez A, et al. Surgical complications of posterior urethral valve ablation: 20 years experience. J Pediatr Surg 2010; 45: 2222–26

VI

SECTION VII

Acute Kidney Injury

31 Management of Acute Kidney Injury

Acute renal failure (ARF) or acute kidney injury (AKI) is a complex disorder having several etiologies and occurs in a variety of settings with clinical features ranging from mild elevation in serum creatinine to anuric renal failure. In most instances, an acute decline in kidney function is secondary to tubular injury that leads to functional or structural changes in the kidney.

Pre-Renal and Renal Azotemia

The etiology of ARF is classified as prerenal, intrinsic renal or postrenal. The clinical usefulness of differentiating pre-renal from renal azotemia is the potential of appropriate fluid therapy in reducing raised blood levels of creatinine in the former. A number of indices aid in differentiating pre-renal from renal azotemia, the most useful being determination of the fractional excretion of sodium (Table 31.1).

Definition and Staging of Acute Kidney Injury (AKI)

AKI is considered to be present when there is an abrupt (within 48-hr) reduction in kidney function, defined as an absolute increase in serum creatinine of either ≥ 0.3 mg/dL *or* a percentage increase of $\geq 50\%$ *or* reduction in urine output (documented oliguria of <0.5 mL/kg/hr for >6-hr). These criteria include both an absolute and a percentage change in creatinine to accommodate variations related to age, gender

Table 31.1: Indices to differentiate pre-renal azotemia from intrinsic renal failure

	Pre-renal azotemia	Intrinsic renal failure
Urinary sodium (mEq/L)	<20	>40
Urinary osmolality (mOsm/kg)	>500	<300
Blood urea-creatinine ratio	>20	<20
Urine-plasma osmolality ratio	>1.5	<1.0
Fractional excretion of sodium* (%)	<1	>3

$$*FENa\ (\%) = \frac{urine\ sodium \times serum\ creatinine}{serum\ sodium \times urine\ creatinine} \times 100$$

Acute Kidney Injury

Table 31.2: Staging of Acute Kidney Injury (AKI)*: Criteria proposed by the AKI Network (AKIN) and the pediatric modified RIFLE classification

AKIN Stage	Serum creatinine criteria	Urine output criteria
1	Increase in serum creatinine of >0.3 mg/dL or >150% to 200% (1.5- to 2-fold) from baseline	Less than 0.5 mL/kg per hour for >6-hr
2	Increase in serum creatinine to more than 200% to 300% (>2- to 3-fold) from baseline	Less than 0.5 mL/kg per hour for >12-hr
3**	Increase in serum creatinine to more than 300% (>3-fold) from baseline (or serum creatinine of >4.0 mg/dL with acute increase of >0.5 mg/dL)	Less than 0.3 mL/kg per hour for 24-hr, or anuria for 12-hr
RIFLE Class	**Serum creatinine criteria**	**Urine output criteria**
Risk (R)	Decrease in estimated creatinine clearance by ≥25%	Less than 0.5 mL/kg per hour for >8-hr
Injury (I)	Decrease in estimated creatinine clearance by ≥50%	Less than 0.5 mL/kg per hour for >16-hr
Failure (F)**	Decrease in estimated creatinine clearance by ≥75% or <35 mL/1.73 m²/minute	Less than 0.3 mL/kg per hour for 24-hr, or anuria for 12-hr
Loss (L)	Persistent failure >4 weeks	
End stage (E)	Persistent failure >3 months (end stage renal disease)	

*Only one criterion (creatinine or urine output) should be fulfilled to qualify for a stage
**Patients receiving renal replacement therapy (RRT) are considered in stage 3 (AKIN) or F (pRIFLE)

VII

and body mass index and reduce the need for a baseline level of serum creatinine. It is however necessary that the diagnosis be made following estimation of at least two creatinine values within 48-hr. If the diagnosis of AKI is based on the urine output criterion alone, urinary tract obstruction and other reversible causes of oliguria (hydration status and diuretic use), should be excluded.

Patients meeting the definition of AKI are staged from stage 1 to 3 (Table 31.2). This staging system corresponds to the RIFLE criteria proposed previously. The **R**isk, **I**njury and **F**ailure classes match to stages 1, 2 and 3 respectively. **L**oss and **E**nd stage kidney disease were removed from the staging system, since they represent outcomes. Given the variability in indications and resources for commencing renal replacement therapy, patients receiving such therapy are classified as stage 3 AKI.

Etiology

The chief causes of AKI include acute tubular necrosis secondary to hypovolemia, sepsis and nephrotoxic agents; acute glomerulonephritis; and hemolytic uremic syndrome (Table 31.3).

Newborns are at high risk of AKI. Important causes include: *(i)* perinatal hypoxemia, associated with birth asphyxia or respiratory distress syndrome; *(ii)* hypovolemia secondary to dehydration, intraventricular hemorrhage, heart disease and post-operatively; *(iii)* sepsis with renal hypoperfusion; *(iv)* increased insensible losses (due to phototherapy, radiant warmers), twin-to-twin transfusions and placental hemorrhage; *(v)* nephrotoxic medications, e.g. aminoglycosides, indomethacin; maternal intake of ACE inhibitors, nimesulide; *(vi)* congenital anomalies of the urinary tract, e.g. posterior urethral valves, cystic kidneys; *(vii)* renal vein throm-

Table 31.3: Causes of acute kidney injury

Prerenal failure

Hypovolemia: dehydration, blood loss, diabetic ketoacidosis
Third space losses: septicemia, nephrotic syndrome
Congestive heart failure
Perinatal asphyxia
Drugs: ACE inhibitors, diuretics

Intrinsic renal failure

Acute tubular necrosis
Prolonged prerenal insult (see above)
Hemolytic uremic syndrome: diarrhea associated (D+) and atypical (D-) forms
Glomerulonephritis (GN)
    Postinfectious GN
    Systemic disorders: SLE, Henoch-Schönlein syndrome, microscopic polyangiitis
    Membranoproliferative GN
Medications: aminoglycosides, radiocontrast, NSAIDs
Exogenous toxins: diethylene glycol
Intravascular hemolysis, hemoglobinuria
Tumor lysis syndrome
Interstitial nephritis (drug-induced, idiopathic)
Bilateral renal vessel occlusion (arterial, venous)

Postrenal failure

Posterior urethral valves, urethral stricture
Bilateral pelviureteric junction obstruction
Ureteral obstruction: stenosis, stone, ureterocele
Neurogenic bladder

ACE angiotensin converting enzyme; NSAIDs non-steroidal anti-inflammatory drugs; SLE systemic lupus erythematosus

bosis, e.g. in infants of diabetic mothers, dehydration, polycythemia and catheterization of umbilical veins; and *(viii)* delayed initiation and inadequacy of feeding.

Evaluation

A careful history provides clues to underlying cause of ARF. In a child with oligoanuria, it is important to assess for prerenal factors that lead to renal hypoperfusion. A history of diarrhea, vomiting, fluid or blood loss should be sought and an assessment of fluid intake in the previous 24 hr made.

Table 31.4 enlists the investigations in patients with ARF. Ultrasonography is the ideal imaging tool because of its non dependence on renal function. It allows visualization of the pelvicalyceal system, and assessment of the renal size, structural anomalies and calculi.

Kidney Biopsy

Indications for a kidney biopsy in a patient with ARF are:

1. Rapidly progressive glomerulonephritis; or non-resolving glomerulonephritis
2. ARF associated with a systemic disease, e.g. systemic lupus erythematosus, Henoch-Schönlein purpura

Acute Kidney Injury

VII

Table 31.4: Investigations in acute kidney injury

Blood
  Complete blood counts
  Urea, creatinine, electrolytes, calcium, phosphate, pH, bicarbonate
Urine
  Urinalysis; culture
  Sodium, osmolality, fractional excretion of sodium
Chest X-ray
Abdominal ultrasonography

Investigations to determine cause (indication)

Peripheral smear examination, platelet and reticulocyte count, complement (C3), LDH levels; stool culture (suspected hemolytic uremic syndrome)
Antistreptolysin O, C3, antinuclear antibody, antineutrophil cytoplasmic antibody (acute or rapidly progressive glomerulonephritis)
Doppler ultrasonography (suspected arterial or venous thrombosis)
Renal biopsy (specific diagnosis feasible)

3. Interstitial nephritis, where a precise diagnosis may allow institution of specific therapy
4. Patients with a clinical diagnosis of acute tubular necrosis or hemolytic uremic syndrome if significant renal dysfunction persists beyond 2–3 weeks
5. Underlying cause of ARF not apparent on clinical features and investigations

Patients with azotemia (blood urea >150–200 mg/dL, creatinine >3–4 mg/dL) are at risk of bleeding following renal biopsy. These patients should be dialyzed, either by peritoneal or hemodialysis, prior to the procedure. Hypertension should be controlled; platelet count and bleeding, clotting and prothrombin time should be normal. IV (0.3 µg/kg) or nasal (2–3 µg/kg) desmopressin, administered 60–90 minutes prior, is useful in reducing the risk of bleeding.

MANAGEMENT

Management includes treatment of life-threatening complications, maintenance of fluid and electrolyte balance and nutritional support. Specific management of the under-lying disorder is possible in a minority (Table 31.5). Patients with urinary tract obstruction should be managed urgently. Definitive surgery is performed after AKI has been treated.

Complications

In patients with AKI and oligoanuria, attention is directed towards the diagnosis and management of life-threatening complications (Table 31.6). These include hyperkalemia, pulmonary edema, hypertensive emergencies, severe acidosis and anemia. Clinical evaluation includes measurement of blood pressure, search for signs of congestive heart failure, fluid overload, acidosis and anemia. An electrocardiogram and X-ray chest are done.

Principles of Supportive Care

Fluid and Electrolyte Balance

Fluid and electrolyte intake should be carefully regulated. The daily fluid requirement amounts to insensible water losses (300–400 mL/m^2), urinary output and extrarenal fluid losses. It is usually possible to administer the

Table 31.5: Management of common conditions causing acute kidney injury

Prerenal acute kidney injury	Administer crystalloids; stop therapy with diuretics, NSAIDs, ACE inhibitors; inotropes (for cardiac failure and hypotension)
Acute tubular necrosis	Supportive care; discontinue nephrotoxic drug
	Treat cause of circulatory failure
Glomerulonephritis	Supportive care; occasionally, antibiotics or immunosuppressive medications
Hemolytic uremic syndrome	Supportive care; plasma infusions, plasma exchange
Vasculitis	Immunosuppressive medications; plasma exchange
Interstitial nephritis	Discontinue offending drug; steroid therapy
Renal artery, vein occlusion	Anticoagulation; thrombolysis or surgery
Urinary tract obstruction	Bladder catheter or nephrostomy; treatment of obstruction

required amounts of fluid by mouth. Ongoing treatment is guided by intake-output analysis, daily weight, physical examination and serum sodium.

Diet

Patients with AKI have increased metabolic needs and are usually catabolic. Adequate nutritional support is preferred with maximization of caloric intake. Volume restriction is necessary during the oliguric phase but often imposes limits on the caloric intake. A diet containing 1.2–2 g/kg of protein in infants and 0.8–1.2 g/kg in older children, and 60–80 Cal/kg should be given. The latter requirement is achieved by adding liberal amounts of carbohydrates and fats to the diet. Once dialysis is initiated, dietary protein, fluid and electrolyte intake should be increased.

Infections

Infections (respiratory and urinary tract, peritonitis and septicemia) are an important causes of death. Procedures should be performed with aseptic techniques, IV lines carefully watched, and skin puncture sites cleaned and dressed. Long-term catheterization of the bladder should be avoided. Features that suggest systemic infection include persistent hypotension, hyperkalemia and a disproportionate rise of blood urea compared to creatinine. If infection is suspected, appro-priate specimens are taken for culture and antibiotics started.

Medications

Drugs that increase severity of renal damage, delay recovery of renal function or reduce renal perfusion, e.g. aminoglycosides, radio-contrast media, NSAIDs, amphotericin B, ACE inhibitors and indomethacin, should be avoided. Standard charts are used for modifying the dose and dosing interval of antibiotics, depending on the severity of renal injury (Appendix 3 and 4).

While diuretics may transiently improve urine output, there is no evidence that their use improve either renal function or the prognosis of intrinsic renal failure. They may be useful in instances where high urine flow is required to prevent intratubular precipitation as with intravascular hemolysis, hyperuricemia and myoglobinuria.

Dopamine

Dopamine at low doses causes renal vasodilatation and may induce a modest natriuresis and diuresis. There is however no beneficial effect of dopamine infusion on the outcome of AKI, and its use for prevention or treatment of acute tubular necrosis is not recommended. Infusion of dopamine might be associated with tachycardia, arrhythmias, and myocardial and tissue ischemia. The role of other

Acute Kidney Injury

VII

Table 31.6: Management of complications

Complication	Treatment	Remarks
Fluid overload	Fluid restriction: insensible losses (400 mL/m²/d); add urine output & other losses; 5% dextrose for insensible losses; N/5 saline for urine output	Monitor other losses and replace as appropriate, consider dialysis, prefer oral to IV route
Pulmonary edema	Oxygen; frusemide 2–4 mg/kg IV	Monitor using CVP; consider dialysis
Hypertension	Symptomatic: Sodium nitroprusside 0.5–8 μg/kg/min infusion; frusemide 2–4 mg/kg IV; nifedipine 0.3–0.5 mg/kg oral or sublingual Asymptomatic: Nifedipine, amlodepine, prazosin, labetalol, clonidine	In emergency, reduce blood pressure by one-third of the desired reduction during first 6–8 hr, 1/3 over next 12–24 hr and the final 1/3 slowly over 2–3 days
Metabolic acidosis	Sodium bicarbonate (IV or oral) if bicarbonate levels <18 mEq/L	Watch for fluid overload, hypernatremia, hypocalcemia; consider dialysis
Hyperkalemia	Calcium gluconate (10%) 0.5–1 mL/kg over 5–10 min IV Salbutamol 5–10 mg nebulized Sodium bicarbonate (7.5%) 1–2 mL/kg over 15 min IV Dextrose (10%) 0.5–1 g/kg and insulin 0.1–0.2 U/kg IV Calcium or sodium resonium (Kayexalate) 1 g/per day PO	Stabilizes cell membranes; prevents arrhythmias Shifts potassium into cells Shifts potassium into cells Requires monitoring of blood glucose Given orally or rectally, repeated every 4 hrs
Hyponatremia	Fluid restriction; if sensorial alteration or seizures give 3% saline 6–12 mL/kg over 30–90 minutes	Hyponatremia is usually dilutional; 12 mL/kg of 3% saline raises sodium by 10 mEq/L
Severe anemia	Packed red cells 3–5 mL/kg; consider exchange transfusion	Monitor blood pressure, fluid overload
Hyperphosphatemia	Phosphate binders (calcium carbonate, acetate; aluminum hydroxide)	Reduce dietary phosphate from milk products, high protein diets

CVP central venous pressure, IV intravenous, PO per orally
Modified from Pediatric Nephrology; 5th edn, 2011. Eds. Srivastava RN, Bagga A.

medications, including fenoldopam, atrial natriuretic peptide and calcium channel blockers is investigational.

Monitoring

Accurate record of intake and output and weight is maintained. Laboratory tests are done depending upon the patient's condition, progression of AKI and presence of complications. Careful physical examination is done at least twice a day, or more frequently if necessary.

Renal Replacement Therapy (RRT)

ARF requiring dialysis can be managed with a variety of modalities, including peritoneal dialysis, intermittent hemodialysis, and continuous hemofiltration or hemodiafiltration. The choice of dialysis modality is influenced by several factors, including the goals of dialysis, the unique advantages and disadvantages of each modality and institutional resources.

Indications for initiating RRT include severe or persistent hyperkalemia (>7 mEq/L), fluid overload (pulmonary edema, severe hypertension), uremic encephalopathy, and severe metabolic acidosis (TCO$_2$ <10–12 mEq/L), hyponatremia (120 mEq/L or symptomatic) or hypernatremia. The decision to institute dialysis should be based on an overall assessment of the patient keeping in view the likely course of ARF.

Intermittent Peritoneal Dialysis (IPD)

The initial renal replacement therapy of choice in sick and unstable patients is often IPD. It is popular because of the ease of initiation and effectiveness in children of all ages, including neonates. Peritoneal access can be obtained using a stiff catheter and trocar. While peritoneal dialysis can be effectively performed with these catheters, these should be removed after 48–72 hr, beyond which the risk of infection is very high.

The risk of injury to the viscera and infections is considerably less with soft silastic (Tenckhoff or Cook) catheters, which therefore can be used for prolonged periods. The standard (double-cuff) Tenckhoff catheter needs to be placed surgically, while the temporary (peel-off) catheter can be inserted bedside. The Cook catheter is inserted using a guide wire by the Seldinger technique.

A video on insertion of trocar-based and peel-off catheters and troubleshooting during peritoneal dialysis is enclosed.

The dialysis prescription depends upon the clinical condition. The fill volume varies from 30–50 mL/kg (800–1200 mL/m^2). Commercially available dialysates are lactate based with a dextrose concentration of 1.7%. A higher concentration of dextrose (2.5–3%) facilitates ultrafiltration. The initial dialysis cycles are of short duration (20–30 minutes). Patients who are sick and have severe lactic acidosis are dialyzed using a bicarbonate dialysate.

If the duration of ARF is prolonged and there is a need for renal replacement therapy, chronic peritoneal dialysis may be performed, either manually (continuous ambulatory peritoneal dialysis; CAPD) or with the use of an automated device (continuous cycling peritoneal dialysis; CCPD).

Hemodialysis

Hemodialysis is more efficient for correction of fluid and electrolyte abnormalities and should be the renal replacement therapy of choice in centers where it is available. However, it is expensive to institute, requires expertise and skilled nursing and is not often available. It is not suited for patients with hemodynamic instability, bleeding tendency and in very young children where vascular access might be difficult.

The equipment required is the hemodialysis machine, pediatric dialyzer with tubings and dialysate fluid (*see* Chapter 40). The semipermeable fibers, used in current dialyzers, are made of cellophane, cuprophane or cellulose acetate. These dialyzers are available in different sizes varying between 0.5–1.5 m². Selection of the dialyzer depends upon patient's body size and its ultrafiltrate properties. An appropriate vascular access is necessary for removing and returning large quantities of blood required for the procedure. This is usually achieved using a double lumen venous catheter inserted into the internal jugular, femoral vein or subclavian vein. Most children are maintained on a hemodialysis regimen of 3–4 hr, three times a week. Sick patients with fluid overload often benefit from daily dialysis initially.

Continuous Renal Replacement Therapies (CRRT) and Newer Modalities

CRRT is any extracorporeal blood purification therapy intended to substitute for impaired renal function over an extended period of time and applied, or aimed at being applied for, 24-hr a day. Various modalities include CAVH (continuous arteriovenous hemofiltration), CVVH (continuous venovenous hemofiltration), continuous venovenous hemodiafiltration (CVVHD) and slow continuous ultrafiltration (SCUF). These therapies are useful when large amount of fluids have to be removed in sick and unstable patients. CVVH is also preferred in ARF secondary to major surgical procedures, burns, heart failure and septic shock especially when conventional hemodialysis or intermittent peritoneal dialysis is not possible.

Continuous hemofiltration provides smoother control of ultrafiltered volume and gradual correction of metabolic abnormalities in unstable patients. Special equipment and trained staff is necessary to provide CRRT in children.

The necessity of daily dialysis emphasizes the need for flexible treatments combining the advantages of CRRT and the feasibility of hemodialysis. One such hybrid therapy is a slow long extended daily dialysis (SLEDD) done daily for an extended but limited period (8–10 hr) using lower dialysate flow rates and at the same time minimizing the cost and technical complexities associated with CRRT.

SUPPORT READING

Ricci Z, Cruz D, Ronco C. The RIFLE criteria and mortality in acute kidney injury: A systematic review. Kidney Int 2008; 73: 538–46

Andreoli SP. Acute kidney injury in children. Pediatr Nephrol 2009; 24: 253–63

Bagga A, Bakkaloglu A, Devarajan P, et al; Improving outcomes from acute kidney injury: Report of an initiative. Pediatr Nephrol 2007; 22: 1655–58

Cerda J, Bagga A, Kher V, Chakravarthi RM. The contrasting characteristics of acute kidney injury in developed and developing countries. Nature Clin Pract Nephrol 2008; 4: 138–53

Walters S, Porter C, Brophy PD. Dialysis and pediatric acute kidney injury; choice of renal support modality. Pediatr Nephrol 2009; 24: 37–38

32 Hemolytic Uremic Syndrome

Hemolytic uremic syndrome (HUS) is a triad of hemolytic anemia, thrombocytopenia and renal impairment. The diarrhea associated (classic) HUS occurs in childhood, is caused by shigatoxin (verotoxin) producing bacteria (*Escherichia coli* 0157:H7, O111, O104:H4; *Shigella dysenteriae*) and is associated with a satisfactory prognosis. More than 90% children recover normal renal function with supportive therapy.

Atypical (non-diarrheal) HUS is a heterogeneous disorder, with less favorable outcome. This condition is distinguished from classic HUS by absence of diarrheal prodrome, a chronic and relapsing course, high mortality and risk of end stage renal disease (ESRD). Conditions that might result in HUS are listed in Table 32.1.

Complement Dysregulation in HUS

An uncontrolled activation of the alternative complement pathway is important in many patients. Defects in the genes for complement regulatory proteins have been identified. These include loss of function mutations in factor H (CFH), membrane cofactor protein

Table 32.1: Classification of HUS and related disorders

Infection induced

Shiga and verotoxin producing bacteria: enterohemorrhagic *E. coli* (EHEC), *Shigella dysenteriae* type 1
Citrobacter, Salmonella, Campylobacter, Bartonella, *Streptococcus pneumoniae*
Coxsackievirus, echovirus, influenza, varicella, HIV, Ebstein Barr virus

Disorders of complement regulation

Genetic disorders of complement regulation
Acquired disorders of complement regulation, anti-factor H antibody

Von Willebrand factor protease, ADAMTS13 deficiency

Genetic disorders of ADAMTS13
Acquired von Willebrand protease deficiency; autoimmune; drug induced

Other causes

Defective cobalamin metabolism
Drug induced: quinine, mitomycin, ticlopidine, clopidogrel, calcineurin inhibitors, oral contraceptives
Systemic lupus, post-transplantation

(MCP, CD46), factor I (CFI), factor H related proteins (CFHR) 1–5 and thrombomodulin, and less commonly, gain of function mutations in factor B and C3. Deficiency of a metalloproteinase with thrombospondin motifs-13 (ADAMTS13) and defective cobalamin metabolism are also pathogenic.

Anti-factor H autoantibodies are reported in 6–10% of patients with atypical HUS. These antibodies reduce the binding of factor H to C3b, thereby enhancing activation of the alternative pathway. Antibodies develop chiefly in young children who carry homozygous deletions of *CFHR1* and *CFHR3* genes. A substantial proportion of Indian children presenting with atypical HUS show presence of these antibodies.

While atypical HUS usually develops in presence of an inherent genetic susceptibility, in many individuals, an environmental insult is required for the syndrome to develop (two-hit hypothesis). Many environmental factors such as infection, pregnancy, and drugs are known to trigger episodes of both diarrheal and non-diarrheal HUS. *A proportion of patients with postdysenteric HUS show evidence of complement dysregulation.*

Diagnosis

The diagnosis of HUS is based on documentation of azotemia, thrombocytopenia (platelets <150,000/mm³) and hemolysis, occurring with or without history of preceding diarrhea or dysentery. Hemolysis is identified as anemia with microangiopathy (fragmented RBCs) on peripheral smear, reticulocytosis, and increased LDH. Renal impairment is often severe, with oligoanuria. The urine sediment is normal and the accompanying proteinuria is often in the non-nephrotic range.

Histology

A kidney biopsy is not necessary for confirming the diagnosis. Histological features of thrombotic microangiopathy (TMA) include: (i) intimal hyperplasia resulting in thickening of arterioles and capillaries, (ii) endothelial swelling and detachment, and subendothelial accumulation of proteins and cell debris and (iii) thrombi in capillary lumina (Fig. 32.1). The subendothelial space is widened, platelet thrombi obstruct vessel lumina and there is mesangiolysis. Unless there is rapid resolution, the lesions progress to global glome-

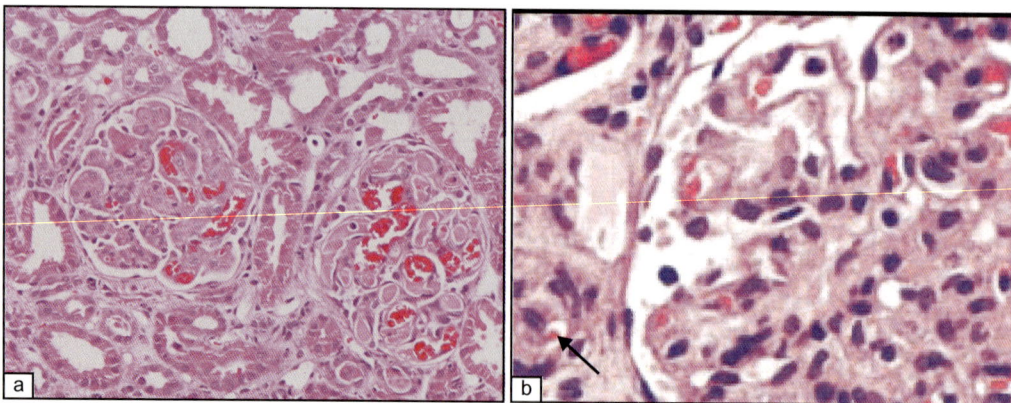

Fig. 32.1: Features of thrombotic microangiopathy showing (a) glomeruli with marked endothelial swelling and capillary lumina occluded with fibrin thrombi, resulting in mesangiolysis; (b) glomerulus showing endothelial swelling and detachment, widened subendothelial space with narrowing of capillary lumina. Arteriole (arrow) shows endothelial swelling and intimal hyperplasia, and platelet thrombi resulting in occlusion of the lumen

rular sclerosis, interstitial fibrosis and tubular atrophy.

While histological changes are most marked in the kidneys, evidence of TMA involving the brain, heart, lungs, gastrointestinal tract and pancreas have been reported.

Evaluation

Investigations aim to identify the underlying etiology.

1. Enterohemorrhagic *E. coli* (EHEC) or *S. dysenteriae* is the likely cause of HUS in patients older than 6 months with history of diarrhea or bloody diarrhea in the 2 weeks preceding the diagnosis. Techniques for detection include stool culture and stool verotoxin analysis (in patients presenting early) and determination of serological response to the bacterial lipopolysaccharide in those presenting late

2. Infection with *S. pneumoniae* (*e.g.*, pneumonia, meningitis, loculated empyema or subdural collection): direct Coombs' test is likely to be positive

3. Systemic causes, such as systemic lupus erythematosus, drugs (calcineurin inhibitors, quinine, antiplatelet agents) and HIV infection should be considered; HELLP syndrome (hemolysis, elevated liver enzymes, low platelet count) of pregnancy should be ruled out

4. Disorder of cobalamin metabolism is suspected in infants with feeding difficulty, hypotonia, lethargy, leukopenia and megaloblastic anemia. Diagnosis requires estimation of plasma and urine homocysteine and methylmalonic acid, and mutation analysis of methylmalonic aciduria and homocystinuria type C genes.

5. Regardless of the diarrheal prodrome, a diagnosis of atypical HUS should be considered in any patient with: age <6 months; insidious onset of symptoms (over >10 days); relapse of HUS (suspec-

ted previous HUS or previous unexplained anemia); HUS post-transplantation; asynchronous family history

Serum levels of complement factor C3 should be estimated. They might be low, however, normal C3 does not exclude a complement disorder and 30–50% patients with complement dysregulation have normal C3 levels.

Blood samples should be taken for estimation of CFH, CFI, CFB, CD46 and anti-CFH antibodies, before instituting plasmapheresis or infusing blood products. In patients with anti-CFH autoantibodies, mutation analysis of genes encoding CFHR proteins should be done. Facilities for whole blood assay for CFH and anti-CFH antibodies are available in many research laboratories across the world. In India, they are available at the All India Institute of Medical Sciences, New Delhi. For details visit *www.ispn-online.org*

In neonates and adolescents presenting with thrombotic thrombocytopenic purpura, congenital deficiency of ADAMTS13 or acquired deficiency due to anti-ADAMTS13 antibodies is suspected. Assay of von Willebrand factor protease (ADAMTS13) activity is required.

MANAGEMENT

Most children with HUS develop some degree of renal insufficiency and approximately two-third require dialysis therapy. Therapy includes the management of acute renal failure and issues specific to HUS. The former includes treatment of fluid and electrolyte disturbances, antihypertensive medications and renal replacement therapy.

Specific management issues in HUS include treatment of hematological complications, avoiding antidiarrheal drugs and monitoring for extrarenal involvement.

Transfusion of packed red blood cells is needed in patients with severe anemia (hemoglobin <6 g/dL). Careful monitoring of blood pressure, urine output and respiratory rate is necessary. Platelet transfusions are limited to children with active bleeding since they might increase microthrombi formation and promote tissue ischemia.

There are no evidence based guidelines on therapy, but there is consensus on the need for prompt *plasmapheresis*, which now forms the standard of care for patients with atypical or recurrent HUS. Blood samples for analysis of complement factors must be taken prior to institution of specific therapies.

Plasmapheresis (Plasma Exchange)

The rationale for plasma exchange is the removal of circulating autoantibodies to complement factor H or the replacement of absent or mutated complement regulators. Plasma exchange should begin as soon as possible, preferably within 24-hr of the diagnosis of atypical HUS, without awaiting a biopsy diagnosis or results of complement studies.

Plasma exchange is performed using either plasma filtration or a centrifugal separator, according to institutional practice. In each session, replacement of 1.5 times the plasma volume (60–75 mL/kg) is done with fresh frozen plasma (*see* Chapter 45).

There are no guidelines on the frequency of plasma exchanges. A rational approach is to perform 1.5 times volume exchange daily for 5 days, or until there is *hematological remission* (platelets >150,000/mm^3 for 2 weeks; no hemolysis on peripheral smear; LDH <300 U/L). This is followed by plasma exchange on alternate day (4–6 exchanges); twice weekly (4–6 exchanges); and then weekly (4 exchanges).

In case of recurrence of activity, therapy may be intensified. The outcome and results of complement testing should be reviewed thereafter to decide regarding need for further plasma exchange. Plasma exchange is not necessary if the clinical features suggest congenital ADAMTS13 deficiency or early onset cobalamin C disorder.

Plasma Infusions

Infusions of fresh frozen plasma are sometimes administered in place of plasma exchange. Care should be taken to avoid fluid overload. The indications for plasma infusions are:

1. Non-availability of facility for plasma exchange, or delay in its institution
2. Difficulty in achieving vascular access
3. Diagnosis of congenital ADAMTS13 deficiency

Fresh frozen plasma is administered at 25–30 mL/kg/day until hematological remission, followed by infusion on alternate days (3–4 infusions), twice weekly (3–4 infusions) and then weekly.

Anti-Factor H Autoantibody Associated HUS

These patients are likely to benefit from plasmapheresis followed by therapy with *intravenous immunoglobulin* (IVIG) and immunosuppression.

Following 3–5 sessions of daily plasmapheresis, IVIG (2 g/kg over 2 days) is administered. The child should not receive plasmapheresis in the 24 hours following IVIG.

Prednisolone is given at a dose of 1 mg/kg/day for 4 weeks, followed by 1 mg/kg on alternate days and then tapered by 0.25 mg/kg every 2 weeks to 0.1–0.2 mg/kg for 12 months following disease remission.

IV cyclophosphamide (500 mg/m^2) is administered 10–15 days following administration of IVIG. Six doses are given every 3–4 weeks, while monitoring for adverse effects. After induction with IV cyclophosphamide, maintenance immunosuppression is continued with *azathioprine* (2 mg/kg/d) or *mycophenolate mofetil* (500–750 mg/m^2) for 12–months.

The above guidelines for therapy of factor H autoantibody associated HUS are based on anecdotal experience from case series, and not from well designed prospective studies. The decision to institute therapy must be taken after appropriate counseling of patients and their families.

Other Agents

The use of *eculizumab,* a high affinity monoclonal antibody targeted against C5, is reported to benefit patients with HUS associated with activation of the complement cascade. Results of an ongoing clinical trial are likely to influence future usage of this agent in patients with complement related HUS. Promising results have also been reported with this medication in recent epidemics of EHEC associated HUS. Other recent potential therapies include factor H concentrate, synthetic complement regulators and rituximab.

Monitoring

Hematological relapse is defined as recurrence of microangiopathic hemolytic anemia and thrombocytopenia, after these parameters have normalized for at least 2 weeks. Screening for relapses (blood counts, LDH, creatinine, urinalysis) is done frequently, particularly following infectious illnesses. Periodic estimation of blood pressure, estimated GFR and urinalysis is necessary to detect disease progression.

Outcome and Kidney Transplantation

Short term outcomes including achievement of hematological remission, degree of renal dysfunction (estimated GFR), proteinuria and hypertension should be assessed at 2–3 months following disease onset. The long term prognosis for patients with atypical HUS is guarded, with acute mortality of 25% and progression to ESRD in 50%.

An unsatisfactory outcome is predicted in those with mutations in the genes encoding complement factors H or I. Patients with autoantibodies to factor H respond well to plasma exchange and immunosuppression. While patients with abnormalities in the transmembrane regulator CD46 are less likely to respond to plasma exchange, their long-term outcome is better.

Renal transplantation is associated with 50% rate of recurrence in the allograft. The risk is higher in patients with mutations in the CFH or CFI, with 80% of patients losing their graft to recurrent disease within 2 years, in contrast to patients with mutations in the CD46 where post-transplant recurrence is rare. Combined liver and kidney transplantation is recommended in the former patients. Patients with autoantibody-induced HUS who require renal transplantation need plasma exchanges and immunosuppressive therapy before and after transplantation.

SUPPORT READING

Dragon-Durey MA, Blanc C, Garnier A, et al. Anti-factor H autoantibody-associated hemolytic uremic syndrome: review of literature of the autoimmune form of HUS. Semin Thromb Hemost 2010; 36: 633–40

Zipfel PF, Heinen S, Skerka C. Thrombotic microangiopathies: new insights and new challenges. Curr Opin Nephrol Hyperten 2010; 19: 372–78

Ariceta G, Besbas N, Johnson S, European Pediatric Study Group for HUS: Guideline for the investigation and initial therapy of diarrhea negative hemolytic uremic syndrome. Pediatr Nephrol 2009, 24: 687–96

Chronic Kidney Disease and Hypertension

33 Principles of Management

Chronic kidney disease (CKD) is defined as kidney damage lasting for at least 3 months, characterized by structural or functional abnormalities of the kidney with or without decreased glomerular filtration rate (GFR). These abnormalities include pathological abnormalities and markers of kidney damage, including abnormalities on urinalysis (hematuria, proteinuria), biochemistry or imaging (e.g. hydronephrosis, single kidney).

Classification

Five stages of CKD are recognized based on the level of kidney function as assessed by estimated GFR (Table 33.1). The classification allows severity to be classified in a standard manner, and enables uniform application of clinical practice guidelines. Since renal maturation increases from infancy to reach adult values at the age of 2 years, CKD stages apply to children beyond >2-yr-old.

Evaluation and Management

Identification and evaluation in children with early stages of CKD has two purposes. General measures can be instituted to retard progression of CKD, and specific treatment allows one to correct a potentially reversible cause. Children with conditions listed in Table 33.2 are at risk of progressive CKD.

The initial evaluation is aimed at determining the underlying cause and complications, and assessment of the nutritional and metabolic status. Important investigations

Table 33.1: Stages of chronic kidney disease (CKD)

Stage	GFR, mL/min/1.73 m²	Description
1	90	Kidney damage with normal or increased GFR
2	60–89	Kidney damage with mild reduction of GFR
3	30–59	Moderate reduction of GFR
4	15–29	Severe reduction of GFR
5	< 15, or dialysis*	Kidney failure

*Patients on dialysis are denoted as CKD stage 5D
GFR glomerular filtration rate

Table 33.2: Conditions predisposing to chronic kidney disease

Vesicoureteric reflux associated with recurrent urinary infections; reflux nephropathy
Obstructive uropathy
History of acute kidney injury
History of acute glomerulonephritis, nephrotic syndrome
History of Henoch-Schönlein purpura, systemic lupus erythematosus, systemic vasculitis
Proliferative glomerulonephritis
Steroid resistant nephrotic syndrome
Diabetes, hypertension
Renal dysplasia, hypoplasia
Low birth weight infants
Urolithiasis, nephrocalcinosis
Family history of polycystic kidneys, genetic renal conditions

that should be performed in children with CKD, at presentation and periodically thereafter, are listed in Table 33.3.

Figure 33.1 provides an overview of the important aspects of management in children with CKD. Based on results of screening, children require evaluation for co-morbidities. Close follow up with periodic monitoring is essential to detect hypertension, proteinuria and deteriorating renal function.

Preventing Disease Progression

The natural history of CKD in children varies by age at onset and etiology. The course of disease involves a period of improving renal function during infancy, a period of stable renal function, followed by deterioration of function toward end-stage renal disease (ESRD). The rate of progression is variable. It may include a rapid decline soon after infancy, decline at an early pubertal age, or a steady, slow decline of renal function.

Determinants of Progression

Proteinuria and hypertension are not only markers of renal damage in children with CKD, but can also lead to structural and functional nephron damage. Additional factors that may have a role in disease progression in CKD include the renin-angio-tensin system, the genetic background, anemia, altered mineral bone homeostasis, dyslipidemia, inflammation and oxidative stress.

Management

Important measures aimed at retarding progression of CKD include control of hypertension and proteinuria, dietary counseling and prevention of acute kidney injury.

Hypertension and Proteinuria

Management of hypertension and proteinuria are important in retarding progression of CKD. Indications for intervention include presence of significant proteinuria (>10 mg/m^2/hr, >1+ protein on dipstick or >1 g/1.73 m^2/day) or hypertension. The preferred agent is an angiotensin converting enzyme (ACE) inhibitor, such as enalapril or ramipril. Patients should be evaluated for hyperkalemia every 2–3 months. Concurrent administration of potassium sparing diuretic, NSAIDs and potassium supplements is avoided.

While most guidelines advise reduction of blood pressure to the 90th percentile, recent reports suggest that control of blood pressure to the 50–75th percentile for age effectively retards disease progression.

Table 33.3: Evaluation of a child with chronic kidney disease

Evaluation at onset; periodically thereafter

Growth (weight for age, height for age, weight for height)
Blood pressure (stage of hypertension), evidence of end-organ damage
Hemogram; peripheral smear
Blood urea, creatinine, uric acid; electrolytes; pH, bicarbonate
Calcium, phosphorus, alkaline phosphatase; parathormone; 25-hydroxyvitamin D
Total protein, albumin; transaminases
Iron studies (ferritin, transferrin saturation)
Urinalysis; spot or timed protein to creatinine ratio
Chest radiograph; electrocardiogram; echocardiography
Radiographs for mineral bone disease (rickets, osteomalacia, osteitis fibrosa cystica)

Evaluation for cause

History and physical examination
Urinalysis; 24-hr urine protein, creatinine

Suspected structural cause

Ultrasonography for kidney, ureters and bladder
Micturating cystourethrography, CT scan with contrast, MR urography
Radionuclide DTPA, MAG-3 scintigraphy

Suspected tubulointerstitial disease

DMSA renal scan
MR urography
Renal histology (in select cases)

Evaluation for glomerular disease

Eye; ear examination
Complement C3; antinuclear nuclear antibodies, antibodies to double stranded DNA, antineutrophil cytoplasmic antibody
Hepatitis B surface antigen; hepatitis C antibody; HIV antibody
Renal histology

Other agents are used if blood pressure control is unsatisfactory. Angiotensin receptor blockers have additional antiproteinuric effects. Dihydropyridines (e.g. nifedipine, amlodipine) are avoided since they might increase proteinuria. Thiazide diuretics are not helpful at creatinine clearance <30 mL/minute/1.73 m². Beta blockers have adverse effects of exercise intolerance, dyslipidemia and hyperglycemia.

Nutrition

Dietary protein restriction has an equivocal role in retarding disease progression. *Protein restriction is not recommended* in children with CKD since it restricts normal growth, with no clear benefits in terms of retarding progression. A balanced diet that provides the recommended dietary allowance for calories and protein should be ensured, with 10–12% of calories through proteins of predominantly

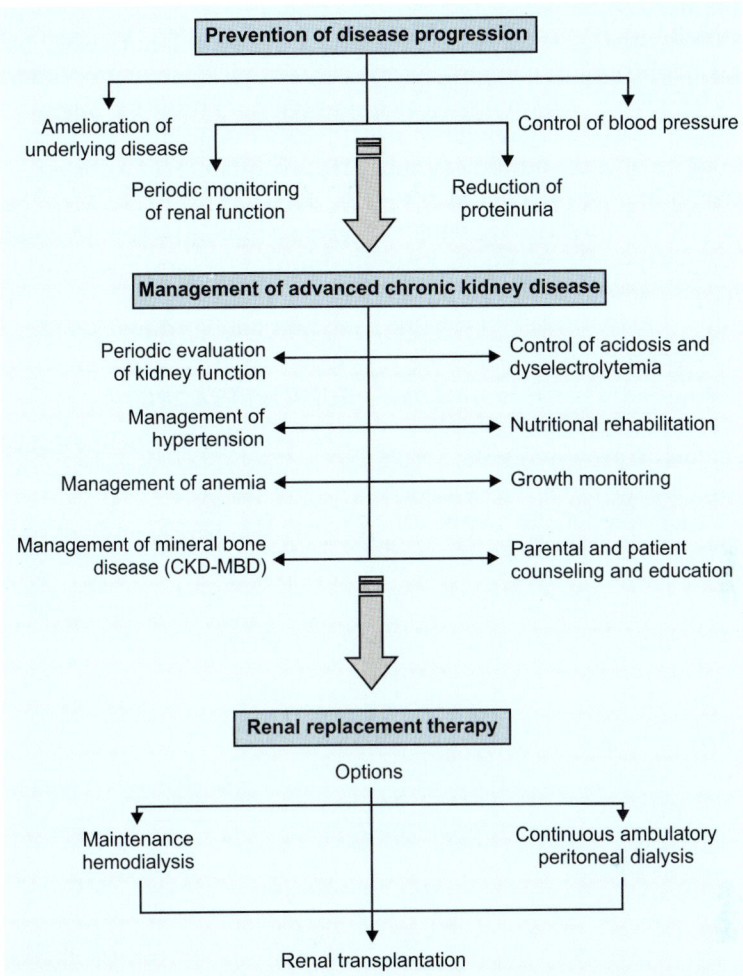

Fig. 33.1: Scheme for evaluation and management of chronic kidney disease (CKD) in children. All children require measures to prevent further disease progression, and evaluation for co-morbidities. Close follow up with periodic monitoring is essential to detect hypertension, proteinuria and deteriorating renal function. Children with CKD stages 3 and beyond require management of co-morbidities such as mineral bone disease and anemia. Renal replacement therapy is indicated when the estimated glomerular filtration rate falls below 8–12 mL/min/1.73 m^2

high biological value (*see* Chapter 36). Children on dialysis need additional protein.

Preventing Additional Renal Injury

An essential component of preventing disease progression is the prevention of added renal insult. The strategies include:

Avoidance of volume depletion: Attention to adequate fluid intake is particularly important during diarrhea, vomiting, fever or sepsis.

Prevention of cortical scarring: Patients with recurrent urinary tract infections and vesicoureteric reflux should receive antibiotic prophylaxis to prevent renal cortical damage.

Chronic Kidney Disease and Hypertension

VIII

Prevention of radiocontrast induced nephropathy: All patients with CKD and AKI are at risk of contrast nephropathy. Patients with advanced CKD (eGFR <30 mL/min/1.73 m²) are at higher risk. The use of imaging procedures that do not involve the administration of radiocontrast should be considered. Strategies to prevent radiocontrast induced injury are discussed in Chapter 37. Magnetic resonance imaging with administration of gadolinium is avoided due to the risk of nephrogenic systemic fibrosis.

Prevention of drug-induced nephrotoxicity: When available, non-nephrotoxic drugs are preferred over nephrotoxic agents. Drug doses are adjusted according to the estimated glomerular filtration rate (eGFR) (Appendix 3). Loading doses may be administered without renal dose adjustment. Maintenance doses are adjusted either by reduction of individual dose or by increasing the dose interval. While the former strategy risks toxicity due to drug accumulation, the latter risks subtherapeutic dosing.

Therapy with NSAIDs and cyclo-oxygenase inhibitors should be avoided. Herbal compounds, and medications containing heavy metals, ephedra and aristolochic acid should not be administered.

SUPPORT READING

Staples A, Wong C. Risk factors for progression of chronic kidney disease. Current Opin Pediatr 2010; 22: 161–69

Whyte DA, Fine RN. Chronic kidney disease in children. Pediatrics Rev 2008; 29: 335–41

34 Mineral Bone Disease

The majority of children with CKD stage 3 or greater have bone disease and mineral disorders. These abnormalities are associated with significant morbidity, including bone pains, fractures, vascular calcification and adverse cardiovascular events.

Definition and Classification

The term renal osteodystrophy should be used in patients with CKD where an alteration of bone morphology is seen on histomorphometry. The constellation of clinical, biochemical, and imaging abnormalities associated with CKD are defined as 'Chronic Kidney Disease-Mineral and Bone Disorder' (CKD-MBD). The alterations in bone metabolism are classified as laboratory (L) or bone (B) abnormalities, and vascular and soft tissue calcification (C).

EVALUATION

Biochemical Abnormalities

Monitoring should begin from CKD stage 2 onwards. Evaluation includes: (i) blood levels of calcium, phosphorus, alkaline phosphatase; (ii) venous pH and bicarbonate; (iii) parathormone (PTH) and (iv) X-rays of wrist with hand and pelvis. Table 34.1 provides the target range for biochemical levels.

Blood biochemistry is determined at baseline and monitored every 6–12 months in children with CKD stages 2 and 3, every 6 months in children with CKD 4, every 1–3 months in CKD 5 and monthly in those on

Table 34.1: Biochemical targets for chronic kidney disease-mineral bone disease

	Calcium mg/dL*	Phosphorus mg/dL	SAP IU/dL	Ca x P product	PTH pg/mL
Age 1–12 years					
CKD 2–3	9.0–10.2	4–6	100–450	<65	35–70
CKD 4	9.0–10.2	4–6	100–450	<65	70–110
CKD 5, 5D	8.8–9.7**	4–6	100–450	<65	200–300
Age >12 years					
CKD 2–3	8.8–10.2	2.5–4.5	40–180	<55	35–70
CKD 4	8.8–10.2	2.5–4.5	40–180	<55	70–110
CKD 5, 5D	8.8–9.7**	3.5–5.5	40–180	<55	200–300

*In hypoalbuminemia, corrected calcium (mg/dL) = observed calcium + 0.8 × [4 – serum albumin in g/dL]
**Hypercalcemia is defined as total blood level >10.2 mg/dL
SAP serum alkaline phosphatase, PTH parathormone, CKD chronic kidney disease

dialysis. Blood calcium and phosphorus levels should be measured every 6–12 months in patients with primary or secondary tubular disorders.

In children with CKD 2–4, estimation of 25-hydroxyvitamin D is recommended once at baseline and repeated if PTH is above the recommended levels while serum phosphorus remains normal. Frequent evaluation is required in patients receiving therapy for laboratory abnormalities, transplant recipients or while on recombinant growth hormone therapy.

Bone Radiographs

These are indicated in patients with clinical features suggestive of rickets, avascular necrosis, slipped proximal femoral epiphyses, or for assessment of skeletal maturation.

Iliac Crest Bone Biopsy with Double Tetracycline Labeling

Bone histomorphometric analysis is an accurate test for determining the type of bone disease associated with CKD, but is not performed routinely. Indications for the procedure include: (i) fractures with minimal or no trauma (pathological fractures); (ii) suspected aluminum bone disease, based upon clinical symptoms or history of aluminum exposure; and (iii) persistent hypercalcemia with PTH levels between 400–600 pg/mL.

Common Abnormalities

These include hypocalcemia, hyperphosphatemia, acidosis and/or elevated alkaline phosphatase; low serum 25-hydroxyvitamin D indicates nutritional deficiency. Levels of 1, 25 dihydroxyvitamin D may be low despite correction of deficiency in patients with CKD 4–5. Secondary hyperparathyroidism is present in advanced CKD.

Radiological changes mimic those seen in rickets. With untreated severe disease, subperiosteal resorption, osteosclerosis, bony deformities or fractures are noted (Fig. 34.1).

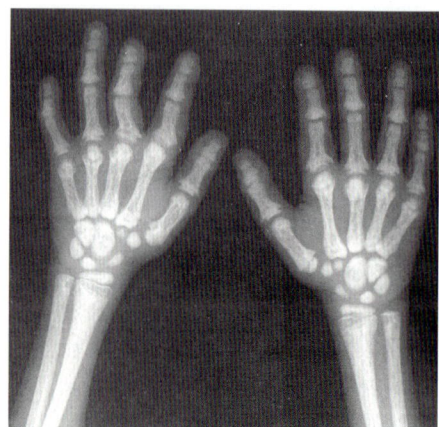

Fig. 34.1: X ray of wrist and hand in a 11-yr-old with primary hyperoxaluria and CKD 5D. There is marked subperiosteal resorption at ends of metacarpals and in proximal and middle phalanges

Bone disease may manifest as growth failure, features of rickets, fractures or body aches

MANAGEMENT

The principles of management of CKD-MBD are similar across all stages of CKD. Dialysis is an additional modality for management of refractory hyperphosphatemia in patients with CKD 5. Table 34.2 summarizes the strategies in management.

Vitamin D Deficiency

Supplements of cholecalciferol (vitamin D3) are recommended if the blood level of 25-hydroxyvitamin D is <30 ng/mL. Dosing is based on the severity of deficiency (Table 34.3). In absence of levels, patients with elevated PTH and alkaline phosphatase may be treated once empirically, provided the serum phosphorus is not elevated. Patients with CKD 5 cannot convert cholecalciferol to its active forms, and thus might not benefit by the above supplementation.

Cholecalciferol preparations available in India contain 60 000 IU per sachet. Most oral preparations of calcium carbonate contain 200 IU of vitamin D per 5 mL of syrup or 400 IU per tablet.

Table 34.2: Treatment strategies for chronic kidney disease-mineral bone disease (CKD-MBD)

	Biochemistry	Therapy
A.	Normal calcium, phosphorus, SAP & PTH	No treatment
B.	Hypocalcemia	Calcium supplements with or without vitamin D
C.	Normal or low calcium, normal phosphorus, high PTH	***CKD 2–4*** Vitamin D deficiency: Therapy with cholecalciferol, later give multivitamin preparation with 400 IU vitamin D Restrict dietary phosphate to dietary recommended intake ***Non response or CKD 5:*** Active analog of vitamin D
D.	Normal calcium, high phosphorus, high PTH	Restrict dietary phosphate to 80% of dietary recommended intake Oral phosphate binder (i) calcium based; (ii) non calcium based ***CKD 5:*** Initiate dialysis
E.	CKD 5; normal or high calcium, normal or high phosphorus, high PTH	Measures as in D above Consider 'low calcemic' vitamin D (doxercalciferol, oxacalcitriol, paricalcitol) Consider cinacalcet Subtotal parathyroidectomy if PTH level >500 pg/mL
On Vitamin D Therapy		
A.	High calcium, high phosphorus, low PTH	Withhold or decrease vitamin D dose Decrease dose of calcium based binder; switch to non-calcium based binder If on dialysis: use low calcium dialysis settings
B.	Normal or low calcium, normal or low phosphorus, high PTH	Increase dose of vitamin D

Table 34.3: Correction of vitamin D deficiency

Blood 25(OH) D	Severity	Cholecalciferol dose, IU		Administration	Duration of therapy
<5 ng/mL	Severe deficiency	Initially	60000	Weekly	4 weeks
		Later	60000	2 times a month	2 months
5–15 ng/mL	Mild deficiency	60000		2 times a month	3 months
16–30 ng/mL	Insufficiency	60000		Once a month	3 months

25(OH)D 25 hydroxyvitamin D

Hyperphosphatemia

Dietary Restriction of Phosphate

Children with elevated PTH despite normal serum phosphorus levels should reduce dietary phosphate to that recommended by dietary reference intake (DRI). Age appropriate DRI are as follows: (i) <6 months old: 100 mg; (ii) 7 months to 1 year old: 275 mg; (iii) 1–8 years old: 500 mg; (iv) 9–18 years old: 1250 mg. If serum phosphorus levels are elevated, dietary phosphate should be restricted further to 80% of the DRI.

Phosphate consumption (mg) may be approximated by the product of daily protein intake (g) and 15. Foods with high phosphorus content include dairy products (milk, yogurt), processed foods, maize, wheat, Bengal gram, green gram, rajmah, soyabean, carrot and groundnut. Cottage cheese, pulses, egg and chicken have lower phosphorus content (*see* Appendix 11).

Dietary intervention is difficult to implement because foods with high phosphate content are also usually rich in protein and calcium. Therefore the use of phosphate binders is an important strategy to restrict dietary phosphate absorption (*see* below).

Phosphate Binders

In patients with CKD 2–4, phosphate binders are required if phosphorus levels are not controlled despite dietary restriction. An ideal binder is one that is effective, palatable, non-toxic, not absorbed, compatible with tube feeding, long acting and inexpensive. No current binder fulfils all requirements. Table 34.4 compares the potency of various types of phosphate binders. All binders require to be given with food. Simultaneous administration of iron preparations is avoided.

Calcium based phosphate binders are used most commonly because they are inexpensive and safe. However, in absence of urinary excretion, their use may be associated with hypercalcemia and ectopic calcification. When taken between meals, they act as calcium supplements. They are administered at a dose of 30–50 mg/kg of elemental calcium, such that the total calcium from all sources (including diet) does not exceed twice the RDA for age (maximum dose 2.5 g). Calcium acetate has lower risk of hypercalcemia and higher phosphate binding capacity than calcium carbonate. Gastro-intestinal effects (nausea, vomiting, abdominal pain, diarrhea, constipation) are common with acetate preparations.

Magnesium carbonate is not used since it causes diarrhea, is less effective than calcium salts, and may lead to hypermagnesemia in children on dialysis.

Sevelamer hydrochloride, a non-absorbable polymer of allylamine hydrochloride,

absorbs phosphate and organic anions while releasing chloride anions in the small intestine. It is used if hyperphosphatemia persists despite maximal doses of calcium based binders, or if hypercalcemia develops. The drug is currently not recommended for infants and young children. Sevelamer cannot be added to tube feeds as it forms an insoluble gel that occludes the lumen. Patients are monitored for acidosis and low serum cholesterol; malabsorption of fat soluble vitamins may occur. *Sevelamer carbonate* is free of the risk of metabolic acidosis. Blood levels of calcium and phosphate are repeated every 4–8 weeks, and PTH every 3–6 months.

Aluminum hydroxide is effective but carries the risk of aluminum toxicity, which manifests as bone disease, anemia and encephalopathy. A single course lasting 4–6 weeks is used in patients with serum phosphorus >7 mg/dL. Concurrent administration of citrate-based products promotes aluminum absorption and should be avoided.

Lanthanum is a trivalent cation that binds phosphate ionically and is active over a wide pH range. While approved for adults on dialysis, it is not licensed for use in children due to concerns of its deposition in skeleton and liver. Other potential phosphate binders include ferric citrate and niacin; experience with these agents is limited.

Dialysis

Phosphate is poorly removed by conventional thrice-weekly hemodialysis or peritoneal dialysis. By 12-hr post dialysis, levels reach 80% of predialysis values. Most patients on dialysis require oral phosphate binders. Short daily or slow nocturnal hemodialysis is effective for removing phosphate. Modifying the dialysis prescription to use calcium neutral dialysate (1.25 mmol/L, 5 mg/dL) allows for prescription of larger doses of calcium.

Table 34.4: Relative efficacy of oral phosphate binders

	Ca absorbed %	Phospho-rus (P) binding (per g)	Ca (mg) absorbed per mg P bound	Pills to bind 100 mg P	Comments
Calcium carbonate* (calcium content 40%) 250, 500 mg	20–30	39 mg	8	5 (2500 mg)**	Dissociates at pH <5; avoid with H2 blockers/proton pump inhibitors; maximal binding at high pH
Calcium acetate (calcium content 25%) 167 mg	20; 40 if between meals	45 mg	3	13 (2197 mg)	Soluble over wide pH; less Ca absorbed for same P binding than CaCO₃; GI adverse effects
Sevelamer hydrochloride 400, 800 mg	0	80	0	3 (1200 mg)	Preferred if hypercalcemia; Metabolic acidosis a side effect
Aluminum hydroxide 200 mg/10 mL	0	22 mg/ 5 mL; 15 mg/ tablet	0		Constipation, bone disease, encephalopathy; avoid >6 weeks

* All preparations contain vitamin D_3 125 IU per 250 mg elemental calcium
** Exceeds daily permissible limit, as calcium administered through food and medications should not exceed 2.5 g

Therapy for Hyperparathyroidism

Active Forms of Vitamin D

Patients with CKD are treated with vitamin D analogs (calcitriol, alphacalcidiol) if hyperparathyroidism persists despite lowering serum phosphorus to below 5.5 mg/dL while serum calcium is normal (<10.2 mg/dL). In patients with CKD 2–4, such therapy should be considered only if these abnormalities persist despite repletion of 25-hydroxy-vitamin D (>30 ng/mL).

The dosing of 1, 25 dihydroxyvitamin D in patients with CKD stage 2–4 is based on body weight: <10 kg: 0.25 µg twice a week; 10–20 kg: 0.25 µg on alternate days; and >20 kg: 0.25 µg daily. In patients on dialysis, the dose is titrated to serum PTH levels, as follows: 300–500 pg/mL: 7.5 ng/kg (maximum 0.25 µg/d); 500–1000 pg/mL: 15 ng/kg (maximum 0.5 µg/d); and >1000 pg/mL: 25 ng/kg (maximum 1 µg/d). The benefits of pulse oral or IV calcitriol for the control of hyperparathyroidism in children are unclear.

Close monitoring and frequent dose adjustments are required during therapy. Serum calcium and phosphate should be measured monthly initially and every 1–3 months thereafter.

For patients with persistent hyperparathyroidism (PTH >500 pg/mL) and high normal serum calcium (10.2–10.5 mg/dL), therapy with a low-calcemic vitamin D analog is preferred. These include doxercalciferol (oral 1–3.5 µg daily; IV 4–6 µg thrice a week after hemodialysis) and paricalcitol (2–4 µg thrice a week).

Parathyroidectomy

This is indicated if serum PTH >1000 pg/mL, with persistent or recurrent hypercalcemia with or without persistent hyperphosphatemia, which is refractory to measures described above. Rare indications include patients with evidence of metastatic calcifications or calciphylaxis. An ultrasound and nuclear scintigraphy are performed to evaluate the parathyroid glands. Subtotal parathyroidectomy or total parathyroidectomy with autotransplantation is performed.

Cinacalcet

Calcimimetics increase the sensitivity of the calcium sensing receptor in the parathyroid glands to ionized calcium by allosteric binding. Therefore, administration of cinacalcet causes a dose dependent decrease in plasma PTH levels (up to 80%) that is useful in patients with refractory hyperparathyroidism. Adverse effects include nausea, vomiting and hypocalcemia. The drug is not approved for use in children in absence of safety information, particularly in relation to its impact on longitudinal growth.

Abnormalities in Serum Calcium

Calcium Supplements

If hypocalcemia (blood calcium <8.4 mg/dL) is noted, elemental calcium is prescribed at 30–50 mg/kg/day, to be given between meals or on an empty stomach.

Change in Dialysate Calcium Concentration

In patients receiving calcium-based binders, its dialysate concentration is targeted to 2.5 mEq/L or 5 mg/dL. In patients not receiving these binders, the dialysate calcium is kept at 2.5–3.0 mEq/L (1.25–1.5 mM/L or 5–6.25 mg/dL).

Severe Bony Abnormalities

Lower extremity angular deformity should be surgically corrected if the deformity is progressive or severe, as defined by interference with gait, or by the presence of a mechanical axis deviation of >10° between the femur and tibia. Control of secondary hyperparathyroidism is required prior to

surgical correction. Symptomatic proximal femoral slipped epiphyses should be surgically stabilized if recommended target values for PTH are not achieved within 3 months.

Recombinant Human Growth Hormone (rhGH)

Causes of growth failure among children with CKD include: (i) malnutrition due to nutrient deprivation, undue dietary restrictions and anorexia; (ii) fluid and electrolyte disturbances; (iii) metabolic acidosis; (iv) anemia of chronic disease; and (v) hormonal disturbances, including impaired PTH and vitamin D metabolism, abnormalities of the gonadotropic hormone and altered growth hormone and insulin related growth factor axes. Failure is particularly marked in children with onset of disease in young age, syndromic illness, and if parents have short stature. The onset of puberty and pubertal growth spurt are delayed by 1–2 years in children with advanced CKD.

Therapy with rhGH should be considered in children with CKD with short stature (height below 3rd percentile) and significantly decreased growth rate (height velocity below the 5th percentile) refractory to management of malnutrition, metabolic acidosis, renal osteodystrophy and supplementation of electrolyte losses. Eligible children should have appropriate radiographs before initiation of therapy to confirm bone age and that epiphyses are open, and exclude the presence of active rickets or slipped capital femoral epiphysis. Prerequisites for therapy include: (i) serum PTH level ≤2 times the target upper limit for CKD stages 2–4, or ≤1.5 times the target upper limit for CKD stage 5; (ii) serum phosphorus ≤1.5 times the upper limit for age; and (iii) exclusion of active rickets.

Therapy is administered subcutaneously at a daily dose of 4 IU/m²/day (0.05 mg/kg/day or 12 mg/m²/day) for at least 12 months. Adequate response is indicated by improvement in growth velocity by ≥ 2 cm/year above baseline. Subsequently, therapy may be withheld to observe catch up growth in a proportion of patients. Levels of calcium, phosphorus, alkaline phosphatase and PTH are monitored once in 3 months in CKD 2–4 and monthly in CKD 5. Therapy with rhGH is withheld if features of high turnover disease or slipped capital femoral epiphysis develop, or if the serum PTH rises beyond 400 pg/mL in CKD 2–4 and 900 pg/mL in CKD 5. Bone age is performed annually. GH therapy should be stopped once the epiphyses are closed.

SUPPORT READING

K/DOQI Clinical Practice Guidelines for bone metabolism and disease in children with chronic kidney disease. Am J Kidney Dis 2005; 46: S1–123

Rees L, Shroff RC. Phosphate binders in CKD: chalking out the differences. Pediatr Nephrol 2010; 25: 385–94

Tonelli M, Pannu N, Manns B. Oral phosphate binders in patients with kidney failure. N Engl J Med 2010; 362: 1312–24

www.kidney.org/professionals/KDOQI/guidelines_pedbone/index.htm

35 Anemia of Chronic Kidney Disease

Anemia refers to a reduction of the absolute number of circulating red blood cells. A hematocrit of 30–36 is associated with normal appetite, satisfactory exercise capacity and better quality of life. Guidelines from Expert Groups suggest that hemoglobin levels in patients with CKD should be maintained between 11–12 g/dL. Evaluation for anemia is initiated at hemoglobin level <11 g/dL in children with CKD.

Etiology

Anemia is noted when the renal function declines to reach CKD stage 3 or more. Its chief cause is decreased erythropoiesis due to lack of erythropoietin production by renal peritubular cells. Other causes include uremic marrow suppression, iron and folate deficiency, myelofibrosis secondary to hyperparathyroidism and aluminum accumulation through antacids and hemodialysis. Hemolysis and blood losses also contribute.

Evaluation

Table 35.1 shows a plan for evaluation of anemia. Red cell morphology offers important clues to the etiology. Peripheral smear may show hypochromic microcytic cells, normocytic normochromic anemia (anemia of chronic disease, e.g. renal failure, hypothyroidism) or macrocytosis (folate, vitamin B12 deficiency). Peripheral smear enables the detection of nucleated red cells, target cells (thalassemia, hemoglobin SC), sickle forms

Table 35.1: Evaluation for etiology of anemia

Hemoglobin level; leukocyte, platelet counts
Peripheral smear for red cell morphology
Reticulocyte count (normal ≤1%), corrected for anemia
Red blood cell (RBC) count, RBC indices
Red cell distribution width
Iron studies
    Plasma iron (normal 50–175 µg/dL)
    Total iron binding capacity (TIBC, normal 250–370 µg/dL)
    Plasma ferritin (normal 100–250 ng/mL)
    Transferrin saturation (normal 20–50%)*
Parathormone level
Venous blood gas
Liver function tests

Unexplained anemia

Stool for occult blood
Hemoglobin electrophoresis
Bone marrow aspirate, biopsy
Blood folate, vitamin B12 levels
Osmotic fragility test
Blood lead level

* Transferrin saturation, % = $\dfrac{\text{Plasma iron}}{\text{TIBC}} \times 100$

(sickle cell disease), microangiopathy (hemolytic uremic syndrome), spherocytes and bite/blister cells (G6PD deficiency).

Reticulocytosis suggests hemolysis or blood loss, while decreased reticulocyte response is seen with iron deficiency, anemia of chronic disease and marrow hypoplasia. Red cell distribution width is increased in iron deficiency but is normal in thalassemia.

Metabolic acidosis and hyperparathyroidism may cause bone marrow suppression. Hyperbilirubinemia or increased serum lactate dehydrogenase are noted with hemolytic anemia and hemolytic uremic syndrome.

MANAGEMENT

Target

The aim of treatment is to achieve a hemoglobin level of 11 to 12 g/dL. Targets for iron status are plasma ferritin level of >100 ng/mL and transferrin saturation of >20%. If anemia is not severe (<6 g/dL), these can be achieved with oral or parenteral iron therapy and erythropoietin administration. Fig. 35.1 provides an overview for management of anemia in children with CKD.

Therapy with Iron

Features suggestive of iron deficiency include microcytic and hypochromic red cells on peripheral smear, mild thrombocytosis, low mean corpuscular volume (MCV) and mean corpuscular hemoglobin concentration (MCHC), and wide red cell distribution width. Low levels of plasma iron (<20 ng/mL), ferritin (<100 ng/mL) and transferrin saturation (<20%) are characteristic.

Therapy with oral iron is initiated at a dose of 2–6 mg/kg/day. Oral iron is available as ferrous salts; sulfate preparations are the most effective. While carbonyl iron preparations may have better gastrointestinal tolerance, their bioavailability is 70% of sulfate salts. Oral iron is best absorbed when taken on empty stomach. The bioavailability decreases if given with phosphate binders, antacids, or H_2 blockers.

Correction of iron deficiency is associated with increase in reticulocyte count (within 1 week) and hemoglobin concentration (1 g/dL per month). Inadequate response to iron therapy for more than 3 months requires re-

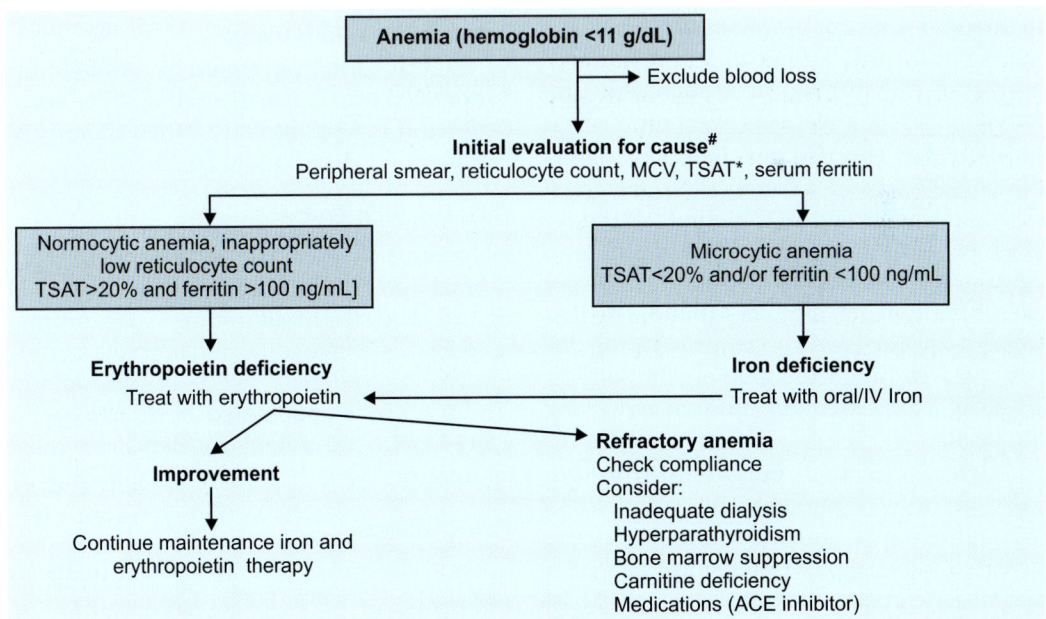

There is no indication for routine estimation of blood levels of vitamin B_{12} and folate unless there is presence of macrocytes on smear. Routine supplementation with folic acid is indicated in all patients with CKD and anemia.

*TSAT (percentage transferrin saturation) = serum iron/total iron binding capacity

Fig. 35.1: Approach to a patient with anemia and chronic kidney disease

evaluation of the cause. If iron deficiency is persistent, it is necessary to ascertain compliance and assess for gastrointestinal adverse effects. Normal serum ferritin with low (<20%) transferrin saturation and persistence of hypochromic RBC (>10%) suggest functional iron deficiency.

Therapy with *parenteral (IV) iron* is indicated if adequate iron stores cannot be maintained with maximum oral dose (6 mg/kg/day) or compliance is questionable. Regardless of anemia and iron status, parenteral iron therapy is initiated when the patient begins maintenance hemodialysis, since oral preparations are insufficient at maintaining iron stores in presence of frequent procedure related blood losses.

Preparations for parenteral therapy include iron dextran, polynuclear ferric hydroxide sucrose or iron sucrose and sodium ferric gluconate. Iron dextran is administered at 4 mg/kg per dose (maximum 100 mg; 100 mg elemental iron per 5 mL) and polynuclear ferric hydroxide sucrose or iron sucrose is given at 2 mg/kg or 0.1 mL/kg per dose (maximum 7 mg/kg or 0.35 mL/kg). Iron sucrose is preferred in view of better side effect profile.

Just prior to infusion, iron sucrose is diluted 20-fold with normal saline, and given slowly over 30 minutes. The first (test) dose is given at half the calculated dose. Iron dextran is given by slow IV push at a rate not exceeding 1 mL (50 mg) per minute. The first (test) dose for iron dextran is 10 mg for patients weighing <10 kg, 15 mg for patients 10–20 kg, 20 mg for older children and 25 mg for adults.

Adverse effects of parenteral iron therapy include hypersensitivity reactions (bronchospasm, angioedema, urticaria, pruritus, flushing, hypotension), and pain and muscle spasms of chest or back. Most effects resolve within 1–2 hr; severe or persistent symptoms require treatment with diphenhydramine or chlorpheniramine and steroids.

The dose required for correction of iron deficiency is calculated as:

Total iron deficit (mg) = Weight in kg x (target Hb - actual Hb in g/dL) × 2.4 + depot iron in mg

The depot iron is 15 mg/kg body weight for children <35 kg, and 500 mg for >35 kg.

In order to treat iron deficiency and replenish stores, patients should receive 3 infusions per week at the close of hemodialysis sessions for the first ten sessions. Subsequently, once-weekly dosing with parenteral iron is sufficient for maintenance hemodialysis.

Monitoring

Transferrin saturation and ferritin are estimated at diagnosis of anemia, during evaluation for inadequate response to therapy and if anemia recurs. These levels should be evaluated every 3–4 months in patients on parenteral iron to detect overdosing. Estimation is delayed by two weeks if the last IV dose of iron exceeds 1 g, and by one week if it is between 200 and 500 mg.

Therapy with iron should be withheld for 3 months if transferrin saturation >50% and/or ferritin is >800 ng/mL. When therapy is resumed, the dose should be 33–50%.

Therapy with Erythropoietin

Anemia of chronic disease is suggested by normal iron profile (plasma ferritin level >100 ng/mL, transferrin saturation >20%), normal or low reticulocyte count and normocytic normochromic red cells. While erythropoietin (rhEPO) use is anticipated in children with CKD 4 or 5, concomitant iron deficiency must be treated.

Preparations

Epoetin alfa and epoetin beta are available in strengths of 1000, 2000, 4000 and 10000 units. Administration of erythropoietin beta is associated with higher and delayed peak concentration and greater reticulocyte response.

Darbepoetin alpha is a novel erythropoiesis stimulating protein, which has a prolonged half life due to the presence of five N-linked carbohydrate chains (two more than rhEPO). Darbepoetin is as efficacious as rhEPO in treatment of anemia associated with CKD, and the extended half-life of darbepoetin provides the advantages of less frequent dosing, enhanced compliance and convenience. Pegylated forms of rhEPO (e.g. methoxypolyethylene glycol epoetin beta) are not approved for use in children.

Dosing

Therapy with rhEPO is begun at 150 units/kg body weight, split into two doses every week. Increments are made to reach 250 units/kg per week (maximum dose 400 units/kg). The dose is increased in times of stress, such as infection or surgery. Erythropoietin may be replaced by darbepoetin; 200 IU of former is equivalent to 1 μg of the latter.

Route

Erythropoietin is given by intravenous (IV), subcutaneous (SC) and intraperitoneal (IP) routes. IP administration is cumbersome, requires higher doses, and given when the abdomen is dry. IV administration is convenient in patients on maintenance hemodialysis, since the medication is given at close of the dialysis session into the venous port. The SC route uses comparatively lower doses and requires less frequent dosing, q weekly or twice weekly. Doses are administered into the arm, thigh or anterior abdominal wall using a small (29 G) needle, with regular rotation of injection sites.

Adverse effects

Therapy may be associated with development or worsening of hypertension, seizures, hyperkalemia or hyperphosphatemia, and rarely, thrombosis of the vascular access. Hypertension is managed by increasing the dose of antihypertensives and/or decreasing the dose of rhEPO. Prior epilepsy is not a contraindication to therapy.

Monitoring of Response

The hematocrit is measured every 2 weeks until the target is reached, then every 4 weeks. There is a rise in reticulocyte count by the end of 1–3 weeks, which peaks at 3–8 weeks.

The dose of rhEPO is titrated upward or downward by 25–50% in case of an inadequate increase in hemoglobin (<1 g/dl in 4 weeks) or an excessive rise in hemoglobin (>2 g/dl in 4 weeks), respectively.

A lack of response to adequate doses of rhEPO (300 U/kg/week) should prompt evaluation for another cause of anemia. Iron deficiency is the usual cause, which responds to iron supplements. Other causes include chronic or acute infections, blood loss, deficiency of folate, vitamin B_{12}, carnitine and macronutrients, hyperparathyroidism, aluminium toxicity and hemoglobinopathies. Pateints with megaloblastic anemia should receive therapy with vitamin B_{12} (intramusular 1–2 mg over 2–4 weeks, then RDA orally) and folic acid (15 μg/kg/day, maximum 1 mg/day).

Blood Transfusions

Severe anemia (hemoglobin level <6 g/dL) is unlikely to respond to therapy with oral iron and rhEPO. Transfusion of packed red cells is indicated in patients on dialysis and in presence of incipient cardiac failure, shock or sepsis. Patients with anemia refractory to therapy with rhEPO (>300 units/kg per week) also require transfusions. The use of leukocyte poor, packed red cells is preferred in order to avoid sensitization to blood antigens.

SUPPORT READING

K/DOQI; National Kidney Foundation. Clinical practice recommendations for anemia in chronic kidney disease in children. Am J Kidney Dis 2006; 47: S86–108; www.kidney.org/professionals/kdoqi

36 Nutrition in Chronic Kidney Disease

The goal of dietary therapy in patients with chronic kidney disease (CKD) is to maintain an optimal nutritional status without increasing the risks of uremic toxicity and metabolic abnormalities.

Assessment of Growth and Nutritional Status

The parameters that assist in the evaluation of nutritional status include: (i) dietary intake (3-day diet record or three 24-hr dietary recalls); (ii) estimated dry weight and weight-for age percentile or standard deviation score (SDS); (iii) length or height-for-age percentile or SDS; (iv) BMI-for-age percentile or SDS; (v) head circumference-for-age percentile or SDS in children <3-yr-old; (vi) height velocity-for-age percentile or SDS; and (vii) serum albumin, with values <3 g/dL suggesting insufficient protein intake.

Frequency of Assessment

Assessments should be made frequently. The nutritional assessment is performed every 6 months in patients with CKD 2–5 and every 1–3 months in CKD 5D. Assessments are more frequent for children with (i) severe malnutrition, (ii) evidence of growth delay, (iii) decreasing or low BMI, (iv) comorbidities influencing growth or nutrient intake, and (v) recent change in medical status or dietary intake. Infants need a close follow-up to monitor dietary adequacy, feeding tolerance and growth.

MANAGEMENT

Energy Intake

The energy intake should be equivalent to the recommended dietary allowance (RDA) of healthy children (Table 36.1). In order to achieve catch up growth, the requirement for energy intake is 125% of that recommended. The diet should provide 55–60% of calories from carbohydrates, 30% from fats and 10% from proteins (up to 15% in case of protein losing states such as nephrotic syndrome and chronic ambulatory peritoneal dialysis). Oral intake of an energy-dense diet and commercial nutritional supplements should be considered the preferred mode for supplemental nutritional support for children with CKD stages 2 to 5 and 5D.

Examples of locally available energy-dense sources include: parantha (1 piece=175 Cal),

Table 36.1: Dietary reference values for children

Age	Energy, Cal/kg/day	Protein g/kg/day
0–3 months	100–115	2.1
4–6 months	105	1.6
7–12 months	95	1.5
1–3 years	95 (1000–1300*)	1.1
4–6 years	90 (1500–1800*)	1.1
7–10 years	1700–2000*	28*
11–14 years	2100–2300*	42*
15–18 years	2200–2600*	45–55*

* Refers to total daily caloric, protein requirement

ice cream (100 g=193 Cal), banana (1 fruit=90–120 Cal), mango (1 fruit=70 Cal), sooji halwa (25 g=150 Cal), paneer (25 g=77 Cal), buffalo milk (250 mL=292 Cal), milk shake (200 mL~275 Cal). A complete list is available in Appendix 11.

Nutritional supplements include Resource Dialysis, which provides 2 Cal/mL if made in water, and Simyl MCT oil, 1 mL of which provides 7.8 Cal. Table 36.2 provides a list of available supplements.

Supplemental nutritional support (tube feeding) should be considered when the usual intake of a child with CKD fails to meet energy requirements and the child does not achieve expected rates of weight gain and/or growth for age. Oral feeding can continue simultaneous with tube feeds, or tube feeds can be used for night time intermittent nutrition alone. Options for tube feeding include: (i) full cream milk (100 mL) + sugar (1 spoon) + MCT oil (5 mL) provides 145 Cal; and (ii) Resource Dialysis with milk (100 mL=270–290 Cal).

Special Considerations

Gastrostomy feeding should be preferred in children receiving prolonged tube feeding.

In presence of untreated recurrent vomiting (abnormal gastric motility, delayed gastric emptying), the energy intake should be increased by up to 30%.

Intradialytic parenteral nutrition is advised for malnourished children receiving maintenance hemodialysis, who are unable to meet their nutritional needs through oral and tube feeding. While the procedure augments nutritional intake, it is expensive and requires close monitoring.

Rarely, patients on CAPD may require the energy intake to be reduced to compensate for calories derived from dialysate glucose (8–12 Cal/kg/day) if there is excessive weight gain.

Post-transplant energy requirements match those of normal children. Reduction in energy intake is indicated if there is excessive weight gain.

Table 36.2: Commonly used nutritional supplements

Product	Energy, Cal	Protein, g	Fat, g	Ca/ P/ Na/ K, mg
Resource Dialysis (100 g)	486	17.6	23.8	200/ 267/ 148/ 389
Resource Dialysis (21 g = 3 level scoops; added to 33 ml water; makes 50 ml total volume)	102	3.7	5	42/ 56/ 31/ 82
Albumen Care (100 g)	294	65		
Albumen RRT (100 g)	316	70	4	NA
Albumen RRT (10 g serving/pouch, added to food, e.g. 1 serving curd)	31.6	7	0.4	NA
Reno-pro (25 g serving, added to 40 ml water)	116	2.25	5	28/ 35/ 57.5/ 30
Reno-pro High protein (25 g serving, added to 40 ml water)	127	5	5	28/ 10/ 57.5/ NA
Renuris Dialysis (16 g serving, added to 40 ml water)	Low	10	Low	
Novasource peptide (100 g; one scoop is 6.25 g)	400	20	9.2	

Ca calcium, P phosphorus, Na sodium, K potassium

Protein Intake

The diet should provide 100% RDA of protein intake for healthy children of the same chronological age (Table 36.1). Excessive protein intake should be avoided to prevent metabolic acidosis, hyperphosphatemia and accumulation of toxic nitrogen waste products.

The initial dietary protein intake for dialyzed patients should be prescribed at RDA + 0.4 g/kg/day for a patient on hemo-dialysis, and at RDA + 0.7–0.9 g/kg/day for a patient on CAPD. The increment for CAPD losses should be higher for infants and for patients with peritonitis. Protein supplements may be used to augment inadequate oral and/or enteral protein intake.

Locally available or home-made high protein sources include: paneer (25 g=4 g protein), egg (5 g), meat (100 g=21 g), chicken (100 g=26 g), fish (100 g=18 g), cow milk (250 mL=8 g), daal or rajma (25 g=6 g) and soyabeans (25 g=11 g). A complete list is available in Appendix 11. Commercially available protein supplements include Albumen RRT and Resource Dialysis.

Fat

Up to 30% of calories should be derived from lipids. In patients with CKD 5 and those with dyslipidemia, saturated fats should comprise less than 10% of total calories. Essential fatty acids should provide about 3% of calories.

Micronutrients

The recommended dietary intake should be 100% of RDA for vitamins A, B_1, B_2, B_6, B_{12}, C, E and K, and folic acid, copper and zinc (Table 36.3). Children on hemodialysis and those following renal transplantation should receive 100% of the recommended dietary intakes of vitamins and minerals. Patients on hemo-dialysis may be at risk of zinc deficiency. Whenever nutrient intakes are suspected to be inadequate, supplementation with a multi-vitamin preparation should be considered.

Caution should be observed with respect to intake of multivitamins in view of hyper-vitaminosis A, hypercalcemia, anemia and hyperlipidemia. Patients with CKD 2–4 need annual evaluation for vitamin D status and supplementation if deficiency is present. Folic acid (2.5–5 mg) prevents hyperhomocys-teinemia in patients with CKD 4 and 5. Children on peritoneal dialysis need vitamin C (15–60 mg), folic acid (60–500 µg) and pyridoxine (0.2–1.5 mg) supplements to offset dialysis losses.

Table 36.3: Daily reference intakes of nutrients for infants and children

	0–1 year	1–6 years	7–14 years	> 15 years
Thiamine, B_1 (mg)	0.2–0.4	0.5–0.9	1–1.3	1.1–1.5
Riboflavin, B_2 (mg)	0.3–0.5	0.5–1.1	1.2–1.5	1.3–1.8
Niacin, (mg NE)	2–6	6–12	13–17	15–20
Pyridoxine, B_6 (mg)	0.1–0.6	0.5–1.1	1.4–1.7	1.5–2
Folic acid (µg)	25–80	50–200	100–150	180–200
Vitamin B_{12} (µg)	0.3–0.5	0.7–1	1.4–2	2
Biotin (µg)	5–6	8–12	NA	NA
Vitamin C (mg)	30–50	15–45	45–50	60
Vitamin A (µg)	375–500	300–500	700–1000	800–1000
Vitamin D (IU)*	400	400	400	400
Vitamin E (IU)**	4–6	9–10	10–15	12–15
Zinc (mg)	2–5	3–10	10–15	12–15
Copper (µg)	200–220	340–440	300–700	400–1000

*1 µg = 40 IU; **1 mg α tocopherol equivalent = 1.49 IU

Minerals, Electrolytes and Fluids

Calcium: The total intake from nutritional sources and phosphate binders should be between 100–200% of the recommended intakes for age, and not exceed 2.5 g daily.

Phosphorus: In children with CKD stages 3 to 5 and 5D, dietary phosphorus intake should be reduced to 100% of the RDA for age if hyperparathyroidism is present. Dietary phosphorus intake should be reduced further if serum phosphorus concentration exceeds the normal reference range for age. Foods rich in phosphorus include milk and its products, meat, chicken, chocolate, soft drinks, nuts, dried beans and peas, and whole grains (*see* Chapter 34).

Fluid Requirements: Patients with CKD stages 2–5 and polyuria should receive supplemental free water and sodium supplements to avoid intravascular depletion. Fluid intake should be restricted in children with CKD stages 3–5 and 5D who are oligoanuric to prevent complications of fluid overload.

Sodium: Infants with obstructive uropathy often have polyuria needing salt supplements. Sodium supplements should be considered for infants receiving continuous ambulatory peritoneal dialysis. Restriction of sodium intake is considered for patients who have hypertension or prehypertension.

Potassium: Intake should be limited for patients at risk of hyperkalemia. Foods rich in potassium include fresh fruits especially citrus, whole grains, vegetables such as tomatoes, cucumber, cabbage and spinach (*see* Appendix 11).

Enteral Tube Feeding

Nasogastric, transpyloric or gastrostomy tube feeding should be considered in patients who fail to meet their nutritional goals by the oral route alone. Patients with declining growth velocity should be offered enteral feeding, initially by nasogastric tube.

The parents are taught how to administer nasogastric tube feeding at home. A whey-dominant infant formula should be used in patients under 2-yr-old. In infants, one-half of the feed may be given as boluses during the day and one-half as continuous over-night feed. Patients having vomiting and feed intolerance, should receive either

Table 36.4: Recommendations for nutritional management of children with CKD

Nutrient	CKD stage 1–4	Hemodialysis	Peritoneal dialysis
Calories (Cal/day)	100% of recommended dietary allowance (RDA)		
	1 yr: 1000 3 yr: 1300		
	5 yr: 1600 10 yr: 2000		
	10–13 yr: 2400 (boys); 2200 (girls)		
	13–16 yr: 2600 (boys); 2200 (girls)		
Protein	10% of calories; 1–2.5 g/kg body weight; 50% of high biological value		
Fat	30% of calories	30% of calories; <10% from saturated fats	
Fluid (mL)	Unrestricted with normal renal output	Urine output + insensible losses	Less restricted
Sodium	Unrestricted , if not hyper-tensive	Low salt diet	Restricted (2 g/day) if hypertensive
Potassium	Unrestricted	Restrict if high blood level (>5.3 mEq/L)	
Calcium	<2.5 g/day from diet and medications		
Phosphorus	Limit to dietary reference intake if PTH high; 80% if hyperphosphatemia		

small, frequent volumes or continuous feeds, and use of prokinetic drugs. Nissen fundoplication may be considered if vomiting persists. Nasogastric tubes are well tolerated and easy to insert, but may be associated with recurrent vomiting and gastroesophageal reflux; aspiration is a concern, and tubes need frequent replacement. Eating difficulties following withdrawal of nasogastric feeding is an important problem, especially when it is initiated during the first year of life.

Gastrostomy

A percutaneous endoscopic gastrostomy should be created in patients with CKD 4–5 requiring prolonged tube feeding or those with persistent vomiting while on naso-gastric feeds. Gastrostomy tubes or buttons are hidden beneath the clothing. Complications include emesis, exit site infections, leakage and peritonitis. Percutaneous endo-scopic gastrostomy (PEG) insertion following initiation of peritoneal dialysis carries a high risk for fungal peritonitis and potential dialysis failure. An open gastrostomy is preferred in such patients.

Gastrojejunostomy should be considered in children undergoing enteral tube feeding when severe gastroesophageal reflux is not resolved by medical therapy.

Table 36.4 summarizes the broad principles for nutritional management for children with CKD.

SUPPORT READING

Rees L, Shaw V. Nutrition in children with CRF and on dialysis. Pediatr Nephrol 2007; 22: 1689–1702

KDOQI Clinical Practice Guideline for Nutrition in Children with CKD: 2008 Update. Am J Kidney Dis 2009; 53: SUPPL 2: 1–128

www.kidney.org/professionals/KDOQI/guide-lines_ped_ckd/index.htm

37 Supportive Care in Chronic Kidney Disease

Children with chronic kidney disease (CKD) require attention to abnormalities of fluid and electrolytes and careful management of co-morbidities in order to prevent additional renal injury and complications. Some important considerations are discussed here.

Fluids and Electrolyte Imbalance

Careful fluid balance is essential in children with advanced CKD in order to avoid fluid overload. Patients with obstructive uropathy and tubulopathies show polyuria due to tubular dysfunction and benefit from increase in dietary salt intake, access to fluids and frequent monitoring.

Metabolic acidosis is noted when GFR falls below 50%. Chronic acidosis is detrimental since it impairs bone mineralization, blunts the response to eythropoetin, affects albumin synthesis and increases protein catabolism. Blood levels of bicarbonate should be estimated annually in children with CKD 1-2; every 6 months in CKD stage 3; every 3 months in CKD stages 4 and 5; and monthly in patients on dialysis (stage 5D). In patients >2 years of age, bicarbonate levels should be maintained at >22 mEq/L; in neonates and young infants, these levels should be >20 mEq/L. If necessary, alkali supplements are administered (Appendix 6). Elevation of bicarbonate concentration in the dialysate is an alternative in patients on hemodialysis.

Children with CKD stages 4 and 5 are susceptible to hyperkalemia. However, persistent hyperkalemia may occur at higher estimated GFR in patients with obstructive uropathy, reflux nephropathy, interstitial nephritis or renal dysplasia due to tubular resistance to the aldosterone action (type 4 RTA). Intake of potassium rich foods (chocolates, potatoes, green leafy vagitables, citrus fruits) should be restricted. Drugs which may cause hyperkalemia (ACE inhibitors and angiotensin receptor blockers, potassium sparing diuretics, calcineurin inhibitors, digitalis, NSAIDs) should be replaced with alternative agents. While dietary restrictions are usually sufficient, short term use of loop diuretics or potassium binding resins (sodium polystyrene sulfonate) may be considered. Refractory hyperkalemia is an indication for initiating dialysis.

Dyslipidemia

Children with CKD are at increased risk of adverse cardiovascular events due to presence of hypertension, impaired glucose tolerance and dyslipidemia. Hypertension, volume overload and anemia contribute to left ventricular hypertrophy, which causes subendocardial ischemia, myocardial fibrosis and ventricular dysfunction, and increases the risk of arrhythmias.

Atherosclerotic or arteriosclerotic changes, secondary to dyslipidemia, hypertension and uremia, and vascular calcifications contribute to vascular injury. Most patients on dialysis have dyslipidemia, asymptomatic atherosclerosis (measured by abnormal carotid intimal medial thickness), and abnormal endothelial function (suggested by impaired flow-mediated dilation of the brachial artery). Therapy with statins is necessary if the LDL cholesterol is persistently raised above 190 mg/dL, or above 160 mg/dL in presence of risk factors. The goals of therapy are an LDL cholesterol <100 mg/dL and total triglycerides <200 mg/dL.

Contrast Induced Nephropathy

Contrast induced nephropathy (CIN) is an acute elevation of serum creatinine more than 50% above the baseline, occuring 1–3 days after IV administration of the radiocontrast. The creatinine peaks by 3–7 days, and returns to baseline in 10–14 days. CIN is not infrequent, especially in subjects with reduced renal function.

Risk Factors

Patients at risk for CIN include those with: *(i)* pre-existing renal insufficiency; high pre-existing serum creatinine levels; *(ii)* congestive heart failure; *(iii)* dehydration, hyperuricemia; *(iv)* concomitant use of nephrotoxic drugs, e.g. aminoglycoside antibiotics, NSAIDs; *(v)* large doses of contrast media; multiple contrast studies within a short period; and *(vi)* liver cirrhosis or nephrotic syndrome.

Management

Table 37.1 summarizes strategies for prevention and management of CIN. Iso-osmolar contrast agents are preferred. Blood levels of creatinine should be measured before the study and for 48 hr thereafter. Preventive measures consist of volume expansion by peri-procedural infusion of isotonic saline or sodium bicarbonate, and the use of minimum amounts of the contrast. Administration of oral N-acetylcysteine (600 mg twice daily for 2 days) has been shown to be useful in preventing contrast nephropathy, although its benefits are equivocal.

Non-ionic low osmolar monomers are the contrast agents of choice. In addition to their nonionic nature and lower osmolality, they are potentially less chemotoxic than the ionic monomers. Common nonionic monomers are iohexol (Omnipaque), iopamidol (Isovue), ioversol (Optiray) and iopromide (Ultravist).

Gadolinium-related Nephrogenic Systemic Fibrosis

A small proportion of patients with chronic kidney disease stage 4–5 and those with acute renal failure who have undergone magnetic

---

Table 37.1: Prevention of contrast induced nephropathy

Low Risk (eGFR >60 mL/min/1.73 m²)
Optimize hydration status

High Risk (eGFR <60 mL/min/1.73 m²)
Avoid nephrotoxic drugs (aminoglycos des, NSAIDs)
Administer N-acetylcysteine: 600 mg orally q12 hr for 4 doses, beginning before contrast
Maintain intravascular volume (avoid dehydration)
   a. Isotonic saline 10–15 mL/kg beginning 3 hr before, and continuing at least 6–8 hr after procedure, or
   b. Sodium bicarbonate 3 mL/kg/hr starting 1-hr before contrast

Radiographic contrast media: minimize volume; use low- or iso-osmolar contrast agents
Post-procedure
   a. Follow-up serum creatinine 48-hr post procedure, and
   b. Avoid toxic medications until renal functions normalize

resonance imaging using gadolinium as a contrast agent may develop *nephrogenic systemic fibrosis*.

The condition is characterized by progressive fibrosis of the skin and internal organs, similar to those in scleroderma. There is hardening, thickening and erythema of the skin of limbs; pruritus and pain may be noted. Some cases show rapid progression with joint contractures. Systemic involvement results in cardiomyopathy, pulmonary fibrosis, pulmonary hypertension and diaphragmatic paralysis. Skin biopsy shows fibrosis, sometimes with mucin deposition, without inflammatory infiltrates.

Deposits of gadolinium are found in tissues of patients. Patients at risk for developing nephrogenic systemic fibrosis include those with: *(i)* impaired elimination of gadolinium based contrast agents, as in acute kidney injury (AKI) or eGFR <30 mL/min/1.73 m^2; and *(ii)* use of high doses or repeat doses of the contrast.

While NSF may follow administration of any gadolinium based agent, the risk is highest with gadodiamide (Omniscan), intermediate with gadopentetate dimeglumine (Magnevist), and gadoversetamide (OptiMARK) and low with use of Gadobenate (MultiHance) and Gadoteridol (ProHance).

The use of gadolinium based agents should be avoided in patients with impaired kidney function, unless imaging is essential and not available without contrast. If necessary, the lowest dose of contrast based on body weight should be used.

Patients with AKI and CKD stages 4-5, and those on dialysis must be informed of the risks of contrast MRI. If contrast-enhanced MRI is required in a patient on dialysis, patients should receive hemodialysis with high flux dialyzer immediately following the procedure. These patients should be followed and closely monitored for features of nephrogenic systemic fibrosis. No single treatment is effective, although patients show improved symptoms after renal transplantation.

Uremic Platelet Dysfunction

Uremia induces a primary hemostatic defect due to abnormal platelet-vessel wall interaction. This dysfunction induces a bleeding tendency that may or may not be reflected in prolonged bleeding time. Preventive measures should be instituted when an invasive procedure (e.g. renal biopsy, vascular catheter insertion, major surgery) is planned. Active measures are required in presence of ecchymoses, epistaxis, gastrointestinal bleeding or hematuria in a patient with azotemia.

Desmopressin: Desmopressin acts by stimulating release of factor VIII from endothelial stores and increasing vWF activity. The bleeding time and activated partial thromboplastin time are normalized. The medication is given IV at a dose of 0.3–0.4 µg/kg IV (adult dose 20 µg), or intranasally at a dose of 5 µg/kg. The effect of the medication lasts 8 hours, following which the dose may be repeated.

Conjugated estrogens: The mechanism of action is the same as for DDAVP, but the effect lasts 10–15 days. Intravenous administration at 0.6 mg/kg conjugated estrogens decreases active bleeding and the requirement for blood transfusions.

Cryoprecipitate: This is used *(i)* if patient is hemodynamically stable but requires urgent surgery or control of bleeding; *(ii)* after desmopressin has failed; or *(iii)* in patients who are hemodynamically unstable and cannot tolerate whole blood.

Dialysis: performed at serum creatinine >6 mg/dl, improves platelet aggregation.

Recombinant erythropoietin: should be administered if the baseline hematocrit is <30% and iron stores are normal. Administration of this agent reduces bleeding time, because of displacement of platelets such that they are closer to the vascular endothelium.

Preservation of Peripheral Veins

Venipuncture and placement of peripheral venous catheters are commonly required procedures in children with advanced CKD. Indiscriminate venipuncture and inappropriate management of venous access can result in venous occlusion with thrombi, interfering with future placement of vascular access for hemodialysis. Appropriate management of veins is necessary in children with CKD stage 3–5 (eGFR <60 mL/min/1.73 m^2) or serum creatinine >2.0 mg/dL.

An assessment should be carried out prior to placement of any vascular access device, using ultrasound, if required. The dorsal veins of the dominant hand are preferred for venipuncture and for short term venous access for infusion therapies.

Since the forearm veins, upper arm veins and subclavian veins are preferred sites for creation of a hemodialysis fistula, these veins should not be used for venous access procedures, including peripherally inserted central catheters. Where prolonged venous access is essential, one should identify and use alternative long-term venous access to avoid prolonged reliance on peripheral veins. The internal jugular vein is the preferred vessel for central venous access. If central venous catheters inserted *via* the internal jugular vein are intended for long-term use (>4 weeks), these should be placed using a subcutaneous tunnel (Permacath). The use of subclavian vein for central venous access should be avoided.

Counseling

Although management of chronic kidney disease retards disease progression, many pediatric patients develop advanced CKD. Patients and their parents should receive education about the importance of regular monitoring, the likelihood of disease progression and options for renal replacement therapy (*see* Chapter 39). During discussion, it is important to consider all medical and psychosocial factors that may impact the decision making by the family. Early preparation of the family prevents the need of emergency procedures such as temporary dialysis and associated unnecessary morbidities. Counseling regarding options for RRT must begin by the time children reach CKD stage 4. Children with CKD secondary to abnormalities of the lower urinary tract need corrective surgeries (vesicostomy, augmentation cystoplasty, ureteric reimplantation) before transplantation can be considered.

SUPPORT READING

Weisbord SD, Palevsky PM. Strategies for the prevention of contrast-induced acute kidney injury. Curr Opin Nephrol Hyperten 2010, 19: 539–49

Hellman RN. Godolinium-induced nephrogenic systemic fibrosis. Semin Nephrol 2011; 31: 310–16

Gangji AS, Sohal AS, Treleaven D, Crowther MA. Bleeding in patients with renal insufficiency: A practical guide to clinical management. Thrombosis Research 2006; 118: 423–28

McLennan G. Vein preservation: An algorithmic approach to vascular access placement in patients with compromised renal function. JAVA 2007; 12: 89–91

38 Hypertension

Hypertension is an important disorder in children. Firstly, mild asymptomatic hypertension in older children and adolescents often persists (tracks) as essential hypertension in adults. Secondly, symptomatic hypertension is usually secondary, to a renal parenchymal or renovascular condition. These patients require diagnostic evaluation to determine the cause and for appropriate management. Children with hypertension are also at risk of short- and long-term target organ damage involving the brain, kidneys and heart.

Definition and Staging

Normative data on blood pressure, derived from a large multiethnic cohort of children, based on gender, age and height percentiles is shown in Appendix 7. Guidelines have been developed to interpret diastolic and systolic blood pressures, and define hypertension (Table 38.1). Normal blood pressure is defined as systolic and diastolic blood pressure less than the 90th percentile for age, sex and height. Figures 38.1 and 38.2 provide charts for screening and staging of hypertension in boys and girls respectively.

Patients with stage 2 hypertension may present with severe hypertension, or *hypertensive crises*, classified as emergencies or urgencies. *Hypertensive emergencies* are situations that require immediate blood pressure reduction to prevent or limit target organ damage, such as hypertensive encephalopathy, intracranial hemorrhage, acute left ventricular failure with pulmonary edema, papilledema and acute renal failure. Patients with *hypertensive urgencies* show high blood pressure which is desirable to be reduced within a few hours, but there is no evidence of acute end organ damage.

White coat hypertension refers to high office blood pressures in patients who have normal blood pressures in familiar setting. *Masked hypertension* refers to situations where office blood pressures are normal but the child or adolescent is actually hypertensive.

Table 38.1: Definition and staging of hypertension in children	
Pre-hypertension	SBP or DBP 90th–95th percentile or >120/80 mm Hg, even if below 90th percentile in adolescents
Hypertension	SBP or DBP >95th percentile
Stage I hypertension	SBP or DBP between 95th percentile and 99th percentile + 5 mm Hg
Stage II hypertension	SBP or DBP >99th percentile + 5 mm Hg

SBP-systolic blood pressure; DBP-diastolic blood pressure

Chronic Kidney Disease and Hypertension

VIII

Systolic blood pressure

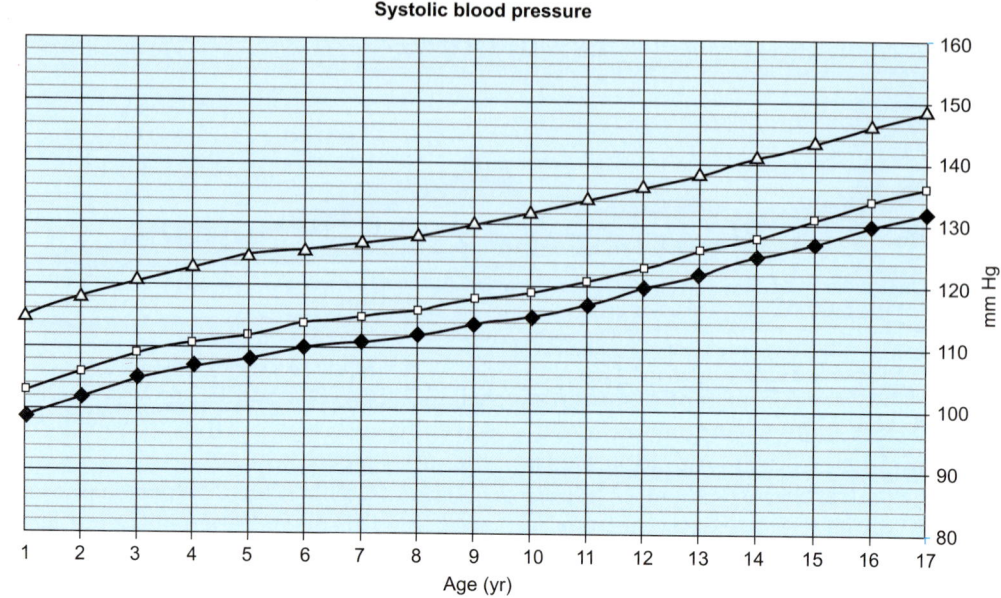

-◆- 90th percentile -□- 95th percentile -△- 99th percentile + 5 mm

Diastolic blood pressure

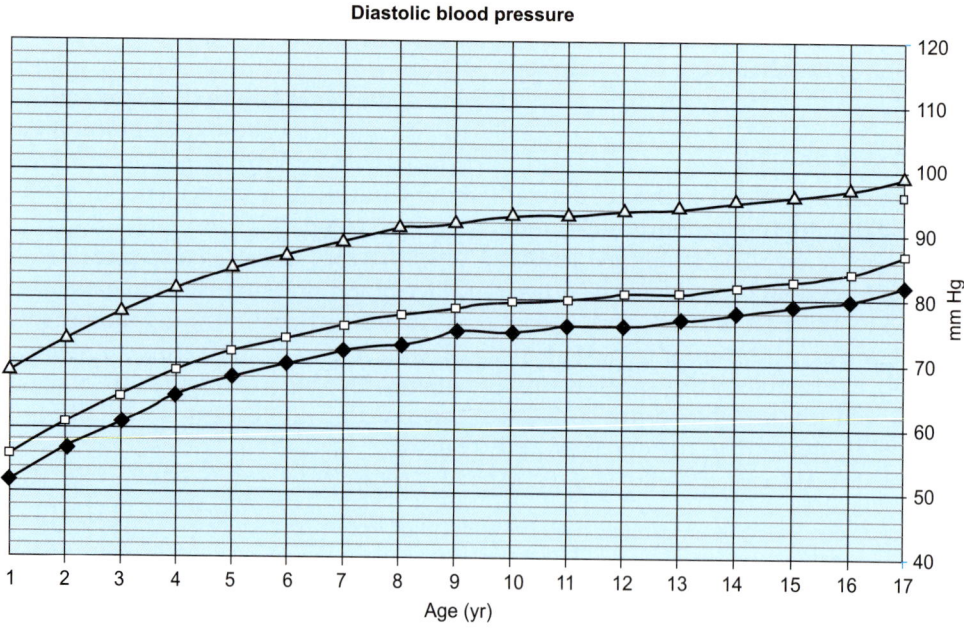

Fig. 38.1: Blood pressure levels for boys at 50th percentile for height. Chart depicting 90th (closed diamonds), 95th (open squares) and 99th + 5 mm (open triangles) percentile values for (*a*) systolic and (*b*) diastolic blood pressures, representing cut off values for the diagnosis of pre-hypertension, stage I and stage II hypertension, respectively, in boys (based on the Fourth US Task Force Report on Hypertension). With permission from Indian Pediatrics 2007; 44: 103–21

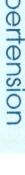

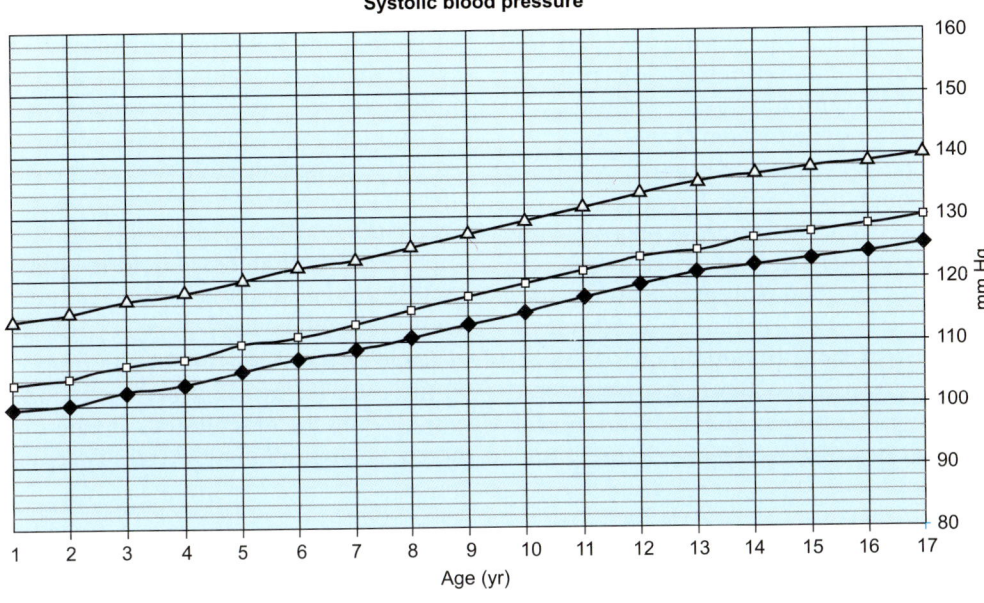

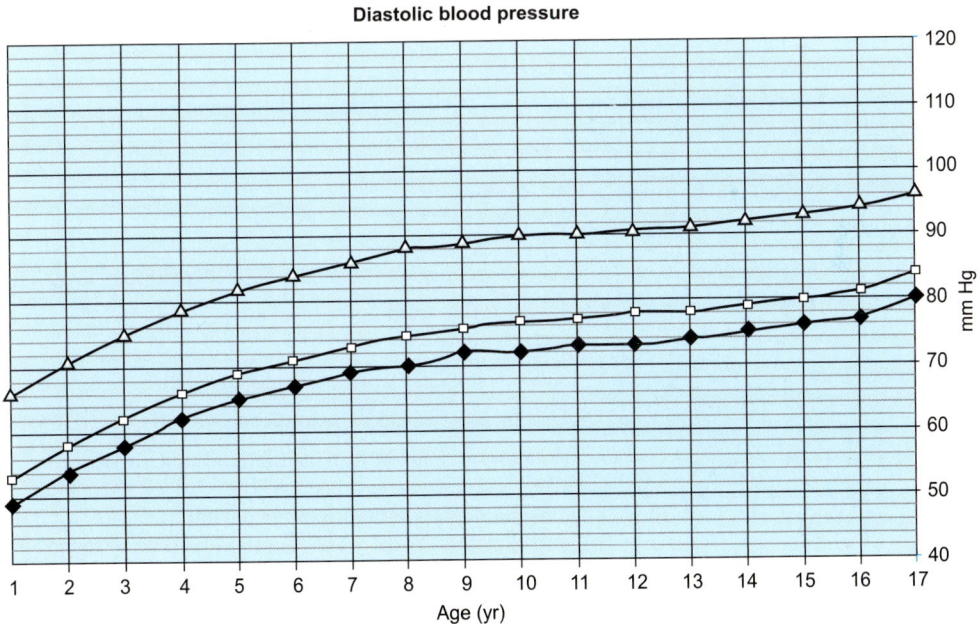

Fig. 38.2: Blood pressure levels for girls at 50th percentile for height. Chart depicting 90th (closed diamonds), 95th (open squares) and 99th + 5 mm (open triangles) percentile values for (*a*) systolic and (*b*) diastolic blood pressures, representing cut off values for the diagnosis of pre-hypertension, stage I and stage II hypertension respectively in girls (based on the Fourth US Task Force Report on Hypertension). With permission from Indian Pediatrics 2007; 44: 103–21

Diagnosis

Blood pressure levels should be measured annually in all children and adolescents more than 3-yr-old, and in younger children who are at risk for hypertension (Table 38.2).

A single elevated blood pressure recording is not enough to diagnose hypertension. The diagnosis should be confirmed by repeating the measurement at least twice in the next 1–2 weeks for stage 1 hypertension, within 2–5 days for stage 2 hypertension (or at the same visit if symptomatic), and every six months for patients with pre-hypertension.

Blood pressure measurements are performed after having the patient rest for 5 minutes, in an upright position with the back supported, and with the cubital fossa at the level of the heart. Infants are evaluated in the supine position. Multiple measurements, at the same or subsequent visits, ensure that results are reproducible and decrease the effect of white coat hypertension. Appropriate sized cuffs (bladder width ≥40% of the mid-upper arm circumference, and length sufficient to cover 80–100% of the arm circumference) should be used.

Table 38.3 outlines the techniques commonly used for measurement of blood pressure. While the auscultatory method using mercury sphygmomanometers is standard,

Table 38.2: Medical conditions that increase risk of hypertension in young children

History of prematurity; very low birth weight; complications requiring NICU care
Congenital heart disease (repaired or non-repaired)
Recurrent urinary tract infections, hematuria or proteinuria
Known renal disease or urologic malformations
Family history of congenital renal disease
Solid organ transplant or bone marrow transplant
Malignancy; neurofibromatosis; tuberous sclerosis; elevated intracranial pressure
Treatment with medications known to raise blood pressure

Table 38.3: Techniques for monitoring blood pressure

Technique	Comments
Mercury sphygmomanometry	*Advantages:* Evidence based; quick to perform; low cost
	Disadvantages: Observer bias; mercury an environmental hazard
Aneroid manometry	*Advantages:* Easily portable; mercury free
	Disadvantages: Needs frequent calibration
Oscillometric devices	*Advantages:* Easy to use; useful in infants; no observer bias
	Disadvantages: Limited reference data; values of systolic and diastolic blood pressure are derived from mean arterial pressure; requires repeated validation; higher cost
Ambulatory blood pressure monitoring	*Advantages:* Diagnosis of white coat, masked hypertension; data on diurnal variability; reliable normative data available
	Disadvantages: Expensive; regular maintenance of equipment; requires patient cooperation

these instruments are being phased out due to environmental concerns. This has resulted in increased use of oscillometric devices, especially in clinic and hospital settings.

Ambulatory Blood Pressure Monitoring (ABPM)

ABPM refers to the continuous recordings of blood pressure over 12- or 24-hr. These records reflect the true blood pressure, are reproducible and correlate with target organ damage. If available, ABPM should be used in addition to clinic blood pressure monitoring in patients with high pretest probability of hypertension (Table 38.4). ABPM devices are programmed to record blood pressure frequently (q 20–30 minutes when awake; q 30–60 minutes during sleep). Data are inspected for inconsistencies, evaluated for reliability and assessed in terms of mean blood pressure load (readings above the ambulatory 95th percentile) and nocturnal dipping (day night difference).

Etiology

Conditions causing transient and persistent hypertension are listed in Table 38.5. Sustained hypertension in children is usually secondary to renal parenchymal disease (60–70%) or renovascular disease (5–10%). A cause is more likely to be identified in younger children and in those with severe

hypertension. Patients with essential hypertension are typically post pubertal and overweight, have stage 1 hypertension and show no target organ damage.

Clinical Features

Patients with hypertension may be detected incidentally or have nonspecific symptoms. Infants may present with irritability, failure to thrive, vomiting, feeding problems, seizures and respiratory distress. Older children may have headache, epistaxis, visual disturbances, vertigo or a decline in school performance. Children with severe hypertension might present with encephalopathy, seizures or congestive heart failure.

EVALUATION

History and examination helps in evaluating the underlying etiology. Blood pressure should be measured in all four limbs to detect asymmetry.

Since the majority of patients with hypertension have an underlying renal parenchymal or renovascular etiology, screening tests should evaluate for these conditions (Table 38.6). A cause for hypertension is found in most instances. Confirmation of diagnosis requires investigations tailored to specific needs. Figures 38.3 and 38.4 illustrate how these investigations can be used to reach a definitive diagnosis.

Table 38.4: Indications for ambulatory blood pressure monitoring	
Intermediate risk of hypertension	Obesity Chronic kidney disease (CKD) stages 1 to 3 Well controlled diabetes Long term treatment with steroids Autonomic dysfunction
High risk of hypertension	End stage renal disease Renal allograft recipients Diabetes with microalbuminuria End organ damage, such as left ventricular hypertrophy
Others	White-coat or masked hypertension Apparent drug resistance Hypotensive symptoms with antihypertensive drugs.

Table 38.5: Causes of hypertension

Transient Hypertension

Renal diseases	*Non renal causes*
Acute glomerulonephritis	Increased intracranial pressure
Interstitial nephritis	Acute intermittent porphyria
Renal artery or vein thrombosis	Guillain-Barré syndrome
Hemolytic uremic syndrome	Anxiety
Acute urinary tract obstruction	Hyperthyroidism
Nephrotic syndrome with relapse	Corticosteroids, cyclosporine, erythropoietin
Acute renal failure	Iatrogenic (fluid, salt overload)

Persistent Hypertension

Renal parenchymal disease	*Primary (essential) hypertension*
Glomerulonephritis (GN): focal segmental glomerulosclerosis, membranoproliferative GN, crescentic GN, lupus GN	Isolated
	Syndrome X (obesity, dyslipidemia, diabetes)
Reflux nephropathy	*Medications*
Obstructive uropathy	Corticosteroids; phenylephrine, pseudoephedrine
Polycystic kidney disease	Erythropoietin, calcineurin inhibitors, theophyl-
Renal dysplasia	line
Post kidney transplant	
Wilms tumor	*Endocrine*
	Cushing syndrome, pituitary tumor
Renovascular hypertension	Congenital adrenal hyperplasia, primary hyperal-
Fibromuscular dysplasia, neurofibromatosis	dosteronism, pheochromocytoma
Renal artery thrombosis	Neuroblastoma
Takayasu aortoarteritis	Hyperthyroidism, hypothyroidism
Cardiovascular	*Monogenic*
Coarctation of aorta	Liddle syndrome
	Apparent mineralocorticoid excess
	Glucocorticoid remediable aldosteronism

All patients with hypertension should also be screened for target organ damage. This includes evaluation of eyes (for hypertensive retinopathy), heart (increased left ventricular mass, diastolic dysfunction) and kidneys (albuminuria).

Management

Non-pharmacological measures are initiated for patients with essential hypertension (Table 38.7). Drug therapy is indicated in patients with: (i) symptomatic hypertension, (ii) stage 2 hypertension, (iii) stage 1 hypertension that persists despite non-pharmacologic measures, (iv) hypertensive target organ damage, and (v) comorbid conditions like diabetes, chronic kidney disease or dyslipidemia. Urgent but careful reduction of blood pressure is essential in patients with hypertensive crises.

Target Blood Pressure

The blood pressure should be lowered to below the 95th percentile, unless comorbidity

Table 38.6: Diagnostic workup for cause and target organ damage

Evaluation for Cause

Step 1: All patients

Complete blood counts
Blood levels
  Urea, creatinine, electrolytes, pH, bicarbonate
  Fasting lipids, glucose, uric acid
Urinalysis, culture
24-hr urinary protein; spot protein to creatinine ratio
Abdominal ultrasonography
Renal artery Doppler

Step 2: Based on clinical and basic evaluation

Recurrent UTI, abnormal ultrasound: DMSA scintigraphy, micturating cystourethrography
Glomerulonephritis: Complement C3, antinuclear antibodies, anti-neutrophil cytoplasmic antibodies;
    kidney biopsy
Renovascular cause: Captopril DTPA scintigraphy; conventional or digital subtraction angiography
Endocrine cause: Plasma renin activity, aldosterone, cortisol
  Urinary catecholamines; if abnormal: CT or MRI for adrenals
  MIBG radionuclide scan
  Serum cortisol, ACTH, thyroid profile
Essential hypertension: Glucose tolerance test, lipid profile, HbA1C

Screening for Target Organ Damage

Retinal fundus examination
Urine spot protein to creatinine ratio
Chest X-ray, electrocardiogram, echocardiography

DMSA-dimercaptosuccinic acid; ACTH-adrenocorticotrophic hormone; MRI-magnetic resonance imaging;
MIBG[131]I-metaiodobenzyl guanidine; HbA1c-glycosylated hemoglobin

is present, in which case the target is below the 90th percentile. An even more strict control of blood pressure, to between the 50th and 75th percentile, is associated with slower decline in renal function in children with chronic kidney disease.

Pre-hypertension: Patients are primarily managed by therapeutic lifestyle modifications (Table 38.7) and evaluated every 6 months. Medications are not required unless the patient has comorbid conditions.

Essential hypertension: Patients with essential hypertension are initially managed with lifestyle modifications (Table 38.7). Pharmacological therapy is administered; therapy with thiazide diuretics and beta-blockers should be avoided. Screening for dyslipidemia and impaired glucose tolerance should be performed every 6–12 months.

Drug Therapy

Table 38.8 gives dosing recommendations for medications used for hypertension. Severe, symptomatic hypertension should be treated with IV antihypertensive medications (Table 38.9).

Therapy is initiated with a single medication from any of the following classes: angiotensin converting enzyme inhibitors (ACEI), beta (β)-blockers or calcium channel blockers (CCB). Drugs with a longer duration of action (once or twice daily dosing) are

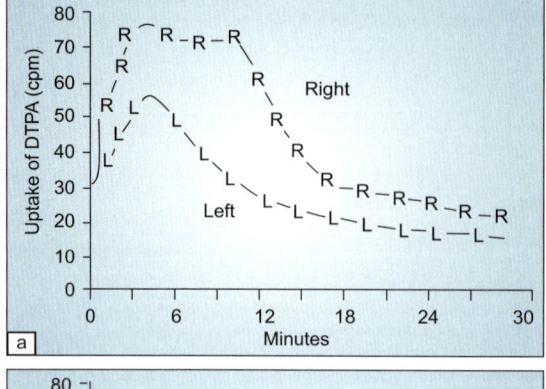

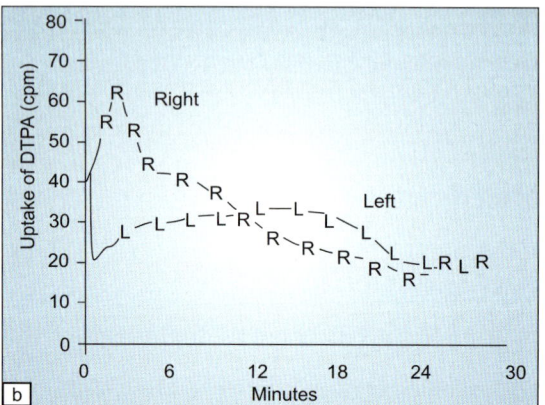

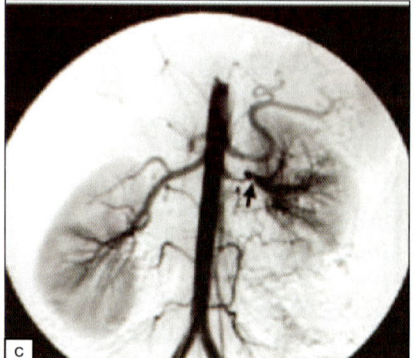

Fig. 38.3: Evaluation for severe hypertension in an 8-yr-old boy suggested bruit over left flank. The left kidney was smaller on ultrasound. DTPA scan showed (a) reduced uptake in left kidney; which (b) reduced further following administration of captopril. Angiography (c) showed stenosis involving proximal part of left renal artery (arrow), confirming the diagnosis of renal artery stenosis

Table 38.7: Therapeutic lifestyle changes
Weight management
Weight reduction in overweight or obese individuals Prevention of excess or abnormal weight gain
Dietary alterations
Increased intake of fresh vegetables, fruits and low-fat dairy Dietary sodium reduction (2–3 g of salt) Portion-size control Decrease in consumption of sugar-containing beverages and energy-dense snacks Regular meals including a healthy breakfast
Exercise
Regular physical activity for 30–60 minutes every day Restrict sedentary activity: television watching, video or computer games to <2 hr/day
Stress reduction

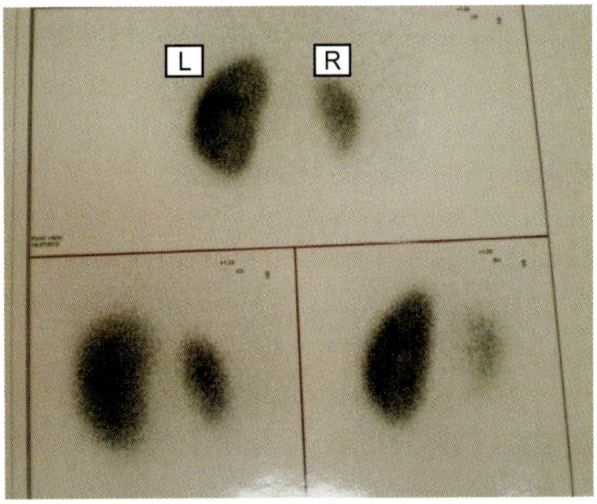

Fig. 38.4: A 10-yr old girl with severe hypertension was found to have a smaller right kidney on ultrasound. Evaluation with ^{99m}Tc-DMSA scan showed multiple renal scars in this kidney, suggesting reflux nephropathy

preferred. Dose adjustment should be made once in 2–3 days.

Once the initial antihypertensive agent has been chosen, a stepped-care approach is followed. It is necessary to begin at the recommended initial dose and increase the dose until the desired blood pressure or the maximum dose is reached. A second or third medication, with complementary mechanism of action, is added if blood pressure control is not achieved. This approach allows for individualization of therapy and facilitates detection of adverse effects.

Calcium channel blockers (CCB): Dihydro-pyridines, e.g. nifedipine, amlodipine, felodi-pine and isradipine have been used. CCB are preferred in low renin or volume expanded states, and where the hypertension is media-ted *via* constriction of afferent arterioles (e.g. cyclosporine induced hypertension). Amlo-dipine is the most frequently used agent. Dihydropyridines increase proteinuria and should be avoided in patients with chronic kidney disease. Adverse effects include headache, flushing, dizziness, tachycardia, fatigue and edema. The sustained release form of nifedipine permits once or twice daily dosing.

Angiotensin converting enzyme inhibitors (ACEI): These include captopril (used in young infants) and enalapril (preferred beyond infancy). Side effects include hyper-kalemia and impaired renal functions; infr-equently, anemia, neutropenia or dry cough may occur. Serum potassium and creatinine should be monitored regularly.

ACEI are preferred in patients with renal disease or diabetes since they cause a reduc-tion of proteinuria, and in left ventricular dysfunction or congestive cardiac failure. ACEI are avoided in children with GFR <30 mL/min/1.73 m^2, contraindicated in pre-sence of bilateral renal artery stenosis, and used with caution in adolescent girls because of the risk of fetopathy (oligohydramnios, hypotension, cardiac defects and renal defects including tubular dysplasia). Newer agents (lisinopril, ramipril, fosinopril) require once daily dosing and have fewer side effects.

Angiotensin receptor blockers (ARB): ARB used in children include losartan, valsartan and irbesartan. The indications, contra-indications and adverse effects (except cough, not seen with ARB) are similar to ACEIs.

Beta blockers: These agents should be avoided in athletes (decrease exercise output) and patients with asthma, congestive cardiac failure or diabetes. Adverse effects include postural hypotension, tachycardia, broncho-spasm, fatigue, depression and increased serum triglycerides.

Cardioselective β-blockers (atenolol, metoprolol) are effective, relatively safe and need to be given once or twice daily. The dose of atenolol needs to be modified in renal impairment. Labetalol, α- and β-blocker, is safe and effective in patients with hyper-tension that is refractory to other medications. Carvedilol, a α- and β- blocker, has also shown efficacy in children with congestive heart failure.

Diuretics: These are used as adjuncts rather than as monotherapy. Diuretics are preferred

Chronic Kidney Disease and Hypertension

VIII

Table 38.8: Antihypertensive agents

Agents	Dose; frequency	Comments
ACE inhibitors, angiotensin receptor blockers		
Captopril	0.3–6 mg/kg/day; tid	Use cautiously if GFR <30 mL/min/1.73 m²; avoid in renal artery stenosis
Enalapril	0.1–0.6 mg/kg/day; qd or bid	Use smaller doses in neonates
Lisinopril	0.06–0.6 mg/kg/day; qd	Monitor serum potassium, creatinine regularly
Ramipril	2.5–6 mg/m²; qd	Hyperkalemia, impaired renal functions; anemia, neutropenia, dry cough infrequent
Irbesartan	4–5 mg/kg/day	
Losartan	0.7–1.4 mg/kg/day; qd	
Valsartan	2 mg/kg/day; qd	
Calcium channel blockers		
Amlodepine	0.05–0.5 mg/kg/day; qd–bid	Extended release (ER) nifedepine must be swallowed whole
Nifedipine (ER)	0.25–3 mg/kg/day; qd–bid	Side effects: Headache, flushing, dizziness, tachycardia; lower extremity edema, erythema
Isradipine	0.15–0.8 mg/kg/day; tid	
Beta-blockers		
Atenolol	0.5–2 mg/kg/day; qd or bid	Atenolol: decrease dose by 50% at GFR <50 ml/min; give on alternate days at GFR <10 mL/min/1.73 m²
Metoprolol	1–4 mg/kg/day; bid	Sleep disturbances with propranolol, metoprolol
Labetalol	10–40 mg/kg/day; bid or tid	Avoid in asthma, heart failure; blunt symptoms of hypoglycemia
Alpha sympathetic agents		
Clonidine	5–25 µg/kg/day; tid or qid	Abrupt cessation may cause rebound hypertension; sedation
Prazosin	0.05–0.5 mg/kg/day; bid or tid	May cause 'first dose' hypotension, syncope
Vasodilators		
Hydralazine	1–8 mg/kg/day; qid	Side effects: headache, palpitations, fluid retention, heart failure.
Minoxidil	0.1–1 mg/kg/day; qd or bid	Pericardial effusion, hypertrichosis
Diuretics		
Frusemide	0.5–3 mg/kg/day; qd or bid	Monitor electrolytes, fluid status
Spironolactone*	1–3 mg/kg/day; qd or bid	Thiazides: dyslipidemia, hyperglycemia, hyperuricemia, hypokalemia, hypomagnesemia
Metolazone	0.2–0.4 mg/kg/day; qd	Loop diuretics: metabolic alkalosis, hypokalemia, hypercalciuria
Hydrochlorothiazide	1–3 mg/kg/day; qd	*Use cautiously with ACEI, angiotensin receptor blockers
Amiloride*	0.4–0.6 mg/kg/day; qd	

qd once daily; bid twice daily; tid thrice daily; qid four times daily

when fluid overload is noted. Adverse effects include fatigue, muscle cramps, nausea, hypokalemia, hyponatremia, metabolic alkalosis and hyperlipidemia. Thiazide diuretics are ineffective at GFR <30 mL/minute/1.73 m². Loop diuretics are potent, but their efficacy decreases with impaired renal function. Potassium sparing diuretics such as spironolactone are useful in conditions associated with mineralocorticoid excess, or as an adjunct to drugs which increase aldosterone levels, such as vasodilators and CCB.

Combination therapy: ACEI and ARB have been used together, but experience is limited in children. Long term combination of thiazides with β-blockers should be avoided because of their association with impaired glucose tolerance.

Specific Recommendations

The choice of medication depends on the cause of hypertension and associated complications.

Acute glomerulonephritis: Restrict fluid and sodium intake; use loop diuretics if congestive cardiac failure, hypertension or severe edema. Use intravenous furosemide and a CCB if severe hypertension with or without encephalopathy is present.

Suspected or confirmed renovascular disease: Initiate therapy with CCB or/and a β-blocker. Avoid use of ACEI or angiotensin receptor blockers if bilateral renovascular stenosis is suspected or confirmed.

Hyperlipidemia: ACEI or CCB are preferred; β-blockers and diuretics should be avoided.

Chronic kidney disease (CKD): ACEI or ARB are preferred in children with proteinuric renal disease. Avoid in those with CKD stage IV–V (GFR <30 mL/min/1.73 m²). Diuretics may be administered to reduce the fluid overload.

Pheochromocytoma: Labetalol or phentolamine (α-blocking agent) are medications of choice; use of β-blocker alone should be avoided since it allows unopposed α-activity that worsens the vasoconstriction.

Postoperative hypertension: This is due to catecholamine surge from activation of the sympathetic nervous system. The treatment of choice is with a α-blocker or labetalol.

Monitoring

Follow-up visits should be scheduled frequently (every 2–4 weeks) until blood pressure control has been achieved, and then less frequently (every 3 months). Home blood pressure monitoring and assessment for medication side-effects are reviewed at each follow-up visit. After 8–12 months of successful blood pressure control, "step down" of therapy may be attempted.

Monitoring for target organ damage should commence at diagnosis of hypertension, and continue at regular intervals. This includes regular echocardiography, retinal fundus examination and urinalysis.

HYPERTENSIVE CRISES

Hypertensive crises are usually caused by noncompliance to medications or poorly controlled chronic hypertension. Treatment is tailored to the extent of end-organ injury and comorbid conditions (Table 38.9).

Hypertensive Emergency

Immediate reduction in blood pressure is required to prevent and limit target organ damage. A potent IV antihypertensive (sodium nitroprusside, nitroglycerine, labetalol or nicardipine) is titrated to produce a controlled reduction in blood pressure. The aim is to decrease blood pressure by up to 25% in the first 8-hr and then gradually to the upper limit of normal (95th percentile) over 24–48 hr. Therapy with oral antihypertensive agents is commenced as soon as the patient can take orally; IV therapy is withdrawn over the next 24-hr.

Sodium nitroprusside is preferred because it is easily available, inexpensive, and has a

Table 38.9: Agents for management of hypertensive crises

Medication	Onset	Duration	Route	Dose	Side effects
Sodium nitro-prusside	30 sec	<10 min	IV infusion	0.5–8 µg/kg/min (made in 5% dextrose)	Nausea, vomiting, headache, tachycardia, cyanide toxicity (dizziness, confusion, seizures, jaw stiffness and lactic acidosis)
Labetalol	5–10 min	3–6 hr	IV infusion IV bolus	0.25–3 mg/kg/hour 0.2–1 mg/kg/dose q 5–10 min (max 40 mg)	Orthostatic hypotension, bradycardia, pallor, abdominal pain, diarrhea
Nicardipine	1–10 min	3 hr	IV infusion IV bolus	0.5–4 µg/kg/min (max 5 mg/hr) 30 µg/kg (max 2 mg/dose) q 15 min	Flushing, reflex tachycardia, phlebitis, nausea, increased intracranial pressure, headache
Esmolol	60 sec	10–20 min	IV infusion	Loading with 100–500 µg/kg over 1–2 min; then maintain at 25–100 µg/kg/min	Bradycardia, orthostatic hypotension, pallor
Nitroglycerine	2–5 min	5–10 min	IV infusion	1–3 µg/kg/min	Methemoglobinemia, headache, tachycardia
Phentolamine	10 min	30–60 min	IV bolus	0.1–0.2 mg/kg (max 5 mg) q 2–4 hr if required	Reflex tachycardia, abdominal pain
Hydralazine	5–20 min	2–6 hr	IV/IM bolus	0.15 mg/kg q 4–6 hr	Reflex tachycardia, prolonged hypotension, nausea, flushing, headache
Nifedipine	10–30 min	1–4 hr	Oral	0.2–0.5 mg/kg (max 10 mg) q 4 to 6 hr	Excessive hypotension, peripheral edema
Clonidine	15–30 min	2–4 hr	Oral	0.05–0.1 mg/dose, may repeat q hr; max 0.8 mg total dose	Somnolence, dry mouth
Minoxidil	30 min	2–5 days	Oral	0.1–0.2 mg/kg per dose (max 10 mg)	Hirsutism, fluid retention; contraindicated in pheochromocytoma

short half-life and a wide dose range that allow easy titration. Cyanide toxicity may be prevented with the concomitant use of sodium thiosulfate or hydroxycobalamin. IV sodium nitroglycerine is less effective, but preferred in patients with myocardial dysfunction. IV labetalol is used as an infusion, or less optimally, as bolus doses every 5–10 minutes. IV nicardipine, esmolol and urapidil are effective, but not available in India.

The use of immediate release nifedipine for hypertensive emergencies has been criticized for its unpredictable effect and association with an increased risk for adverse cardiovascular outcomes in adults. In children, however, nifedipine seems to be effective and well tolerated for decreasing blood pressure, when given at a dose of 0.2–0.5 mg/kg.

The use of IV diuretics should be avoided unless definite evidence of volume overload is present. Volume status can be depleted (due to decreased oral intake and pressure natriuresis), causing stimulation of the renin-angiotensin system, worsening the hypertension. Volume repletion restores tissue perfusion and prevents a precipitous fall in blood pressure.

Hypertensive Urgency

Patients with stage 2 hypertension, no evidence of acute target organ damage and less alarming symptoms (e.g. headache and/or vomiting) can be treated in a non-ICU setting with oral medications over 24 to 48 hr.

Oral medications are administered and titrated initially as an inpatient. Medications with relatively short onset of action that can be used for hypertensive urgency are: nifedi-pine (0.25 mg/kg), clonidine (0.05–0.1 mg/dose), labetalol (0.2–1 mg/kg/dose), isradi-pine (0.05–0.1 mg/kg/dose), hydralazine (0.2–0.6 mg/kg/dose) and minoxidil (0.1–0.2 mg/kg/dose).

Reflex hypertensive crises can develop in patients who have abruptly stopped taking antihypertensives medications, particularly clonidine or β-blockers. Treatment involves restarting previous medications after the initial reduction of blood pressure with labetalol or sodium nitroprusside.

SUPPORT READING

Indian Pediatric Nephrology Group. Evaluation and management of hypertension. Indian Pediatr 2007; 44: 103–21

National High Blood Pressure Education Program Working Group. The Fourth report on the diagnosis, evaluation and treatment of high blood pressure in children and adolescents. Pediatrics 2004; 114 (Suppl): 555–76

Vehaskari VM. Heritable forms of hypertension. Pediatr Nephrol 2009; 24: 1929–37

Lande MB, Flynn JT. Treatment of hypertension in children and adolescents. Pediatr Nephrol 2009; 24: 1939–49

Flynn JT, Tullus K. Severe hypertension in children and adolescents: pathophysiology and treatment. Pediatr Nephrol. 2009; 24: 1101–12

Mitsnefes MM. Hypertension in children and adolescents. Pediatr Clin N Am 2006; 53: 493–512

Lurbe E, Cifkova R, Cruickshank JK, et al. Management of high blood pressure in children and adolescents: recommendations of the European Society of Hypertension. J Hypertension 2009; 27: 1719–42

Renal Replacement Therapy

39 Choice of Modality

In patients with chronic kidney disease, the options for renal replacement therapy (RRT) includes chronic dialysis (hemodialysis or peritoneal dialysis) or renal transplantation. The indications for initiating RRT are based upon a combination of clinical, biochemical and psychosocial assessments. The benefits of early dialysis should be weighed against the risk of complications from chronic dialysis therapy. The following influence the timing of initiation of RRT:

Renal Dysfunction

According to the K-DOQI guidelines, initiation of dialysis should be considered when the glomerular filtration rate (GFR) falls below 15 ml/min/1.73 m^2 body surface area and is strongly recommended when the GFR is <8 ml/min/1.73 m^2.

Clinical Factors

The well being of the patient is more important than the estimated GFR for deciding when dialysis should be started. The presence of fluid overload, hypertension, gastrointestinal symptoms, growth retardation and neurological consequences of uremia influence the decision to initiate RRT.

Biochemical Factors

The presence of laboratory abnormalities, such as hyperkalemia, hyperphosphatemia and acidosis are important considerations.

Options for Renal Replacement Therapy

Renal transplantation is the treatment of choice for children with end stage renal disease (ESRD). While chronic dialysis is life sustaining, it is inferior to renal transplantation in providing adequate renal replacement. Compared to dialysis, transplantation is associated with significant survival advantage, decreased risks of hospitalization and improved quality of life. With the availability of potent immunosuppressive medications and improvements in surgical and urologic techniques, short and long term transplant outcomes have improved considerably.

While awaiting transplantation, RRT may be offered either by hemodialysis (HD) or chronic peritoneal dialysis (PD) (Table 39.1). HD is a more efficient modality for RRT since it allows rapid solute and fluid removal, and precise regulation of volume. HD requires adequate infrastructure, technical expertise and trained personnel. Vascular access may be

Table 39.1: Options for renal replacement therapy

	Peritoneal dialysis	*Hemodialysis*
Complexity of procedure	-	+
Efficiency of solute clearance	Low	High
Need for vascular access	-	+
Anticoagulation required	-	+
Possible use in hemodynamic instability	+	-
Need for nursing support	+	++
Fluid balance achieved	+	Intermittent
Ultrafiltration control	-	+
Ease of optimal nutrition	+	-

difficult to establish in young children. HD is unsuitable for hemodynamically unstable patients and those with bleeding disorders.

Chronic PD allows patients to be managed in the home environment, avoids need for anticoagulation and is hemodynamically less stressful. It allows dialysis in young children, and enables a less restrictive diet resulting in better nutrition.

Patients and their families should be involved in the choice of therapy. Factors that influence decision include patient age, avail-ability of vascular access, native kidney function and relative contraindications to either modality.

SUPPORT READING

Auron A, Brophy PD. Pediatric renal supportive therapies: the changing face of pediatric renal replacement approaches. Curr Opin in Pediatr 2010; 22: 183–88

Bunchman TE. Technical considerations for renal replacement therapy in children. Semin Nephrol 2008; 28: 488–92

40 Hemodialysis

Hemodialysis provides an excellent extracorporeal mode for renal replacement. Advances in technical aspects in hemodialysis and the availability of pediatric size dialyzers and equipment have made it possible to offer hemodialysis to children with end stage renal disease.

Principles

Blood, drawn through a vascular access at a rate of 3–10 mL/kg/minute (maximum 400 ml/min), passes across a blood pump which generates positive pressure and forces it into the dialyzer. Countercurrent dialysis occurs across the semipermeable membrane as the blood entering into one side of the membrane of the dialyzer runs alongside the dialysate on the other side containing pretreated water with varying concentrations of electrolytes, flowing at a rate of 300–500 ml/minute. The blood 'purified' by ultrafiltration and solute removal is returned to the patient circulation (Fig. 40.1). Excess fluid is removed by ultrafiltration, while solutes are removed by diffusion, convection and solvent drag.

Ultrafiltration is the movement of fluid under hydrostatic pressure from the blood to the dialysate compartment. The amount ultrafiltered depends on the pressure difference between the blood and dialysate compartments, the transmembrane pressure. This pressure is controlled by varying the pressure in the dialysate or blood compartments; increasing negative dialysate pressure increases ultrafiltration. Plasma oncotic pressure opposes ultrafiltration, and fluid moves only when transmembrane pressure exceeds the oncotic pressure.

The transfer of solutes depend upon the rates of blood flow and dialysate flow, the solute concentration gradient, the composition of dialysate, and the surface area and the permeability of the dialyzer membrane. The latter is measured in terms of mass transfer coefficient (K_0) of the membrane, times the surface area (K_0A). The efficiency of removal falls rapidly with increasing molecular size, particularly above 300 Da.

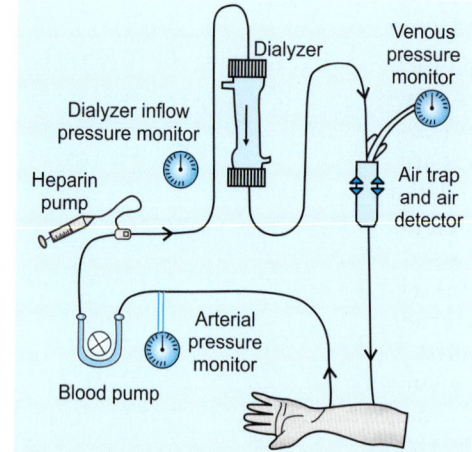

Fig. 40.1: Components of a hemodialysis circuit. Blood lines, dialyzer, blood pumps and monitoring systems are shown. The blood and the dialysate flow countercurrent to each other

Hemodialysis

For small solutes such as urea, the clearance increases with blood and dialysate flow rate, reaching a plateau. For large solutes e.g. vitamin B_{12}, the plateau occurs at much lower flow rates. Thus, while small solutes are flow limited, large solutes are membrane limited, with their clearance related to K_0A. At high rates of ultrafiltration, solute transport increases due to solute drag. Ultrafiltration adds to the clearance value particularly for large solutes, as it is associated with further solute clearance through convective transport, measured as sieving coefficient.

Dialysis Machine

Currently available HD machines allow accurate regulation of ultrafiltrate. Unlike peritoneal dialysis, ultrafiltration and solute removal can be independently controlled. Continuous profiling allows sodium and ultrafiltration to be varied through the session

Vascular Access

A satisfactory vascular access delivers blood flow adequate for the dialysis prescription. Options for chronic hemodialysis include: *(i)* tunneled cuffed catheter; *(ii)* arteriovenous (AV) fistula, and *(iii)* AV graft.

Catheters

Dual lumen 8–13 French catheters are often used. These allow high blood flow rate with low (<2%) risk of recirculation, unless the ports are connected in reverse (20% risk) of circulation.

Percutaneous *temporary dual lumen catheters* are used for acute short term dialysis, and *cuffed central venous catheter (Permacath)* are preferred if chronic HD (>4 weeks) is anticipated. The latter require surgical placement *via* a subcutaneous tunnel to ensure secure placement. Tunneled catheters have lower risk of blood stream infections and last longer (60% for 6 months, 40% for 1 yr). However, they carry risks of thrombosis and vascular stenosis.

Temporary catheters are inserted into the femoral, subclavian or internal jugular veins. The right internal jugular is preferred since its direct angle to the heart achieves high blood flow rates. Subclavian catheters achieve satisfactory flow rates, but venous stenosis and subclavian steal syndrome may occur. Femoral lines are easy to insert with a low risk of complications, but carry risks of sepsis and dislocation, and should not be in place for longer than 7–10 days.

Cuffed catheters are placed in the internal jugular or subclavian vein. The K-DOQI recommends that subclavian access should be used for cuffed catheters only when jugular options are not available. The catheter should not be placed on the same side as a maturing AV access.

Insertion: The use of a portable real-time ultrasound to guide insertion of temporary catheters reduces the risk of complications. Fluoroscopy is mandatory when inserting upper limb cuffed catheters, in order to adjust the catheter tip to the level of cavoatrial junction.

Size: Catheters below 5F are suboptimal and used only in neonate as two single lumen catheters. In others, larger catheters are used according to body weight, as follows: 3–15 kg: 7–8 Fr dual lumen; 16–30 kg: 9–10 Fr ; and >30 kg: 11–12 Fr dual lumen.

Length: The shorter the catheter length, the lower is the resistance to flow, and therefore, the ease of dialysis. Femoral catheters should be long enough to minimize recirculation.

Arteriovenous (AV) Fistula

The AV fistula is created surgically by anastomosing an artery to a vein, resulting in an easily accessible blood vessel with high flow rates. Forearm veins of the non-dominant arm are preferred, beginning distally and moving proximally as access fails. Fistulas include the radiocephalic and brachiocephalic fistula.

A fistula takes about 6–12 weeks to mature, during which the wall of the venous limb

40

becomes dilated and thickened. Hand exercises are advised to enhance the maturity. The maturity is assessed by palpating for a thrill and listening to the bruit over the fistula site. Once a fistula is mature, dialysis can be performed by infiltrating a local anesthestic into the skin, and connecting two needles inserted into the vessel to the arterial and venous ends of the circuit.

Dialysis through an AV fistula allows high and consistent flow rates, and risks of infection and thrombosis are low. Fistulas take long to mature in young children. Complications include thrombosis, infection, steal phenomena and aneurysm formation. Care is taken to avoid applying pressure to the limb (blood pressure cuff; sleeping on the arm); the limb should not be used for venepuncture or IV line. The risk of development of an aneurysm at the needle puncture site can be minimized by rotating the site of insertion of the needles, or by cannulating the fistula with a blunt needle at exactly the same site each time (buttonhole approach).

AV Grafts

These are similar to fistulae except that an artificial graft made of polytetrafluroethylene or Teflon, such as Gore-TexR, is used to join the artery and vein. Grafts are used when the native vessels are small. Forearm loops, linear radiocephalic forearm grafts or upper arm loops are used. AV grafts mature faster and can be used within 1–3 weeks. The risk of vascular stenosis is similar to fistulas, while the risks of infection and thrombosis are higher.

Dialyzers

Hollow fiber dialyzers made of cellulose, modified cellulose or Polysulfone. Their size is dictated by the body surface area; the dialyzer to surface area ratio should be 0.7–1.0. Dialyzers suitable for adults (F8 dialyzer), with a prime volume of 110 ml and surface area 1.8 m^2, are unsuitable except in large adolescents. Table 40.1 lists characteristics of commonly used dialyzers.

Dialyzer clearance (K_D): This is the solute removal rate divided by the dialyzer inflow concentration. K_D is affected by changes in blood flow (Q_B) and dialysate flow (Q_D).

Product of mass transfer coefficient and surface area (K_oA): This is the maximum clearance achieved at infinite blood and dialysate flow rates. K_0A is a function of the membrane since at infinite flow rates the membrane is the only barrier to clearance. The higher this value, the more permeable the membrane. The efficiency of a dialyzer is defined by its urea K_0A. Standard dialyzers have a KoA <300–400, while high-efficiency dialyzers have a KoA >600–700.

Table 40.1: Dialyzers for pediatric use

Dialyzer size	F3	F4	F5	F6
Effective surface area, m^2	0.4	0.7	0.9–1.0	1.3
Ultrafiltration coefficient, mL/hr/mm Hg transmembrane pressure	1.7	2.8	4.0–4.2	5.5
Blood priming volume, mL	28–30	42–44	60–63	82–84
Maximum ultrafiltration, mL/hr	800	1600	2450	3300
Mass transfer area coefficient for urea (KoA) mL/min	290	440	557	670
Urea clearance at blood flow rate (Q_B) 25 mL/min, mL/min	25	25	25	25
Urea clearance at Q_B 200 mL/min, mL/min	125	155	175	183

Ultrafiltration Coefficient (KUf): This is the volume of fluid transferred across the membrane per hr when 1 mm Hg of TMP is applied. Cellulose membranes have lower KUf values than synthetic ones. The KUf of high-flux range between 20–60 mL/mm Hg/hr, low-flux dialyzers have KUf <10 mL/mm Hg/hr, and medium-flux dialyzers between 10–19 mL/mm Hg/hr.

High-efficiency and High-flux Dialyzers

High efficiency dialyzers provide better diffusive clearance, while high flux dialyzers provide convective clearance by solute drag. While the clearance of low molecular weight solutes (urea) is similar, the use of high flux membranes increases clearance rates of large solutes. High flux dialyzers should be considered in larger children who are likely to be on hemodialysis for prolonged duration, patients with amyloidosis, and those requiring rapid removal of large ultrafiltrate.

Dialysis Tubings

Blood lines are available in 3 sizes that vary in their priming volume: *(i)* neonatal 25 mL, *(ii)* pediatric 75 mL and *(iii)* adult 127 mL.

Priming Volume

The extracorporeal circuit volume includes the dialyzer priming volume and the volume of the blood lines. If this volume exceeds 10% of the total blood volume, blood or 5% albumin should be used to prime the blood lines and dialyzer.

Total blood volume (ml) = Weight (kg) × 60 (for adolescent)

Total blood volume (ml) = Weight (kg) × 80 (for child)

The circuit should be primed with blood or 5% albumin for all patients weighing <20 kg.

Dialysate

The solution for dialysis is prepared by mixing a concentrate of electrolytes and water. The base is provided as bicarbonate, since acetate is a vasodilator and may cause hypotension. The constituents of a standard dialysate solution are given in Table 40.2. The precise concentrations of solutes in the dialysate may vary according to specific needs.

The product water used for preparing the dialysate should adhere to standards recommended (Table 40.3). Guidelines are also available for the quality of ultrapure water required for continuous renal replacement therapies.

Blood Flow Rate

The clearance of solutes is related to the blood flow rate,which should be maintained at 3–8 (maximum 10) mL/kg/minute. Changes in blood flow rate affect efficiency of dialysis more than dialysate flow rates or dialyzer size.

Dialysate Flow Rate

The flow rate of the dialysate influences the clearance of solutes, particularly at high flow rates and when using dialyzers with high KoA. The usual rates of flow are 400-500 mL/min in children weighing <20 kg and 600–700 mL/minute in children >20 kg.

Ultrafiltration

The amount of ultrafiltration required is estimated based on the dry weight, the interdialytic weight gain, clinical features and

Table 40.2: Composition of standard dialysate	
pH	7.1–7.3
Dextrose	0–5.5 mmol/L
Sodium	135–145 mEq/L
Potassium	0–4 mEq/L
Calcium	2.5–3.5 mEq/L
Magnesium	0.5–0.75 mEq/L
Chloride	98–124 mEq/L
Acetate	2–4 mEq/L (acetate dialysate)
Bicarbonate	30–40 mEq/L (bicarbonate dialysate)

IX

Table 40.3: Upper limit for definitions of water and dialysate quality

	Bacterial growth, cfu/mL	Endotoxin, units/mL	Cytokine induction
AAMI	<200	<2	+
EuropeanPharmacopeia	100	0.25	–
Ultrapure water	0.1	0.03	–

AAMI Association for Advancement of Medical Instrumentation; cfu colony forming units

vital signs, the goal being to maintain a euvolemic state. Dry weight refers to the post-dialysis weight at which all or most excess body fluid has been removed; this should be adjusted for body growth every 1–2 months.

The initial ultrafiltration rate may be set at 10 mL/kg/hr, and increase as tolerated to a maximum of 0.2 mL/kg/minute, targeting a volume not exceeding 5% of body weight in one session. As an alternative, the hematocrit is continually monitored using special transducers, targeting no more than 8% rise in hematocrit during one session.

Most machines have an obligate ultra-filtration rate of 100 ml/hr. *Isolated ultrafiltration* mode, used in patients with extreme fluid overload, allows fluid removal without simultaneous solute removal.

Length and Frequency of Dialysis

The duration of initial dialysis depends on the amount of urea reduction to be achieved. Calculations for urea reduction and dialysis adequacy are discussed below and detailed in Chapter 42. The aim is for 30% reduction in blood urea nitrogen during the first dialysis (1.5–2 hr); 50% during the second treatment (3 hr) and ≥70% reduction during subsequent treatments (3.5–4 hr).

The first dialysis session is short, in order to prevent occurrence of the disequilibrium syndrome. Mannitol (0.5–1 g/kg/dose IV during dialysis) and phenobarbitone (3–5 mg/kg/dose IV before or after dialysis) are useful in preventing the complication. Some patients require daily dialysis for a few days.

For chronic intermittent HD (IHD), the duration of each session is 3.5–4 hr, three times a week. This frequency allows control of uremic symptoms while being convenient and least disruptive to the lifestyle. With high flux dialyzers, the duration of each session should be 2–2.5 hr.

Anticoagulation

Anticoagulation of the extracorporeal circuit, using unfractionated heparin, low molecular weight heparin or citrate is necessary to prevent clotting of the circuit.

Factors that favor clotting are low blood flow rates, high hematocrit, high ultra-filtration rate, venous access recirculation, use of intradialytic blood products and unsatis-factory priming of the dialyzer. Signs of clotting in the extracorporeal circuit are the presence of dark blood or black streaks in the dialyzer, and foaming within the drip cha-mbers and the venous trap.

Unfractionated Heparin

This is used as continuous infusion or by bolus routes.

Constant infusion: A loading dose of 20 U/kg bolus is administered into the arterial end upstream of the dialyzer. Dialysis is initiated after 3–5 minutes, followed by heparin infusion at 10 U/kg/hr. The infusion is stopped 30–60 minutes before end of the session in case of AV fistulas; for catheters, the infusion is continued till the end of the session.

Bolus route: Following an initial bolus of 40 U/kg, subsequent boluses of 20–25 U/kg are administered every 60 minutes with the dose titrated according to the activated clotting time (ACT). The last bolus is given 30 minutes before closing the dialysis session.

Monitoring: It is important to visually inspect the circuit for clotting and watch for blood leaks. Whole blood ACT is monitored every hour. Blood for ACT monitoring is drawn from the arterial end proximal to any heparin infusion site, and the rate of infusion titrated to keep ACT between 2–3 times normal. With the bolus route, the hourly dose is 20–25 U/kg if the ACT is within 150% of the baseline value. Alternatively, the Lee White clotting time is maintained at 20–30 minutes.

Low Molecular Weight Heparin

Fractionated or low molecular weight heparin (LMWH) may be used in patients with hyperlipidemia or heparin induced hyperkalemia. The agent is given as a single dose of 0.7–1 mg/kg at start of dialysis. Monitoring requires periodic estimation of activated factor X target levels being 1.0 U/ml. The target level is lower in patients at risk of hemorrhage, between 0.2–0.4 U/ml. Disadvantages LMWH include its cost and risk of bleeding, which cannot be antagonized by protamine sulfate.

Saline Dialysis

Dialysis with no anticoagulation is advised in patients with pericarditis, recent surgery, coagulopathy and thrombocytopenia. The dialyzer and tubing are flushed with saline (100 ml in <20 kg; 150 ml >20 kg) every 15–30 minutes. A small dose of heparin (10 U/kg) is given if the ACT is below 1.2 times normal. High blood flow rates are maintained and blood transfusions avoided.

Antibiotic Heparin Lock

The use of an antibiotic lock is associated with decreased risk of catheter related bacteremia. Antibiotic solutions used include vancomycin (2.5 mg/mL), gentamicin or amikacin (1–2 mg/mL) and cefazolin (5–10 mg/mL). The total volume of lock solution depends on the catheter size, and ranges from 2–5 mL. The lock is inserted into both lumina of the catheter at the completion of each dialysis session, and withdrawn completely immediately before the start of the next session. Co-administration of heparin (1000–5000 IU/mL) reduces thrombus formation and catheter related infections.

The use of heparin may stimulate formation of the biofilm; incompatibility with gentamicin and cephalosporins, and risks of systemic heparinization and heparin induced thrombocytopenia are additional concerns. Citrate (final concentration 4%) is suggested as an alternative, but its inadvertent administration carries risk of hypocalcemia and arrhythmias.

Dialysis Prescription

A dialysis prescription requires the following: (i) dialyzer size, type and blood tubing; (ii) blood flow rate (Q_B), (iii) composition of the dialysate; (iv) dialysate flow rate (Q_D); (v) ultrafiltration volume; (vi) anticoagulation regime; (vii) duration of dialysis session; and (viii) frequency of treatment sessions.

The most effective way to increase small solute clearance is to increase blood and dialysate flow rates. For increasing large solute clearance, the choices are to use a membrane that is thin and more porous and has a higher surface area, or a combination of these approaches. A prescription for dialysis is shown in Table 40.4.

Monitoring during Hemodialysis

Table 40.5 summarizes the key components of monitoring during treatment.

Adequacy of Dialysis

The determinants of the dose of dialysis include the patient size, residual native kidney function and the urea generation rate. The adequacy of dialysis is assessed by clinical and biochemical parameters. These include an

Table 40.4: Hemodialysis prescription

Patient dry weight	_____ kg
Body surface area	_____ m²
Dialyzer	_____ surface area = 0.8–1.0 × patient surface area
Priming solution	_____ mL Saline/5% Albumin/Blood
Blood flow rate (Q_B, 3–8 mL/kg/minute)	_____ mL/min
Dialysate flow rate (Q_D)	_____ mL/min
Treatment time (t)	_____ minutes
Ultrafiltrate volume	_____ L (Adjust by dry weight, interdialytic gain)
Heparin dosing*	_____ U

* Loading dose 40 U/kg; maintenance 20 U/kg q hr; adjust to activated clotting time 150–180 sec

evaluation of the hydration, nutritional status, electrolyte and acid/base balance, calcium and phosphorus homeostasis, control of anemia and blood pressure and the overall well being. Objective assessment of dialysis adequacy using urea reduction ratio, Kt/V and normalized protein catabolic rate is described in Chapter 42.

Complications

Table 40.6 summarizes complications observed most commonly during dialysis, their prevention and management.

Type A dialyzer reactions are characterized by dyspnea, sneezing, rhinorrhea, urticaria, diarrhea and abdominal cramps. Chest pain and back pain may be seen in type B dialyzer reaction. Reactions are less frequent with reuse.

Catheter-related Infections

The risk of catheter related blood stream infections (CRBSI) in patients with non-cuffed hemodialysis catheters ranges between 2 to 7 episodes per 1000 catheter-days. Strategies to prevent infections include: *(i)* use of standard aseptic precautions

Table 40.5: Monitoring of a patient on chronic hemodialysis

Evaluation	*Frequency*
Monitoring for adverse events	Continuous throughout dialysis
Vital signs	Half-hourly during dialysis
Routine physical examination	Once, every session
HD access site examination	Once, every session
Blood sugar, electrolytes	Once, every session
Renal, liver function tests	Weekly
Blood counts	Weekly
Dietician consultation	Weekly
Parathormone, Iron studies	Every 3 months
Kt/V	First 4 dialysis sessions; every 3 months
Urea reduction ratio	First 4 dialysis sessions; every 3 months
Normalized protein catabolic rate	Every 3 months
ECG, echocardiogram	Every 6 months
Viral serologies	Once in 6 months
Viral PCR (HBV, HCV)	If transaminases elevated
Blood and catheter cultures	If fever >24 hr

Table 40.6. Complications during hemodialysis

Complication	Cause	Management
Hypotension	Anemia; sepsis; arrhythmia; diastolic dysfunction; high ultrafiltration (UF) rate; underestimation of dry weight Dialysate: low Na⁺; high temperature; acetate buffer; dialyzer reaction; air embolism	*Prevention:* Maintain hemoglobin 10–11 g/dL; avoid pre-HD antihypertensive drugs. Accurate dry weight assessment; use inbuilt UF controller; blood volume monitoring Dialysate Na⁺ 140–145 mEq/L, temperature 35.5 °C; use bicarbonate *Treatment:* Trendelenberg position; Reduce UF to minimum Administer 50–100 mL 0.9% saline; 20% albumin (5 ml/kg) Restart UF at low rate once patient stable
Muscle cramps (2–50%)	Ischemia; hypocalcemia; hypomagnesemia; hypokalemia Risk factors: high UF, hypotension, hypovolemia, low dialysate Na⁺	*Prevention:* Monitor Mg^{2+}, Ca^{2+}, K⁺; increase dialysate Na⁺ Pre-dialysis quinine sulfate (250–325 mg), carnitine (250–500 mg) or oxazepam (5–10 mg) *Treatment:* 50–100 mL 0.9% saline; 3% saline 1–2 ml/kg Hypertonic glucose, mannitol; nifedipine if normotensive; Forced stretching
Nausea, vomiting (10%)	Hypotension; disequilibrium; dialyzer reaction; high dialysate Ca^{2+} or Na⁺	*Prevention:* Avoid hypotension; pre-dialysis metoclopramide *Treatment:* Treat hypotension; antiemetics
Dialysis disequilibrium	Rapid reduction of urea; cerebral edema (headache, disorientation, fits, coma)	Slow blood flow rate or stop dialysis; mannitol 0.5–1 g/kg IV; 3% saline 1–2 ml/kg or hypertonic glucose; manage coma, seizures
Type A (anaphylactic) dialyzer reaction	Ethylene oxide (used for sterilization); filters containing AN69; contaminated dialysis solution; heparin	Stop dialysis; discard dialyser and tubings Cardiorespiratory support; IV antihistamininc, epinephrine, and/or steroids
Type B dialyzer reaction	Complement activation	Nasal oxygen; rule our air embolism, hemolysis and pericarditis Change of dialyzer or reuse may help
Seizures	Hypertension; dialysis disequilibrium	Manage hypertension; load with IV phenytoin or valproate
Itching	Low grade hypersensitivity; uremia	Antihistaminics; target lower calcium phosphorus product; increase dialysis dose

Table 40.7: Diagnosis of catheter related infections

Infection	Definition and diagnosis
Colonization	Significant growth of a microorganism in culture of the catheter tip or catheter hub
Exit site	Erythema, induration, and/or tenderness within 2 cm of the catheter exit site; with or without fever, pus at exit site
Phlebitis	Induration or erythema, warmth, and pain or tenderness around catheter exit site
Probable CRBSI	Bacteremia or fungemia with ≥1 positive culture of blood drawn from the peripheral vein, clinical features of infection (e.g., fever, chills, hypotension), and no apparent source for bloodstream infection except the catheter
Confirmed CRBSI	Probable CRBSI, along with a positive culture result in blood drawn from the catheter, confirming infection with the same organism (species and antibiogram) as present on peripheral blood culture; with or without a ratio of 5:1 for organism colony forming units in culture from catheter versus blood, or a differential time to positivity (culture positivity in sample from catheter occurring ≥ 2 hr earlier than a positive culture from peripheral blood)

CRBSI catheter related blood stream infection

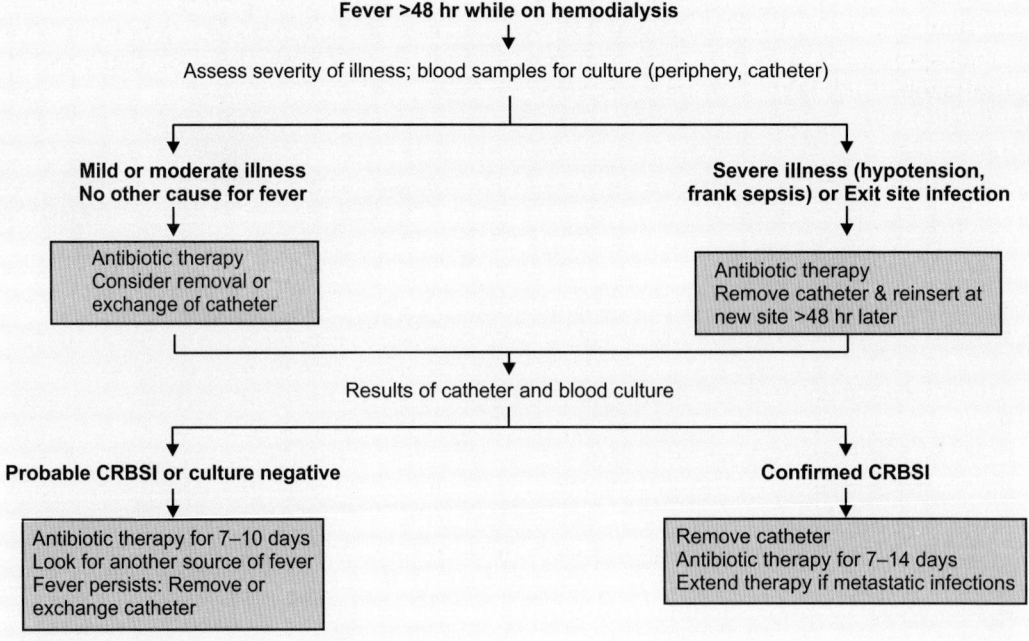

Fig. 40.2: Evaluation and management of catheter related blood stream infections (CRBSI). CRBSI should be suspected in dialyzed patients with fever lasting for >48 hrs, and antibiotic therapy initiated. The catheter must be removed in patients with confirmed CRBSI, except in infection with coagulase negative *S. aureus* (CONS), which may be treated successfully with systemic antibiotics alone. Therapy is modified according to sensitivity pattern of the pathogen and continued for 14 days. Seven days therapy is sufficient in infection with CONS. Patients with septic thrombosis or endocarditis should receive 4–6 weeks of antibiotic therapy. Patients with osteomyelitis are treated for 6–8 weeks

(including hand hygiene); *(ii)* preferring AV fistulas and cuffed (tunneled) catheters to uncuffed catheters in patients on prolonged hemodialysis; *(iii)* use of antibiotic catheter locks; *(iv)* regular exit site dressing with mupirocin or povidone iodine; *(v)* treatment of *S. aureus* carriers with 2% topical intranasal mupirocin and *(vi)* recently, the use of catheters impregnated with antibiotics or antiseptics.

Table 40.7 and Fig. 40.2 summarize the management protocol for catheter related blood stream infections. Antibiotic therapy for catheter-related infection is often initiated empirically. The choice of antibiotic therapy depends on the severity of the patient's illness, the hospital's infection control policy and the pattern of antibiotic resistance reported. Usually, a combination of vancomycin with a third or fourth-generation cephalosporin, such as ceftazidime or piparacillin-tazobactam, is recommended.

The catheter should be removed and cultured if the patient has severe disease, exit site infection or confirmed catheter related infection. A new catheter may be inserted >48 hr after removal of catheter, at a fresh site. If the catheter cannot be removed, it is exchanged for a fresh catheter over a guidewire. If fever persists beyond 72-hr of catheter removal, the patient should be evaluated for metastatic infections.

SUPPORT READING

Chand DH, Valentini RP, Kamil ES. Hemodialysis vascular access options in pediatric: Considerations for patients and practitioners. Pediatr Nephrol 2009; 24: 1121–28

Mermel LA, Allon M, Bouza E, *et al.* Clinical practice guidelines for the diagnosis and management of intravascular catheter-related infection: 2009 Update by the Infectious Diseases Society of America. Clin Infect Dis 2009; 49: 1–45

41 Peritoneal Dialysis

Long-term peritoneal dialysis is an accepted mode of renal replacement therapy. Availability of permanent peritoneal catheters and technical refinements has made the procedure fairly simple. Chronic peritoneal dialysis results in a continuous removal of solute and water, avoiding the rapid fluid and solute shifts that occur during hemodialysis. Hypertension and anemia are better managed than with hemodialysis. The procedure is particularly suitable for infants and small children.

Chronic dialysis can be performed manually (chronic ambulatory peritoneal dialysis, CAPD) or with an automated device (continuous cycling peritoneal dialysis, CCPD). The dialysis system consists of a plastic bag containing the dialysate, transfer set and the permanent peritoneal catheter. The dialysis fluid flows into the peritoneal cavity by gravity and is drained after a dwell of several hours. The connection between the bag and the transfer set is broken 3 to 5 times per day by the care provider at home using a strict, aseptic, non-touch technique.

Peritoneal Dialysis Catheters

The catheter widely used for acute dialysis is the polyurethane trocar catheter. Problems associated with these catheters include bleeding and leakage of fluid around the catheter insertion site. The use of rigid catheters beyond 72 hours increases the risk of peritonitis.

Surgical or laparoscopic placement of 'permanent' peritoneal dialysis catheters made of soft biocompatible plastic, is preferred. The most commonly used PD catheter is the double cuff, soft silastic *Tenckhoff catheter* (Fig. 41.1). Available in pediatric (3–10 kg) and adult sizes (for use in children >10 kg), the catheter is introduced through a subcutaneous tunnel. The presence of Dacron cuff(s) permits secure fixation. The risk of peritonitis is lower if two cuffs are used, the exit site faces downwards, presence of 'swan neck' subcutaneous tunnel and a curled intraperitoneal segment. Omentectomy should be performed at surgery to minimize catheter blockade.

Following a double-cuff Tenckhoff catheter insertion, it is preferable to wait 10–14 days before initiating dialysis in order to increase the longevity of the catheter, reduce leaks and the risk of catheter migration. The catheter may be used early, but with low volume cycles (10–15 ml/kg/cycle) and short dwell; the fill volume is gradually increased over 2–3 weeks.

The single cuff, peel-off Tenckhoff catheter is primarily used for acute dialysis but it can be used for prolonged periods (days-few weeks), and is a feasible option in infants less than 3 kg.

Dialysis Solutions

Peritoneal dialysis solutions usually contain dextrose as the osmotic agent. Non-dextrose containing solutions reduce the risks of hyperglycemia and sclerosis of the peritoneal membrane. These include icodextrin (an isosmotic glucose polymer that produces

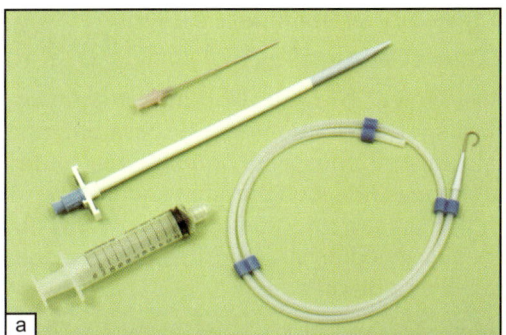

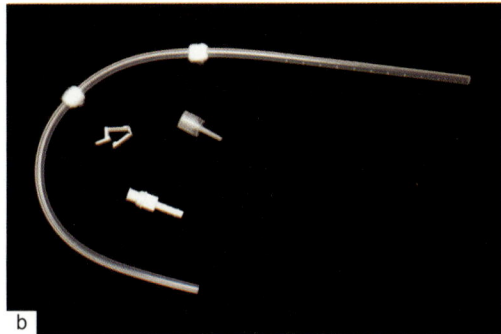

Fig. 41.1: Tenckhoff catheters used for chronic peritoneal dialysis. (a) The single cuff catheter is inserted bedside and is useful for prolonged dialysis for acute renal failure. (b) The double cuff catheter requires surgical placement with creation of a subcutaneous tunnel, and is useful for chronic ambulatory dialysis

Table 41.1: Composition of dialysis solutions

Osmotic agent: glucose/dextrose 1.4–3.9 g/dl; icodextrin 7.5 g/dl; amino acids 1.1 g/dl

Base: lactate 35–40 mEq/L, bicarbonate 34 mEq/L

Sodium 132–134 mEq/L

Calcium 1.25–1.75 mMol/L (2.5–3.5 mEq/L)

Magnesium 0.25-0.75 mMol/L (0.5-1.5 mEq/L)

Chloride 95–103.5 mEq/L

The 7.5% icodextrin dialysate can be used for long nighttime dwell in CAPD patients, long daytime dwell in nocturnal APD patients and in patients with ultrafiltration failure

1000 mL/m² overnight, to be gradually built up to 1100–1200 mL/m². If an increase of the dialysis dose is indicated, these volumes can be increased according to patient tolerance.

Strategies for improving ultrafiltration including increasing the number of peritoneal dialysis cycles, using higher glucose concentrations, increasing the fill volume and overall treatment time and using an icodextrin based dialysate for the long dwell.

Choice of Peritoneal Dialysis Modality

The peritoneal dialysis regimen can be *continuous* (with dialysis solution present in the peritoneal cavity evenly throughout 24 hr) or *intermittent* (with empty abdomen for part of the day, usually during daytime). Peritoneal exchanges can be performed manually as in chronic ambulatory peritoneal dialysis (CAPD) or automated (automated peritoneal dialysis, APD).

Chronic Ambulatory Peritoneal Dialysis (CAPD)

CAPD is performed by three to five daily exchanges (usually four), with a dwell time of 3–4 hrs each during the daytime and a nighttime exchange of 8 to 12 hrs. If an increase of the dialysis dose is indicated the number of exchanges can be increased to five to six per day.

ultrafiltration by colloid osmosis) and a mixture of amino acids. Other solutes in commercially available dialysate are lactate, sodium and calcium (Table 41.1). Heparin (500–1000 U/l), added to the dialysate in children with acute renal failure, prevents clotting of the catheter with fibrin/blood; this is discontinued once the effluent is clear. Heparin does not cross the peritoneal membrane and does not lead to systemic anticoagulation.

Peritoneal Dialysis Prescription

Intraperitoneal Fill Volume

The initial fill volume should be 600 to 800 mL/m² during the day and 800 to

41

Automated Peritoneal Dialysis (APD)

APD is performed with the help of a cycler that delivers peritoneal dialysis fluid. It can be done at night and enables children to carry on daily activities and attend school full time, thus minimizing the burden on lives of patients and their families. Nighttime dialysis in the supine position also allows for large fill volumes thereby increasing dialysis efficacy.

Nightly Intermittent Peritoneal Dialysis (NIPD)

NIPD consists of a series of short nocturnal cycles without a daytime dialysate dwell. Although it has the advantages of no daytime glucose absorption, reduced loss of proteins and amino acids and a better long-term preservation of the peritoneal membrane, it limits solute clearance in patients with low and low-average transporter status. NIPD is useful in children in whom dialysis prescription combined with the residual renal function achieves or exceeds the target solute clearance, and who are without evidence of hyperphosphatemia, hyperkalemia, hypervolemia, or acidosis.

Tidal Peritoneal Dialysis

Tidal peritoneal dialysis is a modality which is used with the cycler device in which the peritoneal exchanges are done on a background reservoir of peritoneal fluid in the cavity thus improving peritoneal dialysis efficiency and reducing inflow and outflow pain.

Adequacy of Peritoneal Dialysis

Clinical Features

Assessment of hydration and nutritional status, electrolyte and acid/base balance, calcium and phosphate homeostasis, control of anemia and blood pressure and the overall well being are important in ascertaining the adequacy of dialysis. Investigations are done at 1–3 month intervals.

Peritoneal Equilibration Test

The peritoneal equilibration test (PET) assesses peritoneal membrane characteristics by measuring the rate at which solutes (creatinine, urea and glucose) come to equilibration between the blood and the dialysate. A standard PET is done 4 weeks following initiation of dialysis (Chapter 42). The ratio of the concentration of dialysate glucose to initial dialysate glucose and urea are calculated at 0, 2 and 4 hrs of the test. These are compared to standard reference results and patients characterized as having a high, high average, low average, or low solute transport. High transport for creatinine (and/or urea) implies its fast removal from blood, whereas high transport for glucose denotes its fast elimination from dialysate, dissipating the osmotic gradient. The dialysis prescription may be modified, based on results of PET (Table 41.2).

Peritoneal Kt/V Urea

Similar to hemodialysis, single pool clearance of urea is useful is estimated adequacy of dialysis (Chapter 42). However, the targets for chronic PD are considerably lower than for intermittent HD. The peritoneal Kt/V urea

Table 41.2: Classification of peritoneal transport

	Ultrafiltration	Clearance	Action required
High transporter	Poor	Adequate	APD
High average	Adequate	Adequate	APD, CAPD
Low average	Good	Adequate	APD, CAPD
Low transporter	Excellent	Poor	Shift to hemodialysis

APD automated peritoneal dialysis; CAPD continuous ambulatory peritoneal dialysis

should be >1.7/week; for patients with significant residual renal function, the total Kt/V from peritoneum and kidneys should exceed 1.7/week. It is recommended that Kt/V be measured within the first month after initiating dialysis therapy and at least once every 6 months thereafter.

COMPLICATIONS

Common complications of continuous peritoneal dialysis are listed in Table 41.3.

Table 41.3: Common complications in chronic peritoneal dialysis
Peritonitis
Exit site infection
Catheter malfunction
Hernia, back pain
Hydrothorax, respiratory difficulty
Loss of protein, amino acids, immunoglobulins
Diabetes, obesity, hyperlipidemia
Peritoneal membrane failure

Peritonitis

This is the chief complication of chronic peritoneal dialysis. Peritonitis rates should not exceed 1 episode every 18 months (0.67/year at risk) at centers involved in care for children with chronic peritoneal dialysis.

Factors associated with reduced risk of peritonitis include *(i)* Patient age: lower rates in older patients; *(ii)* Use of double-cuffed swan neck Tenchkoff catheter with downward directed exit-site; *(iii)* Flush before fill procedure; *(iv)* Prophylactic antibiotics: one dose of IV vancomycin at time of catheter placement; and *(v)* Exit-site care: daily application of mupirocin cream to the skin around the exit site, and *(vi)* Prolonged training for the care providers.

Common organisms causing peritonitis are coagulase negative staphylococcus, *S. aureus* followed by gram negative organisms. Patients present with cloudy effluent, pain and fever. An effluent count of more than 100 leukocytes/mL (after a dwell of at least 2 hours), with >50% neutrophils is suggestive of peritonitis. The peritoneal fluid is examined for turbidity, cell count and culture. The yield from culture is improved on centrifugation of 50 mL peritoneal effluent at 3000 rpm for 15 minutes, followed by resuspension of the sediment in 3–5 mL sterile saline, and inoculation on solid culture plates and blood culture media. For patients presenting with a dry abdominal cavity, 500–1000 mL of the dialysate is infused, allowed to dwell for 1–2 hr, and drained to collect the effluent.

Management

If signs of severe infection (pain and fever) are present, therapy should begin without confirmation of the cell count. Rapid flushes with the dialysate, prior to the initiation of antibiotic therapy, reduces the severity of abdominal pain.

The initial choice of antibiotic therapy should cover both Gram positive and Gram-negative organisms (Fig. 41.2). Vancomycin is advised if: *(i)* history of MRSA colonization or infection, *(ii)* seriously unwell, or *(iii)* history of allergy to penicillins and cephalosporins. Ampicillin is a suitable monotherapy for peritonitis caused by enterococci and streptococci. If the patient is allergic to cephalosporins, aztreonam is an alternative to ceftazidime or cefepime.

Intraperitoneal administration of antibiotics is superior to IV dosing. However, patients having high fever and systemic toxicity should receive IV antibiotics. While intermittent or continuous dosing of intraperitoneal antibiotics is equally effective; the latter is preferred (Table 41.4). Antibiotics are added to the dialysate using sterile technique, through the medication port. Separate syringes are preferred for adding more than one antibiotic. Patients with extremely cloudy effluent might benefit from addition of heparin (500–1000 U/L) into the dialysate, since that prevents occlusion of the catheter due to fibrin.

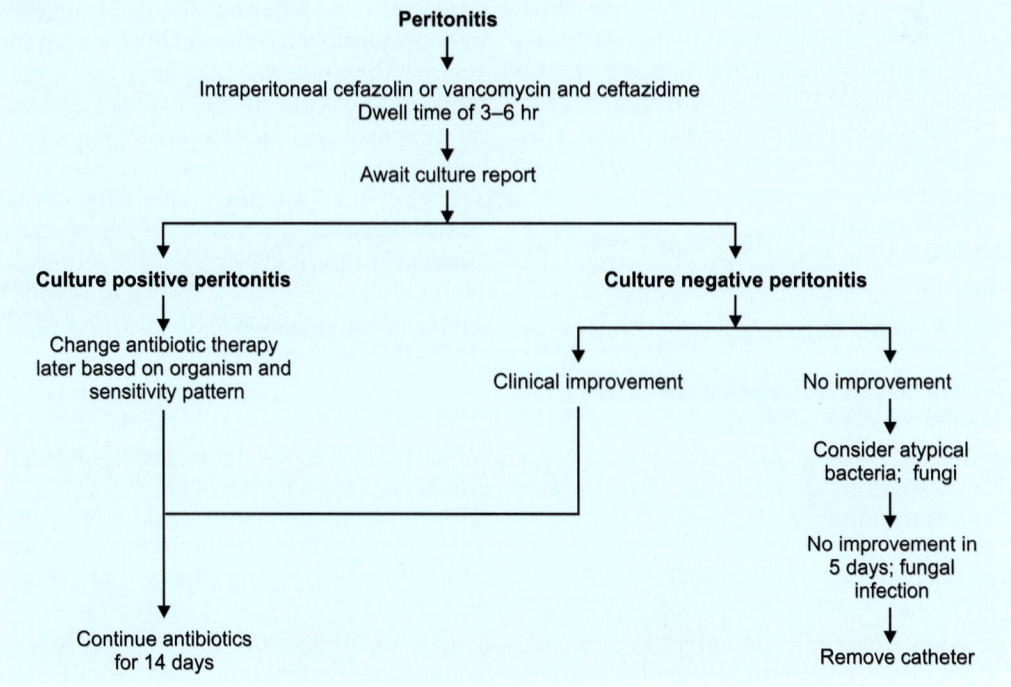

Fig. 41.2: Approach to management of peritonitis

The *loading dose* is given in a full volume exchange (~1100 mL/m^2) with a dwell time of at least 4–6 hr to allow absorption of the antibiotic into the circulation. If a smaller volume is instilled, the concentration must be increased to ensure infusion of an equal mass of antibiotic. *Intermittent dosing* of the antibiotic should be given over >6 hr in one bag per day for CAPD patients, or during a full fill volume daytime dwell for APD patients. The dose of medications requiring renal clearance should be empirically increased by 25% in patients with residual renal function (>100 mL/day urine output).

Assessment of Response

Examination of the effluent after 3-days therapy shows reduced leukocyte count by more than 50%, with shift from predominantly neutrophils to mononuclear cells. Failure of the effluent to clear after 5-days despite appropriate therapy suggests *refrac-tory peritonitis*, often associated with catheter tunnel-related infection (*S. aureus* or *P. aeruginosa*) or fungal peritonitis.

Treatment Duration

Gram positive peritonitis: Three weeks for *S. aureus*; two weeks for all others

Gram negative peritonitis: Three weeks for Pseudomonas, multiple organisms or anerobic organisms; two weeks for other Gram-negative organisms

Fungal peritonitis: Initial therapy with amphotericin or fluconazole for 3 weeks; catheter removal is required

Indications for catheter removal include: (*i*) refractory peritonitis; (*ii*) relapsing peritonitis, occurring within 4 weeks of completion of therapy; (*iii*) refractory exit-site and tunnel infection; and (*iv*)fungal peritonitis.

Re-insertion of a new catheter should be avoided for the next 2–3 weeks. During this

Table 41.4: Antibiotics used for treatment of peritonitis

	Continuous therapy (all exchanges)		Intermittent therapy
	Loading dose	*Maintenance dose*	*(per exchange)*
Vancomycin	1000 mg/L	25 mg/L	15–30 mg/kg q 5–7 d
Teicoplanin	400 mg/L	20 mg/L	15 mg/kg q 5–7 d
Cefazolin	500 mg/L	125 mg/L	15 mg/kg q 24 hr
Cefuroxime	200 mg/L	125 mg/L	15 mg/kg q 24 hr
Cefotaxime	500 mg/L	250 mg/L	30 mg/kg q 24 hr
Ceftazidime	500 mg/L	125 mg/L	1000–1500 mg q 24 hr
Ceftizoxime	250 mg/L	125 mg/L	1000 mg q 24 hr
Cefipime	500 mg/L	125 mg/L	1000 mg q 24 hr
Amphotericin B	–	1.5 mg/L	–
Amikacin	25 mg/L	12 mg/L	2 mg/kg q 24 hr
Gentamicin	8 mg/L	4 mg/L	0.6 mg/kg q 24 hr
Netilmicin	8 mg/L	4 mg/L	0.6 mg/kg q 24 hr
Tobramicin	8 mg/L	4 mg/L	0.6 mg/kg q 24 hr
Azlocillin	500 mg/L	250 mg/L	–
Piperacillin	–	250 mg/L	–
Ampicillin	–	125 mg/L	–
Penicillin G	50000 U/L	25000 U/L	–
Oxacillin	–	125 mg/L	–
Amoxicillin	250–500 mg/L	50 mg/L	–
Ciprofloxacin	50 mg/L	25 mg/L	–
Ampicillin/Sulbactam	1000 mg/L	100 mg/L	2 g q12 hr
Imipenem/Sulbactam	500 mg/L	200 mg/L	1 g q12 hr
Aztreonam	1000 mg/L	250 mg/L	–

ISPD GUIDELINES 2010 UPDATE. Li *et al.* Peritoneal Dialysis International 2010; 30: 393–402

- Vancomycin and ceftazidime are compatible when mixed in a dialysis solution; however, they are incompatible when mixed in the same syringe
- Aminoglycosides should not be added to the same exchange with penicillins
- Administration should be via intraperitoneal route unless specified otherwise
- In patients with residual renal function (>100 mL/day urine output): increase dose by 25%

period, renal replacement therapy may be provided by hemodialysis.

Exit-Site, Tunnel Infections

Purulent drainage and erythema at the exit site indicates the presence of infection. The organisms most often implicated include *S. aureus* and *P. aeruginosa*. Oral antibiotic therapy with a combination of coamoxiclav and ciprofloxacin is recommended. Based on culture results, the therapy may be modified and continued for 2–3 weeks. Patients who are culture negative and fail to show a response to oral medications require therapy with parenteral vancomycin and ceftazidime. If three weeks of antibiotics fail to resolve the infection, the catheter should be replaced as a single procedure, under antibiotic cover.

Mechanical Complications

Mechanical complications are the second most common cause for catheter failure. These include obstruction of the catheter by omentum, migration of the catheter out of the pelvis and blockage of the catheter by fibrin or clots. When omental blockage occurs, laparoscopic removal of the omentum can be considered. In case of catheter migration, repositioning the catheter with interventional radiology techniques or by laparoscopy may be possible.

Occlusion by fibrin or blood clot is common and tissue plasminogen activator (2 mg reconstituted in 40 cc of normal saline and instilled in the catheter for 1 hr) has been shown to be effective in unblocking these catheters.

Dental Prophylaxis

Children with indwelling peritoneal catheters do not require antibiotic prophylaxis for dental treatment, provided there is no other indication, such as congenital heart disease.

Removal of the Peritoneal Catheter Following Transplantation

In children in whom the graft is placed extraperitoneally, the dialysis catheter is usually left in place at the time of transplant, in case it needs to be reused. It should be removed 4-weeks post-transplant, if the graft is functioning well.

SUPPORT READING

http://www.pedpd.org/

ISPD Guidelines recommendations. Consensus guidelines for treatment of peritonitis in pediatric patients receiving peritoneal dialysis. Peritoneal Dialysis International 2000; 20: 610–24

Fischbach M, Warady BA. Peritoneal dialysis prescription in children: bedside principles for optimal practice. Pediatr Nephrol 2009; 24: 1633–42

Chadha V, Schaefer FS, Warady BA. Dialysis associated peritonitis in children. Pediatr Nephrol 2010; 25: 425–40

42 Assessment of Dialysis Adequacy

Clinical parameters such as hydration, nutritional status, electrolyte and acid/base balance, calcium and phosphate homeostasis, control of anemia and blood pressure, and the overall well being provide a subjective assessment of the adequacy of dialysis. An objective assessment of dialysis adequacy links outcomes to adequacy targets. A *satisfactory* dose of dialysis is that below which a significant increase in morbidity and mortality would occur. *Optimal* dialysis refers to the dialysis dose beyond which no further improvement in the patient's clinical well-being can be achieved.

HEMODIALYSIS
Urea Reduction Ratio

This refers to the percentage of urea removed during treatment, calculated as:

Urea reduction ratio (URR) =
$$1 - (\text{urea post HD}/\text{urea pre HD})$$

The URR is often expressed as a percentage; URR during an average session should be ~70%.

Kt/V Urea

The clearance (K) of urea is used to objectively express the delivered dose of dialysis, and helps decide the desired treatment time and prescription for both HD and PD. Clearance of urea follows first order kinetics or single compartment (pool) model.

Single Pool Kt/V

This is an dimensionless index of the total dose per dialysis treatment, taken as the product of urea clearance (K) and the length of the treatment (time, t), to an estimate of body size, taken as the volume of urea distribution (V). It represents the relative volume of the blood cleared of the urea during a session of dialysis. Delivering a Kt/V of 1 means that the total volume of blood cleared during the dialysis session is equal to the urea distribution volume.

$$\begin{aligned} Kt/V &= -\ln[1\text{-URR}] \\ &= -\ln[1-(C_0-C_t)/C_0] \\ &= -\ln(C_t/C_0) \\ &= -\ln R \end{aligned}$$

Where ln natural logarithm, C_0 blood urea before dialysis, C_t blood urea after t time on dialysis, t time on dialysis (in minutes), V body water volume (calculated as $0.6 \times$ body weight), URR urea reduction ratio, R C_t/C_0.

Table 42.2 can be used to estimate the Kt/V from the urea reduction ratio.

The clearance of urea K, at a dialysate flow rate of 500 mL/minute, is calculated from the size of dialyzer, blood flow rate and K_0A, the constant of dialyzer efficiency (Table 42.2). Based on the blood flow rate, either the K or t can be adjusted to maximize the clearance of solutes. Increasing the blood flow rate offers the advantage of augmenting K by increasing Q_B with the advantage of shortening time on dialysis.

Corrections are applied to the Kt/V for urea generated during dialysis (g) and for the clearance of urea associated with ultrafiltration. These adjustments are made as follows:

$$Kt/V = -\log n(R - 0.008t) + (4 - 3.5R)UF/W$$

Table 42.1: Estimation of Kt/V from percentage urea reduction

Percent urea reduction	C_t/C_o	Kt/V
90	0.1	2.302
80	0.2	1.609
70	0.3	1.204
60	0.4	0.916
50	0.5	0.693
40	0.6	0.511
30	0.7	0.357
20	0.8	0.223
10	0.9	0.105

where,

$R = C_t/C_0;$
$C_0 =$ blood urea just before dialysis;
$C_t =$ blood urea just after dialysis,
$t =$ time of HD in hours;
$UF =$ ultrafiltrate in litres; and
$W =$ post-dialysis weight in kg

The single pool (Sp) model is simple to use and gives a satisfactory measure of dialyzer clearance per treatment factored by V. SpKt/V is the standard for evaluating the adequacy of HD. It is recommended that the sp Kt/V should be between 1.4 and 1.8.

Equilibrated Kt/V

The *equilibrated Kt/V* (eKt/V) takes into account the rebound increase in levels of blood urea following the dialysis. The predialysis blood sample is taken from the arterial line and the post-dialysis sample is drawn 30–60 minutes following HD. It is recommended that the eKt/V should be maintained between 1.2 and 1.4.

Standard Kt/V

The standard Kt/V (std-Kt/V) is a weekly expression of the spKt/V, providing the weekly equivalent urea clearance, indexed to body volume. The std-Kt/V takes into account the frequency of dialysis. The std-Kt/V can be calculated mathematically (using the equation provided by Leopoldt) or from Fig. 42.2, based on the spKt/V and dialysis frequency.

Based on body weight, dialysis duration, ultrafiltration volume and pre-HD and post-HD urea levels, calculations for Kt/V can be made online at *www.davita.com*.

Normalized Protein Catabolic Rate

The normalized protein catabolic rate (nPCR) assesses the urea generation rate (g) between two dialysis sessions, and reflects the adequacy of protein intake in patients on

Table 42.2: Dialyzer urea clearance (Fresenius). Value in each cell provides the urea clearance (K) for the particular dialyzer and blood flow rate

Dialyzer			F3	F4	F5	F6	F7
Surface area			0.4	0.7	1	1.3	1.6
K₀A			250	369	402	458	522
		50	49	50	50	50	50
		75	71				
Blood flow rate	(Q_B mL/minute)	100	89	96	97	98	99
		125	103				
		150	114	130	133	137	141
		200	130	154	159	166	173
		250	141	171	178	188	197
		300	149	184	192	203	215

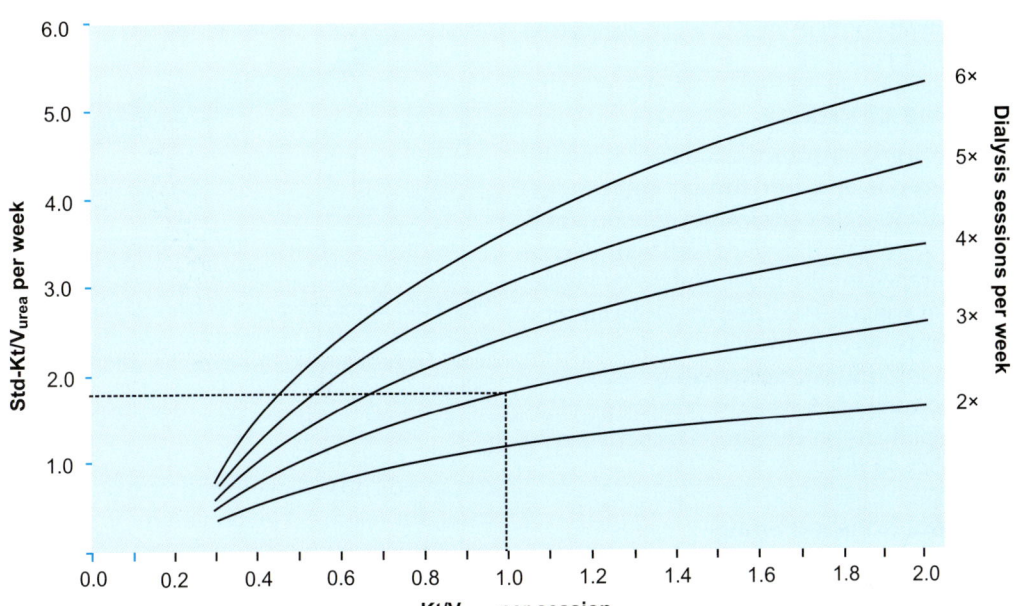

Fig. 42.1: Relationship between weekly std-Kt/V, dialysis frequency and single pool Kt/V per dialysis. (Modified from Daugirdas et al, Eds. in Handbook of Dialysis, Wolters-Kluwer (India) Private Limited, New Delhi 2007, Fourth edition)

maintenance HD. It is calculated as follows:

$nPCR = 5.43 \times g/V1 + 0.17$

where

g = urea generation rate (mg/min)
$\quad$ = $[(C2 \times V2) - (C1 \times V1)]/t$

Where C1 post HD urea (mg/dL), C2 pre HD urea; V1 post HD total body water, V2 pre HD total body water; t minutes from end of HD to beginning of next HD.

The target values for nPCR are >1.0 to 1.2 g/kg/day; values <1.0 g/kg/d are associated with poor nutrition. The clearance of urea into urine should be taken into account in patients with significant residual renal function.

PERITONEAL DIALYSIS

Peritoneal Kt/V urea

Similar to HD, single pool clearance of urea is useful is estimating the adequacy of PD. Patients on PD often have significant residual kidney function, which must be taken into account when evaluating urea and creatinine clearances. It is usual to calculate weekly or standard peritoneal Kt/V, as described below:

Peritoneal Kt = 24-hour dialysate urea/ blood urea

Renal Kt $\quad$ = 24-hour urine urea/blood urea

Total Kt $\quad$ = peritoneal Kt + renal Kt

The timing of the blood sample for estimation of urea is not critical in patients on chronic PD. The product of the total Kt/V and the days of dialysis give an estimate of weekly value of Kt/V. The target for weekly Kt/V should be > 1.8/week. These targets are lower than for intermittent HD. Lower targets are acceptable for PD since it is known that clearances delivered continuously, as with PD, are more efficient than the same amount delivered intermittently.

It is recommended that Kt/V be measured within the first month after initiating dialysis therapy and once every 4–6 months thereafter.

Online measurement of Kt/V can be carried out at *www.pedpd.org*.

Creatinine Clearance

The creatinine clearance is measured as the sum of renal and peritoneal clearances. Discrepancies between clearances of urea and creatinine occure due to less efficient peritoneal clearance for the latter, due to its higher molecular weight. The differences are marked in patients with minimal residual renal function and in low peritoneal transporters. The recommended weekly creatinine clearance in patients on chronic PD is between 50 and 65 L/1.73 m².

Peritoneal Transport Status

Peritoneal membrane transport characteristics vary widely between patients and change during prolonged dialysis, particularly following infections. The peritoneal transport status is an important determinant of dialysis clearances, particularly with automated PD, since short dwells limit solute equilibration between dialysate and plasma. The peritoneal equilibration test (PET) assesses peritoneal membrane characteristics by measuring the rate at which solutes (creatinine, urea and glucose) equilibrate between the blood and the dialysate. A standard PET is done 4 weeks following initiation of dialysis.

Following prolonged overnight dwell (40 mL/kg for 8–12 hr), the dialysate is drained over 20 minutes. Fresh dialysate (1100 mL/m² of 2.5% solution) is infused rapidly over 10 minutes. The levels of glucose, urea and creatinine are estimated in peritoneal fluid samples obtained at 0, 2 and 4 hr. At each time point, approximately 10–20% of dialysate is

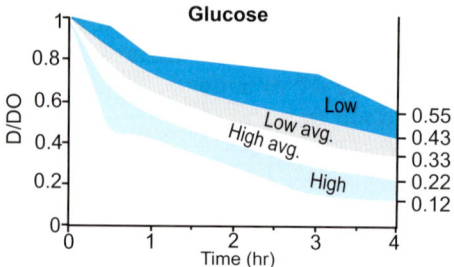

Fig. 42.2: Standard curve for glucose on peritoneal equilibration test, showing ranges of values for high, high-average, low-average and low transporters.

removed, mixed well and 5 mL dialysate taken for testing. The remainder is reinfused peritoneally. In addition, blood samples are taken for urea and creatinine at 2 hr.

The ratio of the concentration of dialysate glucose to initial dialysate glucose at time 0 (D/D0) are calculated at 2 and 4 hours. These ratios are compared to reference results and patients characterized as having a *high, high average, low average* or low solute transport (Fig. 42.2). The dialysis prescription may be modified based on results of PET. Low transporters achieve good clearances with high volume long dwell periods, while high transporters do well with short dwell durations.

SUPPORT READING

Goldstein SL, Sorof JM, Brewer ED. Natural logarithmic estimates of Kt/V in the pediatric hemodialysis is population. Am J Dis 1999, 33; 518–22

Daugirdas JT. Simplified equations for monitoring Kt/V, nPCR, eKt/v and enPCR. Adv Renal Replacement Therapy 1995; 2: 295–304

43 Transplantation

Renal transplantation is the treatment of choice for children with end-stage renal disease (ESRD). Kidney transplants in children in our country are chiefly from related donors, most commonly the parents. Cadaveric transplantation is less frequent.

Indications

The indications for initiating renal replacement therapy are discussed in Chapter 39. Transplantation is considered when estimated glomerular filtration rate (eGFR) falls to <8–12 ml/minute/1.73 m². Most patients preparing for transplantation are already on dialysis.

Transplantation is considered *pre-emptive* when it is carried out without previous dialysis. Preemptive transplantation offers better long-term allograft survival and psychological and financial benefits compared with transplant performed after a period of dialysis. Preemptive transplantation also offers cost advantages since chronic dialysis therapy is expensive.

Contraindications

Contraindications to renal transplant include the presence of acute infection, untreated malignancy and progressive neurological illness. While, human immunodeficiency virus (HIV) infection has been a contraindication, selected children have undergone successful transplantation. Patients with treated malignancies should wait for 2–5 years before being considered for transplantation. Children with end stage kidney disease secondary to primary hyperoxaluria, factor H deficiency and methylmalonic acidemia usually require combined liver and kidney transplant. Chronic infection with hepatitis B or C is not a contraindication, but these children need careful evaluation of liver functions and histology, and might benefit from antiviral therapy prior to transplantation.

The issue of non adherence to therapy, especially in adolescents, should be addressed. Children with multiple congenital anomalies and severe mental retardation pose an ethical dilemma. A multidisciplinary team should evaluate the option of transplantation, with input from ethicists and parents.

Patients with obstructive uropathy may undergo transplantation after correcting the underlying anomaly, and ensuring normal bladder capacity and function.

Socioeconomic factors should be considered before committing to transplantation, in view of financial constraints in providing life-long immunosuppressive medications.

Immunological Factors

Children are excellent candidates for renal transplantation due to lack of significant comorbidities. For technical reasons (to allow anastomoses and to accommodate adult kidney), most surgeons would prefer that the child be at least 1-yr old and weigh 10 kg or more at the time of transplant.

ABO compatibility between donor and recipient is a prerequisite for successful transplantation; the same rules that govern blood transfusion apply to solid organ transplantation. Transplants have occasionally been performed across blood group barriers. Rhesus group matching is not required for successful transplantation.

Genetic differences between individuals are recognized by differences in the composition of major histocompatibility complex antigens *(HLA antigens)* encoded on short arm of chromosome 6 and expressed on surface of nucleated cells. HLA antigens are divided into class I (A, B and C) and class II (DR, DQ, DP). HLA class I antigens are present on all nucleated cells; HLA class II antigens are present on macrophages, dendritic, endothelial and B-cells. T lymphocytes, tubular epithelial and endothelial cells increase expression of class II molecules upon stimulation with cytokines, such as interferon-γ.

Each individual inherits one haplotype from each parent. Siblings can be complete HLA matched, one haplotype matched or completely mismatched, depending upon the recombination of haplotypes. The great degree of polymorphism makes complete HLA matching between two random individuals a rare event. The term HLA mismatches defines the number of non-shared HLA antigens between the donor and recipient. HLA mismatches determine the strength of immunologic reaction in the recipient. While the extent of HLA mismatching has an impact on long term allograft survival, availability of potent immunosuppressive therapy has attenuated the effect of HLA mismatching on allograft survival.

Sensitization refers to the presence of anti HLA antibodies in the recipient at the time of transplantation. The anti HLA antibodies form due to blood transfusions, previous transplants, pregnancies and infections. These antibodies bind to HLA antigens on the allograft endothelium and cause *hyperacute rejection* and immediate graft loss.

Antibodies directed at HLA class I antigens and those that are complement binding are deleterious.

The test, *panel reactive antibodies* (PRA), examines for presence of antibodies in recipient serum against a panel of donor HLA antigens. PRA testing can be done using the lymphocytotoxicity assay, ELISA or flow cytometry. Specific HLA antigens are identified by HLA typing or flowcytometry. Highly sensitized individuals are likely to experience acute rejection episodes even when unacceptable antigens are avoided. In recent years, these patients have been successfully transplanted using desensitization protocols.

PREPARATION FOR TRANSPLANTATION

Patients and their parents should have the opportunity for discussion regarding transplantation, including its benefits, risks, complications, risk of recurrence and costs.

Recipient and Donor Evaluation

Important aspects of evaluation are summarized in Tables 43.1 and 43.2. Pretransplant donor evaluation is aimed to ensure the patient's suitability as a transplant candidate. The cause for ESRD should be determined if possible. The risk of recurrence of some conditions, e.g. focal segmental glomerulosclerosis (FSGS), atypical hemolytic uremic syndrome (HUS) and membranoproliferative GN should be considered. The child should receive age appropriate immunizations. Nutritional status should be optimized. The child and family's ability to comply with medications cannot be underscored, as non adherence is an important cause of graft loss.

A *cross match* is performed between the recipient and the prospective living or deceased donor. The recipient serum is tested against donor T and B cells to detect preformed antibodies. Cross match is done by the lymphocytotoxicity assay; the sensitivity of

Table 43.1: Recipient evaluation prior to Transplantation

History and Physical Examination

Underlying renal disease
Past illnesses, surgery
Concomitant medications
Heart, respiratory rate; blood pressure
Height, weight, nutritional assessment
Systemic examination

Investigations

Blood group; ABO and Rhesus typing
Urinalysis, culture; 24-hr protein
Blood counts; glucose; electrolytes
Renal and liver functions
Calcium, phosphorus, alkaline phosphatase
Lipid profile
Parathormone
Bleeding, clotting times

Screening for infections

Tuberculin test
Antibodies to human immunodeficiency virus, hepatitis C virus, cytomegalovirus, Ebstein Barr virus
Hepatitis B surface antigen; anti-HBs antibody
VDRL

Imaging

Chest X-ray; bone age
Electrocardiogram; echocardiogram
Ultrasound for kidneys, ureters and bladder
Doppler ultrasound for major abdominal vessels
Micturating cystourethrography

Immunology

Human leukocyte antigen (HLA) A, B, C, DR
Cross match (T cell, B cell)
Panel reactive antibody

Consultations

Dental surgery
Pediatric surgery
Dietician
Cardiology
Anesthesia

Immunization

Pneumococcal; hepatitis B; measles, mumps, rubella; varicella

Table 43.2: Donor evaluation prior to transplantation

History and Physical Examination

Relationship to recipient
History of medical illnesses, surgery
Concomitant medications
Heart, respiratory rate; blood pressure
Height, weight, nutritional assessment
Systemic examination

Investigations

Blood group; ABO and Rhesus typing
Urinalysis, culture; 24-hr protein
Blood counts; glucose; electrolytes
Renal and liver functions
Calcium, phosphorus, alkaline phosphatase
Lipid profile
Bleeding, clotting times

Screening for infections

Tuberculin test
Antibodies to human immunodeficiency virus, hepatitis C virus, cytomegalovirus, Ebstein Barr virus
Hepatitis B surface antigen; anti-HBs antibody
VDRL

Imaging

Chest X-ray
Electrocardiogram; echocardiogram
Ultrasound for kidneys, ureters and bladder
CT angiography: Number of renal arteries, veins (delayed film serves as IVP)

Immunology

Human leukocyte antigen (HLA) A, B, C, DR

Consultations

Internal medicine
Nephrology
Cardiology
Psychiatry
Gynecology (female donors)
Anesthesia clearance

this test has increased using ELISA and flowcytometry techniques.

Transplant donors can be living related (parents or siblings older than 18 yr), unrelated, altruistic or deceased donors. An independent physician should evaluate the living donor to ensure that he is medically suitable and emotionally stable. Donor work up includes evaluation of medical history, physical examination and detailed investigations. The renal anatomy is defined by ultrasound and its vasculature by angiography.

Preoperative Period

Examination is repeated to ensure fitness for surgery. Hemodialysis is scheduled on the day prior to transplant, avoiding fluid deficits. Investigations prior to the procedure include blood counts, levels of creatinine and electrolytes, chest X-ray and cultures of possible infection sites (catheter exit site, urine, peritoneal dialysis fluid). A T-lymphocyte cross match is repeated 48-hr before the transplant. Parental consent is taken and center specific protocols followed.

Transplant Procedure

The allograft is placed in the iliac fossa (Fig. 43.1). The renal artery and vein are connected to the common or external iliac artery and vein respectively as end to side anastomosis. In infants and young children (<20 kg) the kidney is placed higher up in the abdomen in the retroperitoneum. Renal artery and vein of the allograft are connected to the side of the aorta and inferior vena cava close to the bifurcation. The ureter is anastomosed to the bladder using ureteroneocystostomy.

Postoperative Period

Monitoring of the central venous pressure (CVP) is essential during surgery and post-operative period, aiming for a CVP level of 10-12 cm water. A high urine flow rate (>2 ml/kg/hr) is desirable on the first two post-operative days. Isotonic fluids (normal saline,

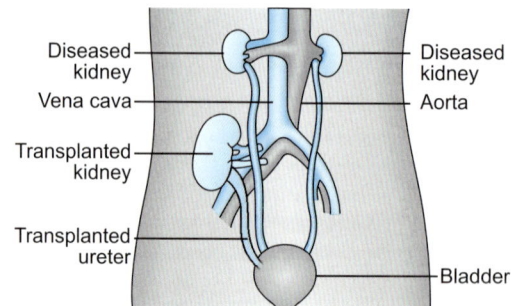

Fig. 43.1: Location of the transplanted kidney

Ringers lactate, dextrose saline) are used to replace urine volume. Potassium is administered at maintenance rates when serum potassium falls below 3.5 mEq/l. Beyond the second day, the hourly IV fluid replacement should be decreased to half the urine output, volume by volume, if the renal function is normal. Options for management of persistent hypertension include sustained release nifedipine (0.5–2 mg/kg/d), ramipril (5–6 mg/m^2/d), amlodepine (0.3–0.6 mg/kg/d), metoprolol (1–2 mg/kg/d) or prazosin (0.1–0.4 mg/kg/d).

IMMUNOSUPPRESSION PROTOCOLS

Patients undergoing the first live-related transplant, with primary disease other than FSGS and panel reactive antibodies (PRA) below 20% are considered as *standard risk*. These patients should receive induction therapy with IV methylprednisolone with or without anti-interleukin (IL)-2 receptor (IL-2R) antibody (daclizumab, basiliximab). This is followed by maintenance therapy with triple immunosuppression comprising of prednisolone, a calcineurin inhibitor (tacrolimus or cyclosporine) and mycophenolate mofetil (MMF) (Table 43.3). Azathioprine can be used as an alternative to MMF.

Patients undergoing retransplantation or if highly sensitized (PRA >20%), and those in whom delayed graft function is anticipated are considered as *high risk*. Such patients should receive induction with antithymocyte globulin (ATG) and IV steroids, followed by maintenance therapy with triple immuno-suppression.

Protocols with Steroid Avoidance

Transplant recipients at *standard risk* may receive immunosuppression with steroid minimization, with protocols that allow steroid avoidance or early withdrawal. In the latter, steroids are used for 5–7 days in tapering doses.

Steroid avoidance protocols, utilize multiple doses of an induction agent (ATG, daclizumab) over the first few months post-transplantation. Tacrolimus and MMF are begun 24-hr prior and continued after surgery. A dose of IV methylprednisolone is given on the morning of the surgery, and a smaller dose the next day. Tacrolimus trough levels are monitored frequently and target higher levels than in standard protocols.

Desensitization Protocols

Highly sensitized patients require desensitization, in order to decrease the risk of antibody mediated rejection. For recipients with living donors, desensitization is begun 6 weeks before the transplant. Therapy includes the use of IV immunoglobulin and rituximab. Donor specific antibodies and PRA are done regularly. Transplantation is done after a negative cross-match is documented. These patients should receive induction with ATG and triple immuno-suppression as per *high risk* protocol. Post-transplant monitoring of donor specific antibodies is recommended.

Drug Level Monitoring

Tacrolimus trough levels are monitored, 4 days after initiating therapy and every 3–4 days until discharge. Blood levels are determined every 2 weeks for the first month, monthly for 6 months, and 3-monthly for one year (Table 43.3). An estimate of tacrolimus availability can also be determined by calcu-lating 'area under the curve' on pharma-cokinetic assays.

Monitoring of cyclosporine levels using 2 hours post-dose (C_2) monitoring is a superior strategy compared to trough levels (C_0) in preventing acute rejection.

Drug Interactions

Interaction with tacrolimus increases drug levels of MMF, necessitating dose reduction of the latter. Acyclovir and ganciclovir increase levels of mycophenolic acid, while antacids reduce levels; simultaneous adminis-tration of these agents should be avoided.

Several drugs alter the metabolism of tacrolimus and cyclosporine. Phenytoin, isoniazid, carbamazepine, phenobarbitone, rifampicin and sodium bicarbonate increase the metabolism and therefore decrease their levels. Cimetidine, fluconazole, itraconazole, ketoconazole, clotrimazole, diltiazem, methyl-prednisolone, erythromycin and verapamil increase drug levels of tacrolimus or cyclo-sporine. Diarrhea increases levels of tacro-limus.

MONITORING

Blood levels of sugar, electrolytes and bicarbo-nate are monitored every 8–12 hr, and later once daily. Blood creatinine, calcium, phos-phate, albumin, electrolytes and blood counts are checked regularly. Levels of calcineurin inhibitors are monitored.

Following discharge, recipients return for evaluation twice weekly for 6-weeks, weekly for 6 weeks, monthly for the first year, and at three months thereafter. If complications are suspected, outpatient visits become more frequent and the patient may require to be hospitalized.

In patients on a steroid free or high risk protocol, regular surveillance by polymerase chain reaction is done for infection with cytomegalovirus, BK virus and Ebstein-Barr virus. Viral monitoring is also required during episodes of allograft dysfunction, presence of

Renal Replacement Therapy

IX

Table 43.3: Immunosuppressive drugs, doses and side effects

Medication	Dose	Side effects
Antithymocyte globulin	10–15 mg/kg/d for 7–14 days	Fever, chills, leukopenia, thrombocytopenia, anaphylaxis
Daclizumab Basiliximab	1 mg/kg at day 0 and 2, 4, 6, 8 weeks 12 mg/m^2 (<35 kg: 10 mg/dose; ≥35 kg: 20 mg/dose) at 0 and 4 days	Minimal; same as placebo
Methylprednisolone	Induction: 10 mg/kg on day 0 Acute rejection. 10 mg/kg/d for 3 days	Fluid retention, risk of infections, hypertension, obesity, cushingoid features, hyperglycemia, growth
Prednisolone	2 mg/kg/d; tapered to 0.5 mg/kg/d in 2 weeks; reduce to 0.1–0.15 mg/kg/d over 3 months	suppression, osteoporosis, gastric ulcers, impaired wound healing, mood changes, cataract
Cyclosporine Tacrolimus	6–8 mg/kg/d at onset; adjust dose according to levels 0.2–0.3 mg/kg/d, adjust dose according to levels	Hirsutism, gum hyperplasia, hypertension, tremors, hyperglycemia, nephrotoxicity, hyperlipidemia, hypomagnesemia
Azathioprine	2 mg/kg/d	Myelosuppression, hepatotoxicity, pancreatitis
Mycophenolate mofetil	1200 mg/m^2/d; decrease to 600 mg/m^2/d in tacrolimus based protocols	Myelosuppression, diarrhea, vomiting
Sirolimus	Initially 6 mg/d, followed by 2–5 mg/d, adjust by levels	Hypertriglyceridemia, mucosal ulcers, pneumonia

Tacrolimus (12-hr targets): first two months 10–12 ng/mL; 3–6 months 8–10 ng/mL; later 4–7 ng/mL
Cyclosporine (2-hr post dose): first month 1500–2000 ng/mL; 1–3 months 1300–1500 ng/mL; 4–6 months 1100 ng/mL; 7–12 months 900 ng/mL; later 800 ng/mL

elevated liver enzymes, leukopenia or thrombocytopenia.

COMPLICATIONS FOLLOWING TRANSPLANTATION

Allograft Dysfunction

Allograft dysfunction remains the chief complication of renal transplantation and its causes depend on the time post transplantation (Table 43.4). *Delayed graft function* is failure of the renal allograft to function immediately post-transplant, with the need for one or more dialysis sessions within a specified period, typically one week. *Acute allograft dysfunction* refers to the impairment of renal function (elevation of plasma creatinine >25% above baseline) noted during the first 6 months post-transplantation. *Chronic allograft dysfunction* refers to rising plasma creatinine observed beyond 6 months; proteinuria and hypertension are occasionally seen.

Delayed Graft Function

An assessment of volume status is essential to confirm or rule out severe hypovolemia. In addition, patients undergo an ultrasound of the allograft, ureter and urinary bladder. Other investigations include Doppler test and DTPA scintigraphy. An allograft biopsy is considered in patients at high risk of allograft rejection (highly sensitized recipients).

Acute Tubular Necrosis

The chief cause for delayed graft function is acute tubular necrosis, risk factors include perioperative hypotension or hypovolemia, trauma to renal vessels during harvesting from donor or placement, inadequate flushing of donor organ, prolonged cold ischemia time and medications.

The therapy of acute tubular necrosis is supportive. This includes: avoiding fluid overload; maintaining hemodynamic stability; providing nutritional support; and avoiding nephrotoxic agents. Dialysis is

initiated, if indicated, taking care to *(i)* avoid intradialytic hypotension, *(ii)* use minimum anticoagulation, and *(iii)* use biocompatible membranes.

Renal artery or renal vein thrombosis usually occurs in the first 72 hr, and is the most common cause of graft loss in the first post-transplant week.

Acute Allograft Dysfunction

Review of clinical features may suggest a cause for allograft dysfunction. Evaluation includes:

1. Urinalysis, culture
2. Complete blood count, peripheral smear for viral infection (leukopenia, thrombocytopenia) or thrombotic microangiopathy
3. Calcineurin inhibitor levels: detect medication-related toxicity, non-compliance
4. Ultrasound abdomen, Doppler to detect a post-renal cause, graft artery stenosis
5. DTPA scintigraphy
6. Biopsy: detect acute rejection, CNI toxicity, viral infection of allograft, recurrence

Acute Rejection

The patient may present with oliguria, hematuria and rising creatinine. Changes on renal scintiscan, ultrasound and Doppler flow studies are non-specific. Renal biopsy is performed in suspected cases. The Banff classification is used to grade histological changes, including interstitial edema, mononuclear cell infiltration ($CD4^+$ and $CD8^+$ T lymphocytes, macrophages and plasma cells) and tubulitis (infiltration of tubular epithelium by lymphocytes) (Fig. 43.2a). Vascular involvement may be seen both with cell-mediated rejection (endothelitis) and humoral-mediated rejection (necrotizing arteritis). Immunofluorescence in patients with antibody mediated rejection shows deposition of C4d in peritubular capillaries (Fig 43.2b).

Renal Replacement Therapy

IX

Table 43.4: Differential diagnosis of allograft dysfunction according to time after transplantation

	Delayed graft function	*Acute allograft dysfunction*	*Chronic allograft dysfunction*
Prerenal	Severe hypovolemia (common) Renal vessel thrombosis Graft embolization, thrombosis, rupture	Hypovolemia (common) Renal vessel thrombosis Transplant renal artery stenosis	Transplant renal artery stenosis
Intrarenal	Acute tubular necrosis (common) Accelerated acute rejection Acute CNI nephrotoxicity Hyperacute rejection	Acute rejection (common) CNI nephrotoxicity Thrombotic microangiopathy Recurrence of primary disease Acute pyelonephritis Acute interstitial nephritis	Chronic rejection, chronic allograft nephropathy Chronic CNI nephrotoxicity Recurrence of primary disease Acute rejection (uncommon)
Postrenal	Urinary tract obstruction or leakage	Urinary tract obstruction or leakage	Urinary tract obstruction

CNI calcineurin inhibitor

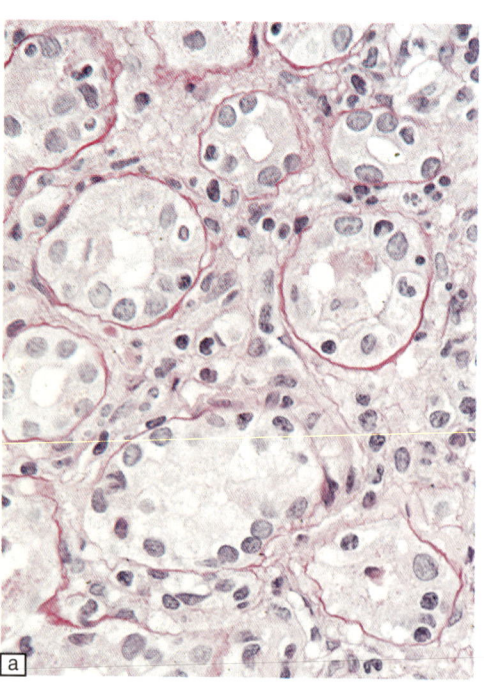 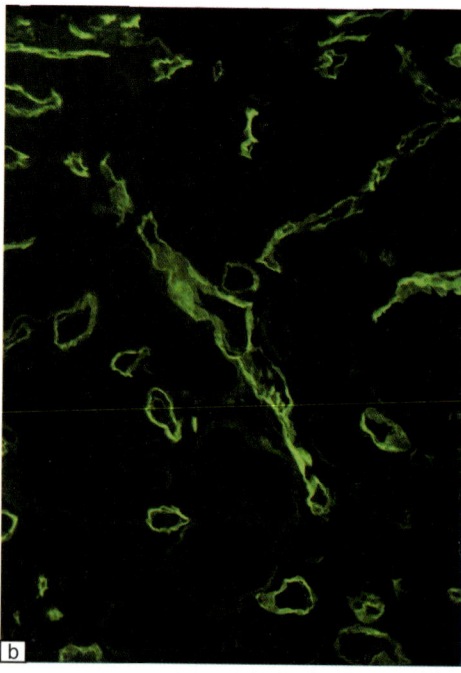

Fig. 43.2: Renal transplant biopsy showing (a) acute cellular rejection: lymphocytes are seen infiltrating the edematous interstitium and tubular epithelium; and (b) antibody mediated rejection: immunofluorescent staining with C4d shows strong linear staining of peritubular capillaries

A short course of high dose steroids, IV methylprednisolone (10 mg/kg per dose for 3–5 days), successfully reverses 70% cases particularly those with milder grades of rejection. Therapy with oral prednisolone is resumed at high dose (1 mg/kg/day) and tapered to maintenance dose over weeks. If blood level of tacrolimus or cyclosporine is low, their dosage is increased.

The use of OKT3 or thymoglobulin (ATG) is reserved for steroid resistant cases or those showing histologically severe rejection (Banff grade IIA or more). *Steroid resistant acute rejection* is defined as a failure of improvement in urine output or plasma creatinine within 5 days of starting pulse treatment. About 80–90% cases are expected to respond to OKT3 or ATG. Important adverse effects of monoclonal or polyclonal antibody treatment are thrombocytopenia, neutropenia, life-threatening infections and lymphoproliferative disease. ATG is preferred, in view of lower incidence of side effects, and the risk of rebound rejection with use of OKT3.

Antibody Mediated (Humoral) Rejection

Patients with antibody mediated rejection should receive therapy with IV immunoglobulin 2 g/kg and alternate day plasmapheresis. Rituximab (375 mg/m² for 4 doses) may be used.

Acute Calcineurin Inhibitor Nephrotoxicity

An acute reversible increases in plasma creatinine may be seen with high levels of calcineurin inhibitors, in a dose- and blood level dependent manner. Renal histology in acute toxicity is often unremarkable, though extremely high levels may result in proximal tubular dilation, isometric vacuolization, giant mitochondria and tubular cell flattening.

Acute Pyelonephritis

Urinary tract infections occur often in the early post-transplantation period, in association with catheterization, stenting and immunosuppression. Patients with urological abnormalities and neurogenic bladder are at risk. Empiric antibiotic treatment is begun without awaiting results of culture. Prophylactic cotrimoxazole in the early post-transplant period is protective.

Recurrence of Primary Disease

Several renal diseases may recur in the post-transplant period (Table 43.5). Recurrence of disease in a previous allograft puts the patient at very high risk for subsequent recurrence. The management of recurrent FSGS is discussed in Section I-C.

Late Allograft Dysfunction
Chronic Allograft Nephropathy (CAN)

An insidiously increasing plasma creatinine, proteinuria and hypertension, noted 6-months post-transplantation is consistent with this diagnosis. Evaluation includes:

1. Renal ultrasound to rule out an obstructive cause
2. Doppler, DTPA scan and angiography if renal artery stenosis is suspected
3. Renal biopsy to establish the diagnosis and assess disease severity

Tubulointerstitial findings include fibrosis, patchy mononuclear cell infiltration and tubular atrophy. Glomerular dropout, collapse or ischemic changes may be noted.

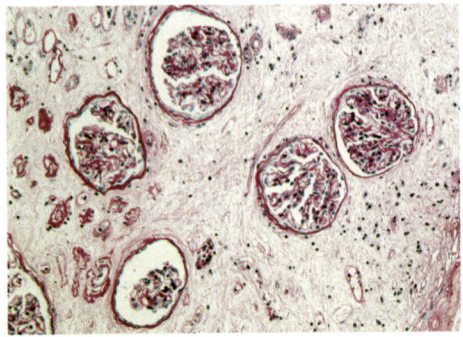

Fig. 43.3: Renal transplant biopsy showing chronic allograft nephropathy. Tubular atrophy and interstitial fibrosis are prominent findings

Table 43.5: Risk of recurrence of native kidney disease after transplantation

Disease in native kidney	Recurrence risk (%)
Alport syndrome	3
Antiglomerular basement membrane (GBM) nephritis	<10
Focal segmental glomerulosclerosis	20–40
Henoch Schonlein purpura	30–80
Hemolytic uremic syndrome	10–50
IgA nephropathy	50
Membranoproliferative glomerulonephritis (MPGN) type II	90
MPGN type I	25
Membranous nephropathy	20
Primary hyperoxaluria type I*	90
Systemic lupus erythematosus**	5–10
Wegener's granulomatosis	5–20

* In the absence of combined liver and kidney transplantation
** Transplantation should be delayed till disease has been quiescent for at least 1 year

Features suggesting chronic transplant glomerulopathy include capillary wall thickening and double contours, increase in mesangial matrix and segmental sclerosis (Fig. 43.3). Vascular changes include thickened arterial intima and disruption or duplication of the internal elastic lamina.

Transplant Renal Artery Stenosis

This is an uncommon and late complication. The stenosis is functionally significant once luminal narrowing is >70–80%. Clues include refractory hypertension, fluctuating renal function, particularly with hypovolemia or ACE inhibition, bruit over the kidney and polycythemia. Color flow Doppler is useful for screening, but definitive diagnosis requires renal angiography. The initial management is percutaneous transluminal angioplasty that has a success rate of 40–75%. Restenosis may require repeat angioplasty or surgical repair.

INFECTIONS

Infections are an important cause of morbidity and mortality after transplantation. In the first month after transplant, infectious complications are related to technical and mechanical problems and include wound infections, urinary tract infections, pneumonia and fungal infections.

Between 1 and 6 months post-transplant, infections include those due to cytomegalovirus (CMV), Ebstein Barr virus (EBV), *Pneumocytis pneumonia* (PCP), HSV, varicella zoster and fungi. Parvovirus B_{19} infection can present as aplastic anemia. CMV and EBV infections may be primary infections or represent viral reactivation. BK virus might cause clinical and histological features mimicking rejection.

Six months after transplantation, the patterns of infections are similar to that in the general population. Patients who develop opportunistic infection in this period are those with high serum creatinine, receiving high doses of steroids or with episodes of rejection, requiring intense immunosuppression.

Hepatitis B and C infections may become a problem in long-term survivors, due to reactivation of these viruses in the recipient or infection acquired in the peritransplant period. Tuberculosis is a serious problem due to high risk of exposure and an immunocompromised state. A high index of suspicion for infections and prompt treatment is necessary.

Immunizations are an important means to prevent vaccine preventable infections. Patients should be vaccinated early in the course of renal failure as response to vaccines gets blunted in the severe organ failure. Influenza, pneumococcal, meningococcal and papillomavirus vaccines should be administered. Family members, close contacts and health care workers should be vaccinated. After transplant, the child and the family members should receive influenza vaccine on yearly basis. Pneumococcal and hepatitis B vaccines are repeated if immunity has waned.

SUPPORT READING

Gulati A, Sarwal M. Pediatric renal transplantation: an overview and update. Curr. Opin. in Pediatr. 2010, 22: 89–96.

Tai E, Chapman JR. the KDIGO review of the care of renal transplant recipient. Pol Arch Med Wewn 2010; 12: 237–42

Filler G, Huang SH. Progress in pediatric kidney transplantation Ther Drug Monit 2010; 32: 250–52

Benfield MR. Current status of Kidney transplantation: Update, 2003. Pediatr. Clin N Am 2003; 50; 1301–34

Specific Therapies

44 Intravenous Pulse Therapies

PULSE CORTICOSTEROIDS

Patients with renal diseases require high dose intravenous (IV) corticosteroids in the following situations:

1. Rapidly progressive glomerulonephritis
2. Systemic vasculitis
3. Systemic lupus erythematosus with impaired kidney function
4. To induce disease remission in difficult nephrotic syndrome
5. Acute allograft rejection

Procedure

The agent used is IV methylprednisolone at a dose of 20–30 mg/kg (maximum 1g); IV dexamethasone (4–5 mg/kg; maximum 150 mg) may be used instead. Either of the medications is dissolved in 150–200 mL of 5% dextrose and infused intravenously over 2–3 hours.

Frequency of Administration

Three to six doses are given, depending on response and side effects. Methylprednisolone is administered daily, while dexamethasone may be given daily or on alternate days.

Adverse Effects

High dose steroids can precipitate or exacerbate systemic infections. Hypertension, fluid retention, hyperglycemia and hypokalemia are common side effects. Dyselectrolytemia may lead to arrhythmias, which may be life-threatening. Neutrophilic leukocytosis may be noted. Steroid induced psychosis and seizures are rare.

Monitoring

Prior to therapy, systemic infections should be excluded. However, the presence of minor upper respiratory tract, gastrointestinal or skin infection is not a contraindication. Hypertension should be controlled using appropriate drugs. Relevant baseline investigations include total and differential white cell counts and blood levels of sugar, urea, creatinine and electrolytes.

During and following therapy, contact with patients of known infectious illnesses should be avoided. Careful monitoring of heart rate, respiratory rate and blood pressure is required every 15–30 minutes. Blood sugar and electrolytes should be estimated daily during therapy.

Specific Protocols

Steroid Resistant Nephrotic Syndrome

While it is usual to administer 3–6 pulses on alternate days to induce remission or confirm steroid resistance, an aggressive protocol is occasionally used (Table 44.1).

Steroid Responsive Nephrotic Syndrome with Significant Steroid Toxicity

The use of 3–6 pulses of corticosteroids allows early achievement of remission with a lower cumulative dose of steroid therapy. To maintain remission, therapy is continued with alternate-day prednisolone 1.5 mg/kg for the next 2 weeks and then tapered.

Lupus Nephritis

Patients with lupus nephritis and moderate to severely impaired renal function (usually class III or IV on histology) benefit with the use of high dose steroids. Intravenous methylprednisolone is given for 3–6 doses before administering prednisolone at a dose of 2 mg/kg/d for 2–4 weeks which is tapered subsequently.

INTRAVENOUS CYCLOPHOSPHAMIDE

The indications for administering high dose (pulse) cyclophosphamide are:

1. Steroid resistant nephrotic syndrome
2. Systemic vasculitis, pauci-immune crescentic glomerulonephritis
3. Lupus nephritis

Procedure

Following admission, the first dose of IV cyclophosphamide is given at a dose of 500–750 mg/m² body surface area, with a maximum dose of 1000 mg. The lower dose (500 mg/m²) is recommended in patients with impaired renal function (creatinine >1.5 mg/dL or GFR <60 mL/min/1.73 m²). The next dose may be increased by 125 mg/m² up to a maximum of 750–1000 mg/m².

Pre-medication

In order to reduce the risk of vomiting, ondansetron is administered IV at a dose of 0.45 mg/kg (5 mg/m², maximum 8 mg) 30 minutes prior to the administration of IV cyclophosphamide. Doses as high as 16 mg/m² (maximum 24 mg) have been used.

Infusion

Cyclophosphamide is diluted in 200–300 mL normal saline or 5% dextrose and infused over 1–2 hours. Care is taken to ensure that the concentration of cyclophosphamide does not exceed 15 mg/mL. Coadministration of sodium-2-mercaptoethane sulfonate (MESNA) reduces the risk of hemorrhagic cystitis. Throughout the administration and for 48 hours after, the patient is encouraged to ensure fluid intake of 2–2.5 L/m² daily. The patient is instructed to pass urine every q 3–4 hr.

Table 44.1: Pulse corticosteroid protocol for steroid resistant nephrotic syndrome

Weeks	Pulse steroids	Oral steroids*
1–2	Alternate day; 6 pulses	Nil
3–4**	Nil	Prednisolone daily
5–12	Fortnightly; 4 pulses	Prednisolone alternate day
13–44	Monthly; 8 pulses	Prednisolone alternate day
45–56	Nil	Prednisolone alternate day

* Prednisolone 2 mg/kg per day for 2 weeks, then 1.5 mg/kg on alternate days for next 4 weeks, 1.0 mg/kg on alternate days for 4 weeks and gradual tapering over the year

** Cyclophosphamide, at a dose of 2 mg/kg daily, is given for a period of 12 weeks usually starting from week 3. Monitoring for leukopenia (<4000/mm³) is required every fortnight.

Specific Therapies

X

Adverse Effects

Adverse effects include hemorrhagic cystitis; nausea or vomiting; bone marrow suppression with neutropenia and leukopenia; infusion related reactions (fever, chills, urticaria); alopecia; exacerbation or precipitation of infections; and hyponatremia and hypomagnesemia.

Monitoring

The total leukocyte count is monitored 10–14 days after each pulse of cyclophosphamide. The next dose is withheld if the total leukocyte count is <4000/mm³. If the leukocyte count is between 4000–5000/mm³, the dose is decreased by 25%. The full dose is given if the leukocyte count is >5000/mm³ and neutrophil count is >2500/mm³.

Systemic infections should be ruled out prior to administration of the medication. Contact with patients with known infectious illnesses should be avoided. The patient should be monitored closely for infections for 1–2 weeks following administration of IV cyclophosphamide.

Management of Complications

Emesis

Ondansetron syrup or tablet (dose 0.15 mg/kg; age 4–11 yr: 4 mg q8–12 hr; age ≥12 yr: 8 mg q8–12 hr) is given for 24–48 hours. Therapy with ondansetron and granisetron (0.01 mg/kg or 10 µg/kg once a day) is safe and superior to chlorpromazine, dimenhydrinate and metoclopramide combined with dexamethasone.

If vomiting is significant, IV dexamethasone (0.5 mg/kg, or 10 to 14 mg/m²) is administered with IV ondansetron before the next dose of IV cyclophosphamide.

Hematuria

Administration of MESNA is indicated if: (i) gross hematuria, dysuria or frequency followed a previous pulse; and (ii) cyclophosphamide dose exceeds 750 mg/m² per dose.

MESNA is given as an IV bolus injection in a dose equal to 20% of the cyclophosphamide dosage (weight by weight in mg) in the same infusion as cyclophosphamide. The IV protocol involves repeat administration of the same dose at 4- and 8-hr (after the dose of cyclophosphamide) in 5% dextrose, normal saline or Ringer lactate, in a concentration not exceeding 20 mg/ml. The total daily IV dose of MESNA is thus 60% of the cyclophosphamide dose.

Alternatively, following addition of the initial dose of MESNA (20% w/w) in the infusion, two more doses are given orally. 2-hr and 6-hr later, orally at 40% of the cyclophosphamide dose (IV-oral-oral protocol). The total dose of MESNA is 100% of the dose of cyclophosphamide. Each oral dose is taken with a full glass of water, or, alternatively, in cola drink or fruit juice. Oral MESNA should be repeated if vomiting occurs within 2-hr of a previous dose.

Patients with persistent gross hematuria benefit by *bladder irrigation,* which is shown to reduce inflammation and decrease intravesical clot formation. This is carried out for 24–36 hr with glycine solution or normal saline. Other therapies include administration of hyperbaric oxygen, oral sodium pentosan polysulfate or intravesical formalin.

Leukopenia

If the total leukocyte count is <4000/mm³ on the scheduled cyclophosphamide day, the dose is withheld, and the prednisolone dosage increased if required. If the repeat leukocyte count is between 4000–5000/mm³, a reduced dose of cyclophosphamide is given.

SUPPORT READING

Sinha A, Bagga A. Pulse steroid therapy. Indian J Pediatr 2008; 75: 1057–66

Mukhtar S, Woodhouse C. The management of cyclophosphamide induced hematuria. BJU International 2010; 105: 908–12

45 Plasmapheresis

Plasmapheresis or therapeutic plasma exchange (TPE) is an extracorporeal blood purification technique performed for multiple indications requiring the removal of large molecular weight substances. The procedure may be performed using centrifugation devices or membrane filters.

While many centers use *centrifugation devices*, their utility is limited by availability, high cost, need for high blood flow rates and removal of large extracorporeal fractions. *Membrane filtration*, using highly permeable filters, is equally efficacious and easier to implement in children, especially in facilities with access to hemodialysis services.

Common indications for therapeutic plasma exchange include:

1. Guillain-Barré syndrome
2. Hemolytic uremic syndrome, thrombotic thrombocytopenic purpura
3. Recurrent or refractory focal segmental glomerulosclerosis
4. Rapidly progressive glomerulonephritis: ANCA associated systemic vasculitis
5. Goodpasture syndrome
6. Myasthenia gravis
6. Systemic lupus erythematosus refractory to standard therapy.

Procedure

Plasmapheresis is performed following placement of a double-lumen dialysis catheter (8–12 French) in the femoral vein or internal jugular vein. Membrane plasma separation is done on a dialysis machine in ultrafiltration or bypass mode. Blood pump flow rates should be kept between 3–8 mL/kg/min and transmembrane pressure between 40–200 mm Hg. The duration of the procedure is usually 1.5 to 2 hr. Systemic anticoagulation with heparin is necessary to avoid coagulation within the filter and IV lines.

Membrane filters include those available through Asahi (Plasmaflo), Fresenius, Gambro and B Braun. The size of the filter used varies by body weight. For children <30 kg, a filter of surface area 0.2 m² (1S) is suitable, and for those weighing >30 kg, a filter of size 0.5 m² (2S) is used.

Usually, 1.5–2 plasma volumes are exchanged, and replaced by an equal volume of plasma or albumin. In patients with fluid overload, the replacement may be 85% of that removed. Plasma volume is calculated as follows:

Plasma volume (mL) = 65 × wt (kg) × (1-hematocrit)

Fluids for replacement include albumin, crystalloids and fresh frozen plasma. The initial 20-30% replacement may be done using crystalloid solutions, *e.g.*, normal saline or Ringer lactate, especially in patients with normal serum albumin. Subsequently 20% albumin is used, diluted with normal saline to prepare 5% solution. Fresh frozen plasma is preferred in patients with hemolytic uremic syndrome, thrombotic thrombocytoepenic purpura, bleeding manifestations, or co-existent hepatic dysfunction.

Specific Therapies

Tabie 45.1: Schedules for therapeutic plasma exchange

Disease	Schedule
Hemolytic uremic syndrome*	Variable duration of treatment 1.5-volume TPE daily till hematological remission (platelet count >150000/mm^3, no hemolysis and LDH <300 U/L); then, alternate day; followed by twice weekly & finally once-weekly
Pauci-immune crescentic glomerulonephritis	1.5–2 volume TPE for 3 days; alternate-day for another 4 days
Focal segmental glomerulosclerosis (pre-transplant)*	1.5 TPE on alternate days for 6 sessions
Guillain-Barre syndrome with impending respiratory failure	1–1.5 TPE daily for 3 days; then on alternate days for 4 sessions

*The preferred replacement fluid is fresh frozen plasma for hemolytic uremic syndrome and albumin for focal segmental glomerulosclerosis

Table 45.1 provides schedules for plasmapheresis for different indications.

Complications

Hypocalcemia: Prophylactic infusion of 1–2 mL/kg calcium gluconate is useful.

Hypokalemia: This may be managed by adding 4 mEq/L KCl to albumin/FFP infusate.

Bleeding: It is useful to measure PT/PTTK before third and subsequent procedure. FFP should be used to partially substitute for the replacement fluid if PT is >1.5 times normal.

Anaphylactic reactions with use of ACE inhibitors: Prekallikrein-activating factors in albumin lead to endogenous bradykinin release. Therapy with ACE inhibitor (TPE) should be discontinued 24–48 hr before plasmapheresis.

SUPPORT READING

Kaplar AA. Therapeutic plasma exchange: Core Curriculum 2008. Amer J Kid Dis 2008; 52: 1180–90

Rahman T, Harper L. Plasmapheresis in nephrology: an update. Curr Opin Nephrol Hypertens 2006; 15: 603–09

Appendices

Appendix 1: Important Formulae

	Formula	Remarks
Estimated glomerular filtration rate (GFR), mL/min/1.73 m²	$GFR = \dfrac{k \times height\ (cm)}{serum\ creatinine\ (mg/dL)}$	k=0.43 Useful in staging chronic kidney disease
Plasma anion gap, mEq/L	$Na^+ - (Cl^- + HCO_3^-)$	Normal value 6–12 mEq/L
Urine anion gap, mEq/L	$Na^+ + K^+ - Cl^-$	Index of urinary NH_4^+ excretion
Plasma osmolality, mOsm/kg	$2 \times (Na^+) + (BUN/2.8) + (glucose/18)$	Normal 280–285 mOsm/kg Osmolality approximates twice plasma Na^+ BUN blood urea nitrogen, mg/dL
Free water deficit, L	Total body water × $\dfrac{(sodium\ concentration - 1)}{140}$	Total body water = 0.6 × wt (kg)
Plasma volume, L	$0.065 \times weight\ (kg) \times (1 - hematocrit)$	Approximately 30–40 mL/kg
Urinary potassium index	$\dfrac{urine\ K^+}{(urine\ K^+ + urine\ Na^+)}$	Value exceeding 0.6 or 60% suggest hypovolemia
Transtubular potassium gradient (TTKG)	$\dfrac{urine\ K^+ \times plasma\ osmolality}{plasma\ K^+ \times urine\ osmolality}$	In patients with normal renal function, the value should be <2.5 in hypokalemia and >7 in hyperkalemia
Fractional excretion of sodium*	$\dfrac{urine\ Na^+ \times plasma\ creatinine}{plasma\ Na^+ \times urine\ creatinine} \times 100$	Value is <1% in volume contraction with appropriate renal Na^+ retention
Corrected serum calcium, mg/dL	Serum calcium + [0.8 × (4.0 – measured albumin)]	Calcium levels require correction in hypoalbuminemia
Change in sodium concentration following infusion of 1 L of a solution, mEq/L	$\dfrac{(infusate\ Na^+ - serum\ Na^+)}{(0.6 \times body\ weight\ in\ kg) + 1}$	Infusate Na^+ is concentration of Na^+ in the fluid infused
Expected bladder capacity, mL	Age 2–12 yr: (age + 2) × 30 Infants: 7 × weight (kg)	

* The fractional excretion of any substance can be calculated similarly

Appendix 2: Conversion from Conventional to SI Units

To convert from conventional to SI unit, multiply by the conversion factor.

	Conventional Unit	Conversion Factor	SI Unit
Albumin	g/dL	10	g/L
Aldosterone	ng/dL	0.0277	nmol/L
Alkaline phosphatase	King Armstrong units/dL	7.1	U/L
Ammonia	μg/dL	0.587	μmol/L
Bilirubin	mg/dL	17.1	μmol/L
Calcium	mg/dL	0.25	mmol/L
	mEq/L	0.50	mmol/L
Carbon dioxide	mEq/L	1.0	mmol/L
Cholesterol	mg/dL	0.0259	mmol/L
Citrate	mg/dL	52.05	μmol/L
Creatinine	mg/dL	88.4	μmol/L
Cystine	mg/dL	4.167	μmol/L
Glucose	mg/dL	0.0555	mmol/L
Iron	μg/dL	0.179	μmol/L
Magnesium	mg/dL	0.411	mmol/L
	mEq/L	0.50	mmol/L
Oxalate	mg/L	11.1	μmol/L
Phosphorus	mg/dL	0.323	mmol/L
Renin	pg/mL	0.0237	pmol/L
Urea	mg/dL	0.357	mmol/L
Uric acid	mg/dL	59.48	μmol/L
Vitamin D			
1,25-Dihydroxyvitamin D	pg/mL	2.6	pmol/L
25-Hydroxyvitamin D	ng/mL	2.496	nmol/L

Appendix 3: Drug Dose Modification in Renal Disease

Drug	Dose for normal renal function	Dose for impaired renal function GFR mL/min/1.73m²			Dose in renal replacement therapy		
		>50	10–50	<10	HD	PD	CRRT
ANTIMICROBIALS							
Acyclovir	10 mg/kg/dose q8 hr iv	5 mg/kg q8 hr	5 mg/kg q12–24 hr	2.5 mg/kg q24 hr	Dose after dialysis	Dose for GFR<10	No data
Amikacin	5–7.5 mg/kg/dose q8 hr iv	90% (1 single dose)	70% (1 single dose)	30% (1 single dose)	50% dose after dialysis	15–20 mg/L/d	Dose for GFR 10–50 and measure levels
Amoxicillin	10–25 mg/kg/dose q8 hr iv, im, po	q8 hr	q8–12 hr	q24 hr	Dose after dialysis	50% q12 hr	No data
Amphotericin B	0.5–1.5 mg/kg/day iv over 6–24 hr	q24 hr	q24 hr	q24–36 hr	No data	Dose for GFR<10	Dose for GFR 10–50
Ampicillin	10–25 mg/kg/dose q6 hr iv, im, po	q6 hr	q6–12 hr	q12–24 hr	Dose after dialysis	50% q12 hr	Dose for GFR 10–50
Azithromycin	15 mg/kg/dose on day 1 (max 500 mg) then 7.5 mg/kg/dose q24 hr on day 2–5 po (max 250mg)	100%	100%	100%	No data	No data	No data
Aztreonam	30 mg/kg/dose q8 hr iv (max 1 g)	100%	50–75%	25%	50% dose after dialysis	Dose for GFR <10	Dose for GFR 10–50
Cefaclor	10–15 mg/kg/dose q8 hr po	100%	100%	100%	Dose after dialysis	100% q8–12 hr	No data
Cefazolin	10–15 mg/kg/dose q6 hr iv, im	q8 hr	q12 hr	q24–48 hr	Dose after dialysis	Dose for GFR 10–50	Dose for GFR 10–50
Cefixime	5 mg/kg/dose q12–24 hr po	100%	85%	50%	Dose for GFR 10–50	Dose for GFR <10	No data
Cefoperazone	25–60 mg/kg/dose q6–12 hr iv, im	100%	100%	100%	Dose after dialysis	No data	No data

Appendices

XI

Drug	Dose for normal renal function	Dose for impaired renal function GFR mL/min/1.73m²			Dose in renal replacement therapy		
		>50	10–50	<10	HD	PD	CRRT
Cefotaxime	25 mg/kg/dose q8–12 hr iv; severe infection: 50 mg/kg/dose q4–6 hr	q6 hr	q8–12 hr	q24 hr	Dose after dialysis	q24 hr	q12 hr
Ceftriaxone	25–50 mg/kg/dose q12–24 hr iv, im	100%	100% q24 hr	50% q24 hr	Dose after dialysis	100%	Dose for GFR 10–50
Ceftazidime	15–25 mg/kg/dose q8 hr iv, im; severe infection: 50 mg/kg/dose q6 hr	q8–12 hr	q24–48 hr	q48 hr	Dose after dialysis	50%	Dose for GFR 10–50
Cefuroxime sodium	25 mg/kg/dose q8 hr iv	q8 hr	q8–12 hr	q12 hr	Dose after dialysis	Dose for GFR <10	Dose for GFR <10
Cephalexin	7.5 mg/kg/dose q6 hr po	q8 hr	q12 hr	q12 hr	Dose after dialysis	Dose for GFR <10	No data
Chloramphenicol	40 mg/kg/dose stat then 25 mg/kg/dose q6–24 hr iv, im, po	100%	100%	100%	No data	No data	No data
Ciprofloxacin	PO: 20 mg/kg/day, q12 hr; IV: 10 mg/kg/day, q12 hr	100%	50–75%	50%	Dose for GFR <10	50% q8 hr	Dose for GFR <10
Clarithromycin	7.5–15 mg/kg/dose q12 hr po	100%	75%	50–75%	No data	No data	No data
Co-amoxiclav	IV: 30 mg/kg q8h	100%	q12 hr	q24 hr	No data	No data	No data
Cotrimoxazole	6–10 mg/kg/day q12 hr	q12 hr	50% q12 hr	50% q12 hr	Dose after dialysis	Dose for GFR<10	Dose for GFR 10–50
Erythromycin	10 mg/kg/dose q6 hr iv, po	100%	100%	50–75%	No data	No data	No data
Fluconazole	6 mg/kg/dose stat then 3 mg/kg/dose q24 hr, iv, po	100%	50%	25%	Dose after dialysis	Dose for GFR <10	Dose for GFR 10–50
Ganciclovir	5 mg/kg/dose q12 hr iv for 2–3 weeks then 5 mg/kg q24 hr iv	q12 hr	q24–48 hr	q48–96 hr	Dose after dialysis	Dose for GFR <10	2.5 mg/kg q24 hr

Drug	Dose for normal renal function	Dose for impaired renal function GFR mL/min/1.73m²			Dose in renal replacement therapy		
		>50	10–50	<10	HD	PD	CRRT
Gentamicin	2–2.5 mg/kg/dose q8 hr iv	100%	2 mg/kg q12 hr	1 mg/kg q24–48 hr	50% dose after dialysis	3–4 mg/L/d	Dose for GFR 10–50 and measure levels
Imipenem–cilastatin	25 mg/kg/dose q6 hr iv	100%	50%	25%	Dose after dialysis	Dose for GFR <10	Dose for GFR 10–50
Itraconazole	2–4 mg/kg/dose q12–24 hr po	100%	100%	50%	Dose for GFR <10	Dose for GFR <10	No data
Levofloxacin	5–10 mg/kg/dose q12–24 hr iv, po	100%	100% q24–48 hr	100% q48 hr	Dose for GFR <10	Dose for GFR <10	Dose for GFR 10–50
Linezolid	10 mg/kg/dose q8 hr	100%	100%	100%	Dose after dialysis	Dose for GFR<10	No data
Lisinopril	0.1–1 mg/kg q24 hr po	100%	50–75%	25–50%	Dose after dialysis	No data	Dose for GFR 10–15
Meropenem	10–20 mg/kg/dose q8 hr iv	100%	50% q12 hr	50% q24 hr	Dose after dialysis	Dose for GFR <10	Dose for GFR 10–50
Metronidazole	15 mg/kg/dose stat then 7.5 mg/kg/dose q8–12 hr iv, po	100%	100%	100%	Dose after dialysis	Dose for GFR <10	Dose for GFR 10–50
Netilmicin	2–2.5 mg/kg/dose q8 hr iv	100%	q12 hr	50% q24 hr	50% dose after dialysis	3–4 mg/L/d	Dose for GFR 10–50 and measure levels
Nitrofurantoin	1.5 mg/kg/dose q6 hr po	100%	Avoid	Avoid	No data	No data	No data
Ofloxacin	5 mg/kg/dose q8–12 hr, iv, po	100%	100% q24 hr	50% q24 hr	50% dose after dialysis	Dose for GFR <10	100%
Penicillin G	50–200 000 U/kg/day, div q4–6 hr	70%; q8–12 hr	50%; q12 hr	20–50%	Dose after dialysis	Dose for GFR <10	Dose for GFR 10–50
Penicillin V	7.5–15 mg/kg/dose q6 hr po	100%	100%	100%	Dose after dialysis	Dose for GFR <10	No data

Appendices

XI

Drug	Dose for normal renal function	Dose for impaired renal function GFR mL/min/1.73m²			Dose in renal replacement therapy		
		>50	10–50	<10	HD	PD	CRRT
Piperacillin	150–300 mg/kg/day, div q6–8 hr	100%	70% q6 hr	70% q8 hr	Dose after dialysis	Dose for GFR <10	Dose for GFR 10–50
Quinine	8.3 mg/kg/dose q8 hr po for 7–10 days	q8 hr	q8–12 hr	q24 hr	Dose after dialysis	Dose for GFR <10	Dose for GFR 10–50
Teicoplanin	10 mg/kg q12 hr for 3 doses, then 10 mg/kg q24 hr	100%	50%	50%	Dose for GFR <10	Dose for GFR <10	Dose for GFR 10–50
Tetracycline	250–500 mg/dose q6 hr po	q8–12 hr	q12–24 hr	q24 hr	No data	No data	Dose for GFR 10–50
Tobramycin	2– 2.5 mg/kg/dose q6–8 hr iv, im	60–90%	30–70%	20–30%	50% dose after dialysis	3–4 mg/L/d	Dose for GFR 10–50 and measure levels
Trimethoprim	3–4 mg/kg/dose q12 hr iv, po	q12 hr	q18 hr	q24 hr	Dose after dialysis	q24 hr	q18 hr
Valganciclovir	450 mg/m²/d or 30 mg/kg/d od	50%	25%	25%	Dose after dialysis	Dose for GFR <10	No data
Vancomycin	10–15 mg/kg q6–8 hr	100%	10 mg/kg q 24 hr	10 mg/kg q48–72 hr	Dose after dialysis	Dose for GFR <10	Dose for GFR 10–50
Voriconazole	6 mg/kg/dose q12 hr on day one, then 4 mg/kg q12 hr	100%	100%	100%	Dose after dialysis	Dose for GFR <10	Dose for GFR 10–50
Antitubercular Drugs							
Ethambutol	25 mg/kg/dose q24 hr po	q24 hr	q24–36 hr	q48 hr	Dose after dialysis	Dose for GFR <10	Dose for GFR 10–50
Isoniazid	10 mg/kg/dose q24 hr iv, im, po	100%	100%	100%	Dose after dialysis	Dose for GFR <10	Dose for GFR <10
Pyrazinamide	20–35 mg/kg/dose q24 hr po	100%	100%	50–100%	40 mg/kg 24 hr prior each session of dialysis	100%	No data
Rifampicin	10–15 mg/kg/dose q24 hr po	100%	50–100%	50–100%	No data	Dose for GFR <10	Dose for GFR <10
Streptomycin	20–30 mg/kg/dose q24 hr im	q24 hr	q24–72 hr	q72–96 hr	50% dose after dialysis	20–40 mg/L/day	Dose for GFR 10–50 and measure levels

Appendix 3

Drug	Dose for normal renal function	Dose for impaired renal function GFR mL/min/1.73m²			Dose in renal replacement therapy			
		>50	10–50	<10	HD	PD	CRRT	
Anticonvulsants								
Carbam-azepine	2–10 mg/kg/dose q8 hr po	100%	100%	100%	Dose after dialysis	No data	No data	
Phenobarbital	5 mg/kg/dose q24 hr iv, im, po	q8–12 hr	q8–12 hr	q12–16 hr	Dose after dialysis	50% dose	Dose for GFR 10–50	
Clonazepam	0.05–0.5 mg/kg/day	100%	100%	75%	Dose after dialysis	Dose for GFR <10	Dose for GFR 10–50 and measure levels	
Lamotrigine	2 mg/kg/day for 2 weeks, then 5 mg/kg/day for 2 weeks, then 5–15 mg/kg/day	100%	100%	75%	Dose after dialysis	Dose for GFR <10	Dose for GFR 10–50 and measure levels	
Levetiracetam	10–60 mg/kg/day q8 hr	50%	50%	50%	Dose after dialysis	Dose for GFR <10	Dose for GFR 10–50 and measure levels	
Phenytoin	5–8 mg/kg/day	100%	100%	100%	Dose after dialysis	Dose for GFR <10	Dose for GFR 10–50 and measure levels	
Topiramate	3–9 mg/kg/day q8–12 hr	50%	50%	25%	Dose after dialysis	No data	Dose for GFR 10–50 and measure levels	
Valproate sodium	10–60 mg/kg/day	100%	100%	100%	Dose after dialysis	Dose for GFR <10	Dose for GFR 10–50 and measure levels	
Miscellaneous								
Acetamino-phen	10–15 mg/kg/dose q4–6 hr po	q4 hr	q6 hr	q8 hr	No data	No data	Dose for GFR 10–50	
Acetazolamide	5–10 mg/kg/dose q6 hr po	q6 hr	q12 hr	Avoid	No data	No data	Avoid	
Acetylsalicylic acid	10–15 mg/kg q6 hr po	q4 hr	q4–6 hr	Avoid	Dose after dialysis	No data	Dose for GFR 10–50	

XI

Appendices

XI

Drug	Dose for normal renal function	Dose for impaired renal function GFR mL/min/1.73m²			Dose in renal replacement therapy		
		>50	10-50	<10	HD	PD	CRRT
Amlodipine	0.05-0.2 mg/kg q24 hr po	100%	100%	100%	No data	No data	Dose for GFR 10-50
Atenolol	1-2 mg/kg/dose po q12 hr	100%	50%	30-50%	50% dose after dialysis	No data	Dose for GFR 10-50
Azathioprine	1-3 mg/kg/dose q24 hr iv, po	100%	75%	50%	Supplement 0.25 mg/kg	No data	Dose for GFR 10-50
Betamethasone	0.01-0.2 mg/kg/dose q24 hr po	100%	100%	100%	No data	No data	Dose for GFR 10-50
Captopril	0.1-1 mg/kg/dose q8 hr po	100%	75%	50%	20-30%	No data	Dose for GFR 10-15
Cetirizine	0.25 mg/kg/dose q12-24 hr po	100%	50%	25%	No data	No data	No data
Chlorambucil	0.1-0.2 mg/kg/dose q24 hr po	No data	No data	No data	No data	No data	No data
Chloroquine	10 mg/kg/dose q24 hr po for 3 days, or 4 mg/kg/dose q12 hr im for 3 days	100%	100%	50%	No data	No data	No data
Cyclophosphamide	600 mg/m²/dose q24 hr iv	100%	100%	75%	Dose after dialysis	No data	Dose for GFR 10-50
Cyclosporine A	1.5-2.5 mg/kg/dose q12 hr po	100%	100%	100%	No data	No data	100%
Dexamethasone	0.1-0.25 mg/kg/dose q6 hr iv, po	100%	100%	100%	No data	No data	Dose for GFR 10-50
Digoxin	15 µg/kg/dose for stat and 5 µg/kg/dose 6 hr later, then 3-5 µg/kg/dose q12 hr po	100%	25-75%	10-25%	No data	No data	Dose for GFR 10-50
Dobutamine	1-20 µg/kg/dose q6-8 hr po	100%	100%	Avoid	No data	No data	Dose for GFR 10-50
Enalapril	0.1-1 mg/kg/day, q12-24 hr	100%	75%	50%	20-25%	No data	Dose for GFR 10-50

Drug	Dose for normal renal function	Dose for impaired renal function GFR mL/min/1.73m²			Dose in renal replacement therapy		
		>50	10–50	<10	HD	PD	CRRT
Insulin	0.05–0.2 U/kg/dose sc	100%	75%	50%	No data	No data	Dose for GFR 10–50
Methyldopa	3 mg/kg/dose q8 hr po	q8 hr	q8–12 hr	q12–24 hr	Dose after dialysis	No data	Dose for GFR 10–50
Methylpred- nisolone	0.5–1 mg/kg/dose q6–24 hr iv, im, po	100%	100%	100%	No data	No data	Dose for GFR 10–50
Metoclopr- amide	0.15–0.3 mg/kg/dose q6 hr iv, im, po	100%	75%	50%	No data	No data	50–75%
Nitroprus- side	0.5–10 µg/kg/min infusion	100%	100%	100%	No data	No data	Dose for GFR 10–50
Omeprazole	0.4–0.8 mg/kg/dose q12–24 hr po	100%	100%	100%	No data	No data	No data
Ondansetron	0.1–0.2 mg/kg/dose q6–12 hr po	100%	100%	100%	No data	No data	Dose for GFR 10–50
Prazosin	5 µg/kg test dose, then 0.025 – 0.1 mg/kg/dose q6 hr po	100%	100%	100%	No data	No data	Dose for GFR 10–50
Prednisolone	2 mg/kg/dose q24 hr po	100%	100%	100%	No data	No data	Dose for GFR 10–50
Ranitidine	2–4 mg/kg/dose q8–12 hr po	75%	50%	25%	50%	No data	Dose for GFR 10–50
Spironolac- tone	6.25– 25 mg/dose q12 hr po	q6–12 hr	q12–24 hr	Avoid	No data	No data	Avoid
Warfarin	0.05 – 0.2 mg/kg/dose q24 hr po	100%	100%	100%	No data	No data	No data

HD hemodialysis; PD peritoneal dialysis; CRRT continuous renal replacement therapy

The dosage modifications given above are an approximation. Each patient should be monitored for signs of drug toxicity.

In acute renal failure, the decline in glomerular filtration rate is virtually total so patients should be dosed as if they have a renal function of <10 mL/min/1.73 m²

Appendix 4: Drugs Requiring No or Minimal Modification in Renal Failure

Drug	Dosage (per day)	Frequency, route	Comments
Diuretics			
Amiloride	0.2–0.6 mg/kg	24 hr, po	Monitor serum potassium levels
Bumetanide	0.01–0.02; maximum 0.3 mg/kg	12–24 hr, po	Avoid if allergic to sulfonamides
Chlorthalidone	0.25–2 mg/kg	24 hr, po	Use cautiously in patients with hepatic or severe renal disease; may cause alkalosis, pancreatitis
Hydrochlorothiazide	1–4 mg/kg; maximum 100 mg	12–24 hr, po	
Frusemide	IV: 1–2 mg/kg; maximum 8–10 Bolus: 1–2 mg/kg, then 0.1–1 mg/kg/hr	6–12 hr, po IV 24 h	Injectable preparation can be given orally; use with caution in hepatic disease; ototoxicity in presence of renal disease, may cause hypercalciuria or renal stones
Metolazone	0.1–0.4 mg/kg	12–24 hr, po	Dyselectrolytemia, marrow suppression, hyperuricemia; more effective than thiazides with reduced creatinine clearance
Spironolactone	1–3 mg/kg	12–24 hr, po	Use with caution with ACE inhibitors, cimetidine; hyperkalemia common with GFR <30 mL/min/1.73 m²
Triamterene	2–4 mg/kg; max 6	8–12 hr, po	
Immunosuppresive Drugs			
Azathioprine	1–2 mg/kg	24 hr, po	Monitor white cell counts, liver functions
Chlorambucil	0.1–0.2 mg/kg	24 hr, po	Marrow suppression, seizures
Cyclophosphamide	2–3 mg/kg 500–750 mg/m²	24 hr, po single dose, IV	Use with steroids; monitor cell counts; hemorrhagic cystitis and vomiting occur more with IV therapy
Cyclosporine	3–6 mg/kg	12 hr, po	Monitor liver/renal functions, drug levels; multiple drug interactions; hypercholesterolemia, hypertension, hirsutism, gum hyperplasia
Immunoglobulins	2 g/kg	Over 3–5 days, IV	Flushing, tachycardia, chills, fever, headache, aseptic meningitis
Levamisole	2–3 mg/kg	48 hr, po	Leukopenia, rash, fever; rarely, seizures

Drug	Dosage (per day)	Frequency, route	Comments
Methylprednisolone	15–30 mg/kg	24–48 hr, IV	Dilute in saline or 5% glucose; infuse over 1–2 hr
Mycophenolate mofetil	1000–1200 mg/m²	12 hr, po	Gastrointestinal symptoms; diarrhea; monitor leukocyte counts
Prednisolone	1–2 mg/kg; maximum 80 mg	8–48 hr, po	Steroid toxicity with long-term use
Tacrolimus	0.1–0.3 mg/kg	12 hr, po	Monitor renal function, blood sugar; headache, seizures, diarrhea
Vitamin D Analogs			
Alphacalcidol	0.25–2 µg	24–72 hr, po	Monitor serum calcium and phosphorus; avoid concomitant use of magnesium antacids; contraindicated in hypercalcemia; calcitriol most potent
Calcitriol	0.25–2 µg	24–72 hr, po	
Cholecalciferol	4000–40 000 IU	24 hr, po	
Doxercalciferol	2.5–5 µg	24 hr, po	Synthetic form of vitamin D, lower risk of hypercalcemia
Phosphate and Potassium Binders			
Aluminium hydroxide	50–150 mg/kg	6–8 hr, po	10 mL provides 200 mg elemental aluminum; may cause constipation; interferes with absorption of digoxin, isoniazid, iron. One tab binds 15–30 mg phosphorus
Calcium carbonate	20–65 mg/kg	8 hr, po	May cause constipation, nausea, vomiting, headache, confusion, hypercalcemia and hypophosphatemia; 1 g binds 39 mg phosphorus
Calcium acetate	667 mg (elemental calcium = 167 mg)	2–4 tabs q8 hr	1 g binds 45 mg phosphorus
Polystyrene sulfonate	1–3 g	8 hr, po/pr	Bowel obstruction may occur; each g resin exchanges 1–2 mEq potassium
Sevelamer hydrochloride	400 mg, 800 mg 2–4 tablets with meals	8 hr, po	Gastrointestinal side effects (nausea, abdominal pain, constipation), metabolic acidosis 400 mg tablet binds 32 mg phosphorus
Sevelamer carbonate	400 mg, 800 mg 2–4 tablets with meals	8 hr, po	Does not cause acidosis
Miscellaneous			
Albumin	0.5–1 g/kg	IV	Infuse over 1–4 hr with frusemide; watch for heart failure, hypertension

Drug	Dosage (per day)	Frequency, route	Comments
Cinacalcet	0.25 mg/kg maximum, dose 180 mg/d	od	Allosteric activators of the calcium sensing receptor (CaSR), used for treatment of secondary hyperparathyroidism
Chloral hydrate	25–50 mg/kg/dose	prn, po	Avoid in renal failure or hepatic disease
dDAVP desmopressin	0.2–0.6 mg	po	For nocturnal enuresis
	10–40 μg	intranasal	
	0.05–0.1 mg	po	For diabetes insipidus
	5–20 μg	intranasal	
	2–4 μg/mg	intranasal	Prevention of bleeds; administer 2 hr before procedure
Diazepam	0.04–0.2 mg/kg/dose	IV	Hypotension and respiratory depression may occur. Do not dilute in IV fluids; give no faster than 1 mg/min
Imipramine	4–7 yr: 10–25 mg	Bedtime for noctur-nal enuresis, po	Do not exceed 2.5 mg/kg/day; avoid concomitant terfena-dine
	8–11 yr: 25–50 mg		
	>11 yr: 50–75 mg		
Ketamine	1–2 mg/kg (over 1–2 min)	IV/IM	Co-administration of diazepam reduces emergence reactions
Midazolam	0.05–0.1 mg/kg; repeat to maximum of 0.2 mg/kg	IV	Administer over 2 minutes; flumazenil is antidote for respi-ratory depression
Oxybutinin	0.5–0.8 mg/kg; maximum total dose 15 mg	8–12 hr, po	Anticholinergic effects; contraindicated in GI obstruction or megacolon
Tamsulosin	0.4–0.8 mg	24 hr, po	Dry mouth, flushing, blurry vision, constipation, heat intol-erance
Tolterodine	1–2 mg	12 hr, po	

Appendix 5: Composition of Intravenous Fluids

Fluids	Osmo-lality, mOsm/kg	Na^+, mEq/L	K^+, mEq/L	Cl^-, mEq/L	Base, mEq/L	Mg^{2+}, mEq/L	Ca^{2+}, mEq/L	Dextrose, g/L
Crystalloids								
Normal saline	308	154	0	154	0	0	0	0
Ringer lactate	274	130	4	109	28 (lactate)	0	3	0
0.45% saline with 2.5% dextrose	293	77	0	77	0	0	0	25
0.18% saline with 4.3% dextrose	299	38	0	38	0	0	0	43
5% dextrose	278	0	0	0	0	0	0	50
Colloids								
5% albumin	260–320	130–160	<1	130–160	0	0	0	0
Fresh frozen plasma	300	140	4	110	25 (bicarbonate)	0	0	0
Dextran 40 or 70	310	154	0	154	0	0	0	0

Appendix 6: Alkali and Phosphate Supplements

Preparation	Composition (per 1000 mL)	Remarks
Bicitra	100 g sodium citrate 60 g citric acid	1 mL = 1 mEq base
Polycitra	110 g potassium citrate 100 g sodium citrate 66.8 g citric acid	1 mL = 2 mEq base = 1 mEq Na$^+$ = 1 mEq K$^+$
Polycitra K	220 g potassium citrate 66.8 g citric acid	1 mL = 2 mEq base
Shohl solution	140 g citric acid 90 g sodium citrate	1 mL = 1 mEq base
Joulie solution	136 g dibasic sodium phosphate 58.8 g phosphoric acid	1 mL = 30 mg inorganic phosphorus
Neutral phosphate	1.0 g sodium dihydrogen phosphate 3.67 g dibasic sodium phosphate	60 mL = 1000 mg inorganic phosphorus
Sodium bicarbonate	Solution (7.5%) 325, 650 mg tab	1 mL = 0.9 mEq base 325 mg = 4 mEq base
Calcium carbonate	250, 500 mg tab	1000 mg = 22.3 mEq base

Appendix 7A: Normal Values for Blood Pressure Centiles in Boys

Age (yr)	BP percentile	Systolic BP (mm Hg) Height percentile							Diastolic BP (mm Hg) Height percentile						
		5th	10th	25th	50th	75th	90th	95th	5th	10th	25th	50th	75th	90th	95th
1	50th	80	81	83	85	87	88	89	35	35	36	37	38	39	39
	90th	94	95	97	99	100	102	103	49	50	51	52	53	53	54
	95th	98	99	101	103	104	106	106	54	54	55	56	57	58	58
	99th	105	106	108	110	112	113	114	61	62	63	64	65	66	66
2	50th	84	85	87	88	90	92	92	39	40	41	42	43	44	44
	90th	97	99	100	102	104	105	106	54	55	56	57	58	58	59
	95th	101	102	104	106	108	109	110	59	59	60	61	62	63	63
	99th	109	110	111	113	115	117	117	66	67	68	69	70	71	71
3	50th	86	87	89	91	93	94	95	44	44	45	46	47	48	48
	90th	100	101	103	105	107	108	109	59	59	60	61	62	63	63
	95th	104	105	107	109	110	112	113	63	63	64	65	66	67	67
	99th	111	112	114	116	118	119	120	71	71	72	73	74	75	75
4	50th	88	89	91	93	95	96	97	47	48	49	50	51	51	52
	90th	102	103	105	107	109	110	111	62	63	64	65	66	66	67
	95th	106	107	109	111	112	114	115	66	67	68	69	70	71	71
	99th	113	114	116	118	120	121	122	74	75	76	77	78	78	79
5	50th	90	91	93	95	96	98	98	50	51	52	53	54	55	55
	90th	104	105	106	108	110	111	112	65	66	67	68	69	69	70
	95th	108	109	110	112	114	115	116	69	70	71	72	73	74	74
	99th	115	116	118	120	121	123	123	77	78	79	80	81	81	82

Appendices

XI

Age (yr)	BP percentile	Systolic BP (mm Hg) Height percentile							Diastolic BP (mm Hg) Height percentile						
		5th	10th	25th	50th	75th	90th	95th	5th	10th	25th	50th	75th	90th	95th
6	50th	91	92	94	96	98	99	100	53	53	54	55	56	57	57
	90th	105	106	108	110	111	113	113	68	68	69	70	71	72	72
	95th	109	110	112	114	115	117	117	72	72	73	74	75	76	76
	99th	116	117	119	121	123	124	125	80	80	81	82	83	84	84
7	50th	92	94	95	97	99	100	101	55	55	56	57	58	59	59
	90th	106	107	109	111	113	114	115	70	70	71	72	73	74	74
	95th	110	111	113	115	117	118	119	74	74	75	76	77	78	78
	99th	117	118	120	122	124	125	126	82	82	83	84	85	86	86
8	50th	94	95	97	99	100	102	102	56	57	58	59	60	60	61
	90th	107	109	110	112	114	115	116	71	72	72	73	74	75	76
	95th	111	112	114	116	118	119	120	75	76	77	78	79	79	80
	99th	119	120	122	123	125	127	127	83	84	85	86	87	87	88
9	50th	95	96	98	100	102	103	104	57	58	59	60	61	61	62
	90th	109	110	112	114	115	117	118	72	73	74	75	76	76	77
	95th	113	114	116	118	119	121	121	76	77	78	79	80	81	81
	99th	120	121	123	125	127	128	129	84	85	86	87	88	88	89
10	50th	97	98	100	102	103	105	106	58	59	60	61	61	62	63
	90th	111	112	114	115	117	118	119	73	73	74	75	76	77	78
	95th	115	116	117	119	121	122	123	77	77	78	79	80	81	81
	99th	122	123	125	127	128	130	130	85	86	86	88	88	89	90
11	50th	99	100	103	104	105	107	107	59	59	60	61	62	63	63
	90th	113	114	115	117	119	120	121	74	74	75	76	77	78	78
	95th	117	118	119	121	123	124	125	78	78	79	80	81	82	82
	99th	124	125	127	129	130	132	132	86	86	87	88	89	90	90
12	50th	101	102	104	106	108	109	110	59	60	61	62	63	63	64
	90th	115	116	118	120	121	123	123	74	75	75	76	77	78	79
	95th	119	120	122	123	125	127	127	78	79	80	81	82	82	83
	99th	126	127	129	131	133	134	135	86	87	88	89	90	90	91

Age (yr)	BP percentile	Systolic BP (mm Hg) Height percentile							Diastolic BP (mm Hg) Height percentile						
		5th	10th	25th	50th	75th	90th	95th	5th	10th	25th	50th	75th	90th	95th
13	50th	104	105	106	108	110	111	112	60	60	61	62	63	64	64
	90th	117	118	120	122	124	125	126	75	75	76	77	78	79	79
	95th	121	122	124	126	128	129	130	79	79	80	81	82	82	83
	99th	128	130	131	133	135	136	137	87	87	88	89	90	91	91
14	50th	106	107	109	111	113	114	115	60	61	62	63	64	65	65
	90th	120	121	123	125	126	128	128	75	76	77	78	79	79	80
	95th	124	125	127	128	130	132	132	80	80	81	82	83	84	84
	99th	131	132	134	136	138	139	140	87	87	89	90	91	92	92
15	50th	109	110	112	113	115	117	117	61	62	63	64	65	66	66
	90th	122	124	125	127	129	130	131	76	77	78	79	80	80	81
	95th	126	127	129	131	133	134	135	81	81	82	83	84	85	85
	99th	134	135	136	138	140	142	140	88	89	90	91	92	93	93
16	50th	111	112	114	116	118	119	120	63	63	64	65	66	67	67
	90th	125	126	128	130	131	133	134	78	78	79	80	81	82	82
	95th	129	130	132	134	135	137	137	82	83	83	84	85	86	87
	99th	136	137	139	141	143	144	145	90	90	91	92	93	94	94
17	50th	114	115	116	118	120	121	122	65	66	66	67	68	69	70
	90th	127	128	130	132	134	135	136	80	80	81	82	83	84	84
	95th	131	132	134	136	138	139	140	84	85	86	87	87	88	89
	99th	139	140	141	143	145	146	147	92	93	93	94	95	96	97

Appendices

XI

Appendix 7B: Normal Values for Blood Pressure Centiles in Girls

Age (yr)	BP percentile	Systolic BP (mm Hg) Height percentile							Diastolic BP (mm Hg) Height percentile						
		5th	10th	25th	50th	75th	90th	95th	5th	10th	25th	50th	75th	90th	95th
1	50th	83	84	85	86	88	89	90	38	39	39	40	41	41	42
	90th	97	97	98	100	101	102	103	52	53	53	54	55	55	56
	95th	100	101	102	104	105	106	107	56	57	57	58	59	59	60
	99th	108	108	109	111	112	113	114	64	64	65	65	66	67	67
2	50th	85	85	87	88	89	91	91	43	44	44	45	46	46	47
	90th	98	99	100	101	103	104	105	57	58	58	59	60	61	61
	95th	102	103	104	105	107	108	109	61	62	62	63	64	65	65
	99th	109	110	111	112	114	115	116	69	69	70	70	71	72	72
3	50th	86	87	88	89	91	92	93	47	48	48	49	50	50	51
	90th	100	100	102	103	104	106	106	61	62	62	63	64	64	65
	95th	104	104	105	107	108	109	110	65	66	65	67	68	68	69
	99th	111	111	113	114	115	116	117	73	73	74	74	75	76	76
4	50th	88	88	90	91	92	94	94	50	50	51	52	52	53	54
	90th	101	102	103	104	106	107	108	64	64	65	66	67	67	68
	95th	105	106	107	108	110	111	112	68	68	69	70	71	71	71
	99th	112	113	114	115	117	118	119	76	76	76	77	78	79	79
5	50th	89	90	91	93	94	95	96	52	53	53	54	55	55	56
	90th	103	103	105	106	107	109	109	66	67	67	68	69	69	70
	95th	107	107	108	110	111	112	113	70	71	71	72	73	73	71
	99th	114	114	116	117	118	120	120	78	78	79	79	80	81	81
6	50th	91	92	93	94	96	97	98	52	53	53	54	55	55	56
	90th	104	105	106	108	109	110	111	68	68	69	70	70	71	72
	95th	108	109	110	111	113	114	115	72	72	73	74	74	75	72
	99th	115	116	117	119	120	121	122	80	80	80	81	82	83	83

Age (yr)	BP percentile	Systolic BP (mm Hg) Height percentile							Diastolic BP (mm Hg) Height percentile						
		5th	10th	25th	50th	75th	90th	95th	5th	10th	25th	50th	75th	90th	95th
7	50th	93	93	95	96	97	99	99	55	56	56	57	58	58	59
	90th	106	107	108	109	111	112	113	69	70	70	71	72	72	73
	95th	110	111	112	113	115	116	116	73	74	74	75	76	76	77
	99th	117	118	119	120	122	123	124	81	81	82	82	83	84	84
8	50th	95	95	96	98	99	100	101	57	57	57	58	59	60	60
	90th	108	109	110	111	113	114	114	71	71	71	72	73	74	74
	95th	112	112	114	115	116	118	118	75	75	75	76	77	78	78
	99th	119	120	121	122	123	125	125	82	82	83	83	84	85	86
9	50th	96	97	98	100	101	102	103	58	58	58	59	60	61	61
	90th	110	110	112	113	114	116	116	72	72	72	73	74	75	75
	95th	114	114	115	117	118	119	120	76	76	76	77	78	79	79
	99th	121	121	123	124	125	127	127	83	83	84	84	85	86	87
10	50th	98	99	100	102	103	104	105	59	59	59	60	61	62	62
	90th	112	112	114	115	116	118	118	73	73	73	74	75	76	76
	95th	116	116	117	119	120	121	122	77	77	77	78	79	80	80
	99th	123	123	125	126	127	129	129	84	84	85	86	86	87	88
11	50th	100	101	102	103	105	106	107	60	60	60	61	62	63	63
	90th	114	114	116	117	118	119	120	74	74	74	75	76	77	77
	95th	118	118	119	121	122	123	124	78	78	78	79	80	81	81
	99th	125	125	126	128	129	130	131	85	85	86	87	87	88	89
12	50th	102	103	104	105	107	108	109	61	61	61	62	63	64	64
	90th	116	116	117	119	120	121	122	75	75	75	76	77	78	78
	95th	119	120	121	123	124	125	126	79	79	79	80	81	82	82
	99th	127	127	128	130	131	132	133	86	86	87	88	88	89	90

XI

Appendices

XI

Age (yr)	BP percentile	Systolic BP (mm Hg) Height percentile							Diastolic BP (mm Hg) Height percentile						
		5th	10th	25th	50th	75th	90th	95th	5th	10th	25th	50th	75th	90th	95th
13	50th	104	105	106	107	109	110	110	62	62	62	63	64	65	65
	90th	117	118	119	121	122	123	124	76	76	76	77	78	79	79
	95th	121	122	123	124	126	127	128	80	80	80	81	82	83	83
	99th	128	129	130	132	133	134	135	87	87	88	89	89	90	91
14	50th	106	106	107	109	110	111	112	63	63	63	64	65	66	66
	90th	119	120	121	122	124	125	125	77	77	77	78	79	80	80
	95th	123	123	125	126	127	129	129	81	81	81	82	83	84	84
	99th	130	131	132	133	135	134	136	88	88	89	90	90	91	92
15	50th	107	108	109	110	111	113	113	64	64	64	65	66	67	67
	90th	120	121	122	123	125	126	127	78	78	78	79	80	81	81
	95th	124	125	126	127	129	130	131	82	82	82	83	84	85	85
	99th	131	132	133	134	136	137	138	89	89	90	91	91	92	93
16	50th	108	108	110	111	112	114	114	64	64	65	66	66	67	68
	90th	121	122	123	124	126	127	128	78	78	79	80	81	81	82
	95th	125	126	127	128	130	131	132	82	82	83	84	85	85	86
	99th	132	133	134	135	137	138	139	90	90	90	91	92	93	93
17	50th	108	109	110	111	113	114	115	64	65	65	66	67	67	68
	90th	122	122	123	125	126	127	128	78	79	79	80	81	81	82
	95th	125	126	127	129	130	131	132	82	83	83	84	85	85	86
	99th	133	133	134	136	137	138	139	90	90	91	91	92	93	93

Appendix 8: Normal Values for Serum Creatinine and GFR

Normal values for serum creatinine (mg/dL)*	
Age	*Range, mg/dL*
Cord blood	0.5–1.0
Newborn	0.3–1.0
<3 yr	0.17–0.35
3–5 yr	0.26–0.42
5–7 yr	0.29–0.48
7–9 yr	0.34–0.55
9–11 yr	0.35–0.64
11–13 yr	0.42–0.71
13–15 yr	0.46–0.81
Adult male	0.7–1.3
Adult female	0.6–1.1

*To convert mg/dL to μmol/L, multiply by 88.4

Modified from Ceriotti F, *et al;* IFCC Committee on Reference Intervals and Decision Limits. Clin Chem 2008; 54: 559–66

Normal values for Glomerular Filtration Rate (GFR)	
Age	*Mean GFR ± SD (mL/min/1.73 m^2)*
1 week	41 ± 15
2–8 weeks	66 ± 25
>8 weeks	96 ± 22
2 – 12 years (males and females)	133 ± 27
13–21 years (males)	140 ± 30
13–21 years (females)	126 ± 22

Hogg RJ, *et al.* Pediatrics 2003; 111: 1416–21

Appendix 9: Tubular Reabsorption of Phosphate

Tubular reabsorption of phosphate (TRP) is expressed as follows:

TRP = 100 - FEP

where FEP is fractional excretion of phosphate

TRP may be estimated from 24-hr urine collection and ranges from 85–95% in normal children. However, TRP is influenced by changes in the glomerular filtration rate (GFR) and plasma phosphate.

The renal tubular phosphate threshold maximum per unit volume of glomerular filtrate (TmP/GFR) is the preferred method for assessment of tubular phosphate handling. TmP/GFR may be estimated from plasma phosphate concentration and TRP, using the Walton and Bijvoet nomogram (Fig. A9.1).

Normal values of TmP/GFR are relatively high throughout childhood and adolescence, with postpubertal decline to near–adult levels. These are:

0–6 month: 4–9.5 mg/dL

6 months to 5 yr: 2.9–4.6 mg/dL

5–12 yr: 2.8–4.4 mg/dL

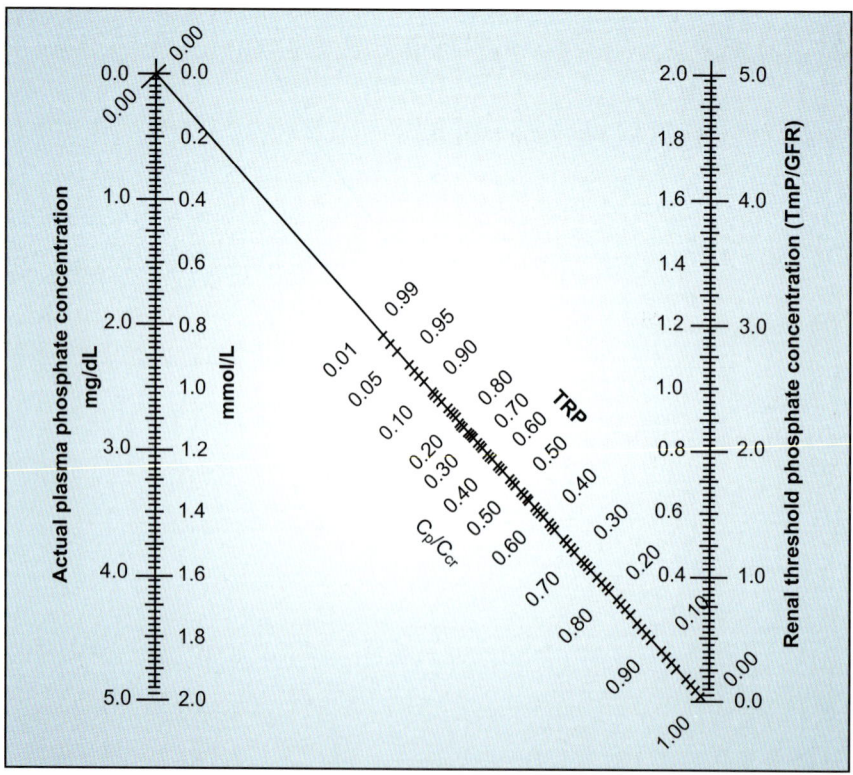

Fig. A9.1: Nomogram for estimation of the renal threshold phosphate concentration

Appendix 10: Bipolar Renal Length on Ultrasound

Age	Mean ± SD (mm)	Range (mm)
1–3 months	50 ± 5.5	39 – 61
4–6 months	56 ± 5.5	44 – 68
7–9 months	61 ± 4.6	54 – 68
1–3 yr	66 ± 5.3	54 – 75
3–5 yr	71 ± 4.5	61 – 77
5–7 yr	79 ± 5.9	66 – 90
7–9 yr	84 ± 6.6	71 – 95
9–11 yr	84 ± 7.4	71 – 99
11–13 yr	91 ± 8.4	71 – 104
13–15 yr	96 ± 8.9	83 – 113
15–17 yr	99 ± 7.5	87 – 116

Modified from Konus DL, *et al.* AJR 1998; 171: 1693–98

Renal length may also be estimated using the following equations:

Age	Renal length (cm)
<1 yr	4.98 + 0.155 age (months)
>1 yr	6.79 + 0.22 age (yr)

Rosenbaum DM, *et al.* AJR 1984; 142: 467–69

Appendix 11: Nutritive Values of Common Food Items

Foods	Quantity	Measure	Energy (Cal)	Carbohy-drate (g)	Protein (g)	Fat (g)	Na+ (mg)	K+ (mg)	Ca²⁺ (mg)	Phospho-rus (mg)
Milk and milk products										
Cow's milk	250 mL	1 glass	167	11	8	10	40	350	300	225
Buffalo's milk	250 mL	1 glass	292	11	12	17	47	225	520	320
Human milk	250 mL	1 glass	160	18.3	3.2	8.5			70	28
Curd	125 g	1 katori	77	4	4	5	40	165	188	110
Paneer	25 g	1 piece	64	3	4	4	60	29		
Butter milk	250 mL	1 glass	39	1	2	3			75	75
Toned milk (Mother Dairy)	250 mL	1 glass	144	11	8	7.5				
Double toned milk	250 mL	1 glass	110	11	8	3.75				
Skimmed milk (fresh)	250 mL	1 glass	72	12	6	0.25			300	220
Ice cream (plain)	100 g	1 cup	203	21	5	11	63	181		
Meat and poultry										
Meat	100 g	4 pieces	130		21	4	33	270	12	193
Chicken	100 g	1 portion	109		26	0.6				
Fish	100 g	2 pieces	118	7	18	2		150		
Egg whole (Hen)	25 g	one								
Cereals and pulses										
Wheat flour (Roti)	25 g	Medium cooked	85	17	3		5	78.7	12	86
Rice	25 g	1 katori cooked	86	19	1.7	0.1	120	20	2.6	
Corn flakes	25 g		94	21	2	0.2	237			

Foods	Quantity	Measure	Energy (Cal)	Carbohydrate (g)	Protein (g)	Fat (g)	Na+ (mg)	K+ (mg)	Ca²⁺ (mg)	Phosphorus (mg)
Bread	25 g	1 medium	61	13	2	0.1	120	20	2.6	
Wheat daliya	25 g	1 katori cooked	89	20	2	0.3	1	87		
Green gram (whole)	25 g	1 katori cooked	80	14	6		7	211	32	80
Lentils	25 g	1 katori cooked	85	15	6	0.1	10	157	18	72
Rajma	25 g	1 katori cooked	84	15	6	0.1			65	102
Bengal gram	25 g	1 katori cooked	87	15	4	1	9	202	50	77
Soyabeans	25 g	1 katori cooked	109	5	11	5			60	170
Sago	25 g	1 katori cooked	88	22						
Vegetable										
Green leafy	125 g	1 katori cooked	42	7.5	2		100	300	73	21
Seasonal vegetables	100 g	1 katori cooked	51	10	2		15	200	60	56
Roots and tubers	100 g	1/2 cup	92	21	2		10	200	10	40
Fruits										
Papaya	100 g	1 slice	32	7	0.6		6	69		
Grapes	100 g	8-9 number	64	16	0.5			70		
Apricot	100 g	2-3 number	52	12	1			430		
Lichi	100 g	4-5 number	60	14	1		104	159		
Pear	100 g	1 medium	52	12	1		6	96		
Watermelon	100 g	1 small	12	3	1		27	160		
Melon musk	100 g	1 slice	12	3			104	340		
Tomato ripe	100 g	2-3 number	20	3.6	1		12	146		
Apple	100 g	1 medium	52	13			28	75		
Orange	100 g	1 medium	48	11	1		4.5	9.3		
Banana	100 g	1 medium	116	27	1		37	88		

Appendices

XI

Foods	Quantity	Measure	Energy (Cal)	Carbohydrate (g)	Protein (g)	Fat (g)	Na⁺ (mg)	K⁺ (mg)	Ca²⁺ (mg)	Phosphorus (mg)
Guava	100 g	1 medium	51	11	1		6	91		
Mausami	100 g	1 medium	40	9	1			490		
Mango	100 g	1 small	74	17	1		26	205		
Lemon	100 g	3-4 number	57	11	1			270		
Miscellaneous										
Cake		1 small piece	114	21	3	2				
Samosa	40 g	1 piece	132	14	1	8				
Pastry	25 g	1 small piece	265	35	2	13				

Commercial nutritional supplements are listed in Table 36.2

Appendix 12: Radiation Dose in Procedures

The conventional unit for radiation dose is the radiation absorbed dose (rad), while the SI unit is gray (Gy), such that 1 Gy = 100 rad. The *dose equivalent* is a measure of biological effect for whole body irradiation. It is expressed in conventional units as rem and in SI units as sieverts; 1 Sv = 100 rem.

Table A12.1 provides a list of dose exposures for various procedures. Imaging by ultrasound and magnetic resonance imaging is not associated with any risk of exposure to radiation.

Table A12.1: Dose exposure associated with radiographic procedures

	Approximate dose equivalent (mSv)	*Equivalent number of chest X rays*	*Compared to natural background radiation for*
Chest X-ray	0.1	1	10 days
X-ray abdomen	1.0	10	3.3 months
Micturating cystourethrography	0.9–1.7	9–17	3–7 months
Intravenous pyelogram	2.5–3.0	25	1 year
Dimercaptosuccinic acid scan	1.0	10	3.3 months
Computed tomography of abdomen and pelvis	10–15	100–150	3–5 years
Computed tomography of head	2	20	6–8 months
Bone densitometry	0.001	–	3 hours

SUPPORT READING
www.radiologyinfo.org; Copyright © 2007 Radiological Society of North America, Inc.

XI

Appendix 13: Vaccination in Kidney Disease

Complete immunization is important in children with end-stage kidney disease as they approach transplantation. Vaccination should begin early in the course of chronic kidney disease and be administered well before transplantation (Table A13.1). Accelerated schedules are less efficacious and may not be sufficiently immunogenic. Immunization with live vaccines is avoided if immunosuppression is due to start within 4-weeks.

Live vaccines are contraindicated in transplant recipients. Immunization in the first six months after transplantation is not recommended. However, the inactivated influenza vaccine may be administered prior to the onset of the influenza season. Other inactivated vaccines including boosters may be given after 6 to 12 months. Additional vaccination may be required for rabies, Japanese B encephalitis, meninigococcus, pneumococcus or typhoid in patients at risk of these diseases.

Use of live vaccines is contraindicated in patients on immunosuppressive medications, as in nephrotic syndrome and systemic lupus erythematosus (Table A13.1). Live vaccines should be avoided in children receiving prednisolone at a dose more than 2 mg/kg or 20 mg total for more than 14 days. The administration of live vaccines should be deferred until the child is off immunosuppressive medications for at least 4 weeks. If essential, these vaccines may be given to patients receiving alternate day prednisolone at a dose <0.5 mg/kg.

Table A13.2 provides an overview of important vaccines.

Table A13.1: Status of vaccines according to clinical situation

Vaccines	Immunosuppression	Dialysis, pre-transplant	Post-transplantation
Diphtheria, pertussis, tetanus	(booster q10 yr)	(booster q10 yr)	(booster q10 yr)
Oral polio	X		X
Inactivated polio		+/−	
Hepatitis B			
Hepatitis A	+/−	If at risk	+/-
Pneumococcccus			(if antibodies wane)
H. influenzae B		+/-	
Meningococcus	+/-	+/-	+/- (if high risk)
Varicella	X (until off immunosuppresion)		X
Influenza (A and B)	+/-		(annually)
Intranasal influenza	X	+/-	X
Typhoid Vi			
Measles, MMR	X		X
Japanese encephalitis	X	If risk of exposure high	X

Recommended, if not immunized previously; +/- optional; X contraindicated; MMR measles, mumps, rubella

Table A13.2: Supplemental vaccines for patients with chronic kidney disease

Vaccine	Doses, Schedule	Comments
Hepatitis B	Three (0, 1 & 2* months) Double dose for patients on dialysis and post-transplant [<18 yr, 1 mL (20 µg); >18yr, 2 mL (40 µg)]	Repeat HBs antibody titers 1–2 months after completing the primary series and annually before and after transplantation Administer booster dose if the anti-HBs titer <10 mIU/mL, up to 3 doses if protective antibody levels do not develop
Tetanus	One	Booster every 10 yr
Pneumococcus PCV PPV23	<2 yr: PCV** (2–4 doses) 2–5 yrs: One dose of PCV, followed 2 months later by PPV23 >5 yr: PPV23 one dose	Both 23-valent (PPV23) and the conjugate (PCV7; PCV 13) vaccines are safe In <2 yr PPV is poorly immunogenic Boosters may be required q3-5 yrs
Mumps measles rubella	One	Given 4 weeks prior to transplantation Administer either simultaneously or 4 weeks apart from other live vaccine
Varicella	Two; 4 weeks apart	Given at least 4-weeks prior to transplantation and 4 weeks after cessation of steroids in patients of nephrotic syndrome
Injectable polio vaccine	Three-four; 2, 6 months & 5 yrs after first d	Recommended for patients of nephrotic syndrome and their siblings

PPV pneumococcal polysaccharide vaccine; PCV pneumococcal conjugate vaccine

* The schedule is accelerated (0, 1, 2 months) in patients planned for transplant or dialysis, compared to normal children (0, 1, 6 months)

** Age <6 months: 3 doses 4-8 weeks apart and booster at 15–18 months; Age 6–12 months: 2 doses 4–8 weeks apart and booster at 15-18 months; Age between 12–23 months: 2 doses 8 weeks apart

SUPPORT READING

KDIGO Clinical practice guidelines for the care of kidney transplant recipients. Am J Transplant 2009; 9 (suppl 3): S41-43

Guidelines for vaccination of solid organ transplant candidates and recipients. Am J Transplant 2004; 4: 160–63

Index

□□□